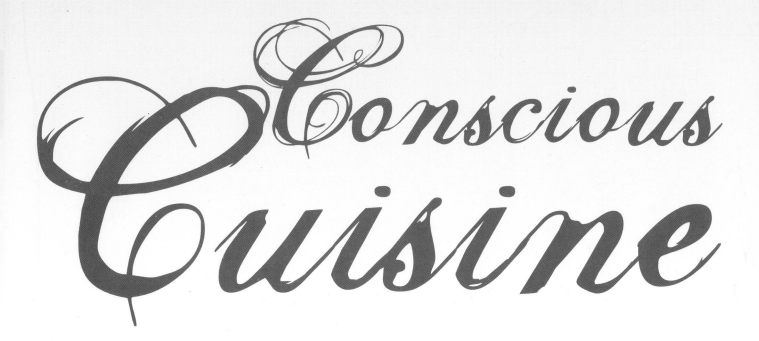

Conscious Cuisine

A New Style of Cooking from the Kitchens of Chef Cary Neff

Cary Neff
Executive Chef

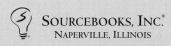

SOURCEBOOKS, INC.®
NAPERVILLE, ILLINOIS

Copyright © 2002, 2005 by Cary Neff
Cover and internal design © 2004 by Sourcebooks, Inc.
Cover photographs © Brooke Slezak
Internal photographs © Brooke Slezak
Photo of Cary Neff © Nancy J. Schroeder
Sourcebooks and the colophon are registered trademarks of Sourcebooks, Inc.

Published by Sourcebooks, Inc.
P.O. Box 4410, Naperville, Illinois 60567-4410
(630) 961-3900
FAX: (630) 961-2168
www.sourcebooks.com

Originally published in 2002
Hardcover edition cataloged as follows:

Neff, Cary.
  Conscious cuisine : a new style of cooking from the kitchens of chef cary neff /
  by Cary Neff.
      p. cm.
  1. Cookery. 2. Diet. I. Title.
  TX715 .N3813 2002
  641.5—dc21
                        2002003135

Printed and bound in China
SNP 10 9 8 7 6 5 4 3 2 1

This cookbook is dedicated to my late father, Herman Neff, who has always been my mentor, hero, and number one fan. He devoted his life for the betterment of his family. Thanks, Dad, I can feel your smile, and a big thumbs-up to you!

I also dedicate the book to my dear friend, Robert T. Allen, whose love and support was unwavering and whose smile was contagious.

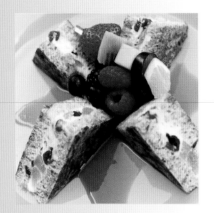

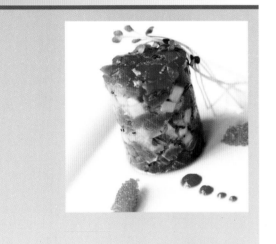

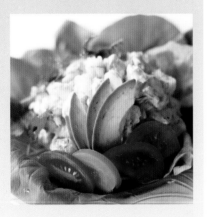

Contents

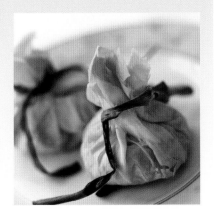

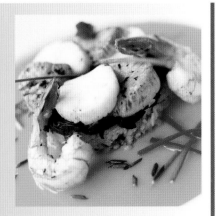

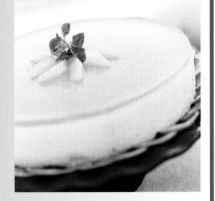

Acknowledgments

Special thanks to my extraordinary culinary team from my years at Miraval. They embraced the task of creating and serving flavorful, nutritious, and wholesome meals. We were more than just a team, we were a fully functional and caring family, where the members supported each other through success and failure.

Special thanks to Patricia Griffin, Steven Bernstein, Bill Cole, Jessica Johnson, J.D. Martin, and Lisa O'Donnell.

Heidi DeCosmo tested and fine-tuned the recipes in *Conscious Cuisine*, in addition to assisting with the book's research, development, and food styling. I can't thank her enough.

Heartfelt thanks to my good friend Chuck Whitthaus who has praised and supported my career for decades.

I tip my toque to consulting editor Jeanette Egan, who somehow made sense of my ideas and helped turn them into a book. Jeanette's profound skill in cookbook writing and recipe testing provided an invaluable asset in the completion of this book.

When preparing the food for this book, I knew I could count on Brooke Slezak's photography to show the food to its best advantage. She is one of the most highly regarded food photographers in the country, and you can see her work in places like *Gourmet*, *Travel and Leisure*, *Food and Wine*, and the *New York Times*. Brooke, thank you for your indefatigable attention to detail and your eye, which is truly magical.

A special thanks to Sourcebooks, my publisher, where CEO Dominique Raccah "discovered" me, had faith in my project, and is helping me to build the future. My editor, Deborah Werksman, is fierce on my behalf and has gone above and beyond the call of duty in extraordinary ways. Susie Benton paid attention to every word and worked tirelessly to make sure every recipe was just right. Megan Dempster personally designed each page of *Conscious Cuisine* with vision and tireless energy. Her bold and clean style is a wonderful complement to my recipes.

I am forever grateful for the love and support of my wonderful wife, Patricia, who has endured the lonesome work hours and demands of being married to a chef; and to my mom, Marie Neff, who has continuously and unfailingly supported my trade and nourished my dreams. I give special thanks to my brothers, Andrew, Dennis, Maurice, and Dwayne, for waving a banner so exuberantly with each of my accomplishments as well as providing a comforting shoulder when needed.

Introduction

Cooking is one of the most memorable, creative, romantic, and caring gestures one person can make for another. Whether it's a simple bowl of cereal for breakfast or a several-course feast to celebrate a special occasion, great food created with love and care nourishes the heart.

The goal of *Conscious Cuisine* is to encourage you to become more conscious or mindful of food. It is a simple act of noticing and embracing the unique flavors, textures, aromas, presentation, and most of all, the healthy benefits that food provides. The abundance and variety of food choices found in America is a blessing and should not be taken for granted. Food fuels our bodies with the necessary nutrients for building a healthy body and sound mind. We have a love affair with food—it is an essential part of all special occasions. Food is used to celebrate weddings, births, graduations, holidays, or gatherings of dear friends. Food has also been abused, with the massive waste of huge restaurant portions, the discouraging increase of obesity and food-related illness, and the adulteration of processed foods to the point where they can only be called "junk" food.

As long as I can remember, I have been infatuated with food. Cooking gives me the opportunity to express my many moods and passions and creativity. Food, more than any other thing, can provide memories that last a lifetime. It warms my heart to be a part of these memories for others.

I began my culinary career over twenty-five years ago. The development of this book started over three years ago and has been indeed a labor of love. Its purpose is to serve as a helpful guideline in preparing delicious foods. For the past seven years, hundreds of requests for recipes and for a cookbook have been made by the guests at Miraval who have seen and tasted the Conscious Cuisine that I originated at Miraval Life in Balance Resort and Spa. This food style has also gained wide appeal from traditional chefs as well as numerous executive chefs from leading hotels, restaurants, and resorts around the country, who have come to study conscious cooking with me. The response of the chefs was a defining moment for me, as it confirmed that Conscious Cuisine is indeed accepted in mainstream American restaurants. It will be just a matter of time before it becomes the new trend in the culinary field.

The Beginning

It was fortunate that I realized I wanted to be a professional chef at the young, impressionable age of sixteen. I chose the hands-on, "in-your-face" instruction of Washburne Trade School in Chicago for my formal training. I worked hard and listened intently to my chef instructors, one of whom soon recommended me for an opening at one of Chicago's finest restaurants, Jimmy's Place. Jimmy's Place was known for its eclectic continental cuisine, its cozy atmosphere, and as the place to see and be seen. Jimmy's was owned and operated by the late Jimmy Rhor, a masterful restaurateur known and respected as a gracious host and for his love of lyric opera. Although Jimmy's Place was my third restaurant job in as many years, this was the most demanding and rewarding of the three. I was paid less to work harder and longer hours; I loved every minute of it.

The head chef of the restaurant was Yoshi Katsaturma. Japanese-born and French-trained, he lived to cook and cooked to live. In Yoshi's kitchen, we made everything from scratch. Although Jimmy's Place was nestled in a northside Chicago neighborhood, I felt as if I were a visitor from another country. Yoshi and the assistant chef spoke Japanese to each other and the two dishwashers spoke Spanish. Yoshi spoke English to me and I communicated with everyone else by pointing and using body gestures and facial expressions. The kitchen roared in rhythm to the dance of pans, heat, and sizzle, but the only voice heard was that of Chef Yoshi. It was here where I learned what being a chef is all about. It means working grueling hours for a perfect composition of food. It means handpicking the freshest and finest ingredients to serve as an expression of the chef. It means the satisfaction of preparing a good meal to create warm memories for someone you'll never see who chose your food over countless other restaurants. Filled with admiration, I was soon hooked on becoming a masterful chef like Yoshi Katsaturma. I'm forever grateful to Chef Yoshi for instilling in my mind the work ethic, attitude, and attention to great detail that epitomizes a good chef—one who cooks passionately in celebration of the glory of good food.

I later worked in various restaurants and hotels perfecting my craft and finding my style. Learning that chefs have the unique opportunity to touch, feel, taste, and prepare foods with the sole purpose of satisfying the customers, I became adept at using food to ignite each of the five senses. I read about food, played with food, and learned about the marriage of different flavors and textures. I studied different countries and cultures and discovered how they celebrate food. I was introduced to interesting and flavorful ingredients and then dreamed of ways to wow diners with my own unique adaptations.

As chefs, we take our experience and knowledge and use them to secure positions and build reputations in the cooking arena of our hearts' desire. It may be classical French, regional Italian, Asian, southwestern, or New American. The culinary arts have forged creative, fun, and inspiring cultural trends and lifestyles that have strongly contributed to the identity of America.

As an aspiring young chef, I never gave a second thought to the excessive amount of fat and calories that I added to the foods I prepared. I took pride in my job as chef saucier (a chef who works the sauté station and prepares all of the soups, sauces, and stocks for the restaurant) and gained a reputation for mastering mouthwatering, flavor-intensive sauces. These sauces made each dish come alive. I finished all of my soups and sauces *au buerre,* adding butter at the end of the preparation. I then whipped them in a blender to create froth and richness, insisting on the finest creams, *crème frâiche*, and high-butterfat whipping creams. I would often reduce the heavy creams to make them richer and thicker before adding them to the sauces or soups. I made conscious efforts to ensure awesome flavor and a memorable dining experience. I viewed my job as one to feed and please. I was not concerned with any social ills that I might have contributed to.

This philosophy served me well as I prospered and advanced in my career. Prior to opening Miraval, I manned the stoves of The 8700 Restaurant at the Citadel. This is a fine dining, southwestern restaurant located in Pinnacle Peak, Arizona. We enjoyed good success at The 8700, earning consistently positive reviews while performing to a consistently full house. Nevertheless, I soon found myself in a creative funk. Although the guests, owners, and staff were all proud and happy with the foods that we produced, I knew there was something more that I could, and should, provide for them and for myself. I looked at the common ingredients that I was using and decided to do something extremely radical.

A New Direction

I pondered the possibilities of creating wonderful foods using typical seasonal ingredients. These foods would be prepared in the same style, with the same presentation and flavor on which I had built my reputation, but this time I would limit or eliminate the use of calorie-laden and high-fat ingredients. I would do the unthinkable. I would cook consciously.

I had forgotten that I was taught to cook consciously with the seasons, to embrace the region in which I lived and worked, and to select only the finest ingredients in preparing foods. To consciously think of the nutritional benefits that my food offered was not something that I spent much time thinking about.

I embarked on creating a menu based on foods that taste great and just so happen to be good for you. Understanding that the notion of a health-conscious, southwestern menu would not be received favorably by most of my audience, it was apparent that I could not tell anyone of my true intent, not even my trusty assistant chef.

I sold the staff, ownership, and marketing executives on a new menu of lighter ingredients in an attempt to follow the public's awareness of better fitness and balance. To my elation, they bought it, and it worked! Our guests were thrilled to learn that the meals they enjoyed were prepared with their wellness in mind. I still offered traditional selections and house favorites that were, let's say, less healthy. I intentionally did not indicate on the menu that some items were healthier. Word quickly spread throughout Arizona about Chef Neff preparing great-tasting foods that were consciously prepared with wellness in mind.

Soon after, fate took over. My mother was diagnosed with fibromyalgia. She was suffering with acute pain in her lower back and knee and quickly became overweight. She found comfort from her pain by eating. Her poor diet created excess weight that caused more pain; a vicious cycle that was horrifically difficult to break. I desperately attempted to suggest foods that would taste great and be healthful. She found that shopping for healthful foods was not only difficult and confusing, it also meant that she had to face the reality of changing her lifestyle. I was now even more intent on creating foods that were healthier and more nutritious. Everything I read insisted that a balanced diet was vital to good health and the relief of numerous illnesses. I found I could play an important role in improving my mother's health and that of so many others.

A Career Change

Within a few weeks, I received a telephone call asking if I would interview at the soon-to-open Miraval Life in Balance Resort and Spa. The offer and the challenge were to develop healthful and balanced gourmet meals for a world-class resort. My responsibilities would also include the orchestration of daily cooking demonstrations and teaching guests how to shop, cook, and eat in a way to achieve wellness. I eagerly accepted the job as Miraval's executive chef and began my journey of defining Conscious Cuisine.

I submerged myself in nutritional literature, studying all sorts of diets that proclaimed good health and weight loss in weeks. It was not long before I discovered that there are no magic diet plans, and the only long-term, proven way of improving one's health coupled with weight loss is a lifestyle featuring exercise and a nutritionally balanced diet.

Conscious Cuisine

Spa cuisine and diet foods in the early '90s were noted for providing nutritionally balanced meals that were low in calories and fat. Unfortunately, most of it was extremely low in taste and enjoyment as well. My goal as the executive chef of Miraval was to use this platform to create a food style that was visually appealing, great tasting, nutritionally balanced, and in step with the current food styles expected by diners today. I titled this style of cooking "Conscious Cuisine," the simple act of being more conscious of the foods we eat in every sense—which gave us the title of this book, *Conscious Cuisine*.

Conscious Cuisine requires a lifestyle change and an understanding of the daily caloric intake that is recommended for your age, height, weight, and gender. Reliable nutritional information is readily available from many government agencies and numerous nutrition books. The change in lifestyle will mean:

- taking the time to decide which foods are the best for you to purchase;
- choosing foods that are the least processed because they retain more of their nutritional value;
- making conscious decisions to balance your meals with foods that taste good to you and are good for you;
- learning some of the countless ways of preparing vegetables and whole grains;
- breaking the habit of focusing each meal on animal proteins and beginning to consciously choose whole foods that provide vitamins and minerals to help combat illnesses;
- making fresh vegetables, legumes, and whole grains a vital part of your diet;
- complementing meals with animal proteins rather than having them as the main ingredient;
- beginning to make conscious choices about when and how often to eat fried, high-fat, or calorie-dense foods;
- remembering that there are no bad foods, just bad portion sizes and frequency of consumption choices.

Conscious cooking soon changed my life and the lives of those around me. For the first time I was questioning the origins of the foods that I ate and served. It was suddenly important to know how my food was grown. Was it organically or conventionally grown, treated with pesticides, growth hormones, steroids, or any other chemical unknown to me? I began to be more conscious of what I wanted from my foods. I was certain that it must be flavorful and fully understood that conscious choices regarding foods could offer healthier benefits and relief to my mom and many others.

Scrumptious foods that offered empty calories were no longer acceptable. The foods that I now served had to be both delicious and nutritious. I began to use more whole grains and the least-processed food products for their ability to provide more of their natural nutrients and unique flavors. I was then able to teach my mom, my wife, and my guests how to shop for produce that was in season, fully ripened, and at its peak of flavor. I taught them the difference and importance of organic foods.

Conscious Cuisine provides you with recipes and techniques that will help you discover new healthful foods, cooking methods, and nutritional awareness. Cooking terminology is explained to help you better understand how professional chefs adapt new recipes with ease. The use of basic cooking terms and techniques has long been a key ingredient for training budding chefs to be more efficient in the kitchen. You too will learn to cook with confidence, creating sinfully delicious foods without the use of excessive fats and calories. I have also included a full nutritional analysis of each recipe to illustrate the nutritional benefits of *Conscious Cuisine*. I'm certain you will enjoy the descriptive and colorful photos that come alive within the pages, demonstrating to you that *Conscious Cuisine* is as visually appealing as it is delicious.

To answer the most frequently asked questions from my guests through the years, I have included information on how to shop seasonally for foods, how to outfit your kitchen with healthful foods, and how to procure hard-to-find natural ingredients.

It is my hope that *Conscious Cuisine* will unleash new ideas for healthier foods for all those who love to cook, from the avid home cook to the aspiring professional. *Conscious Cuisine* will open your senses to new possibilities.

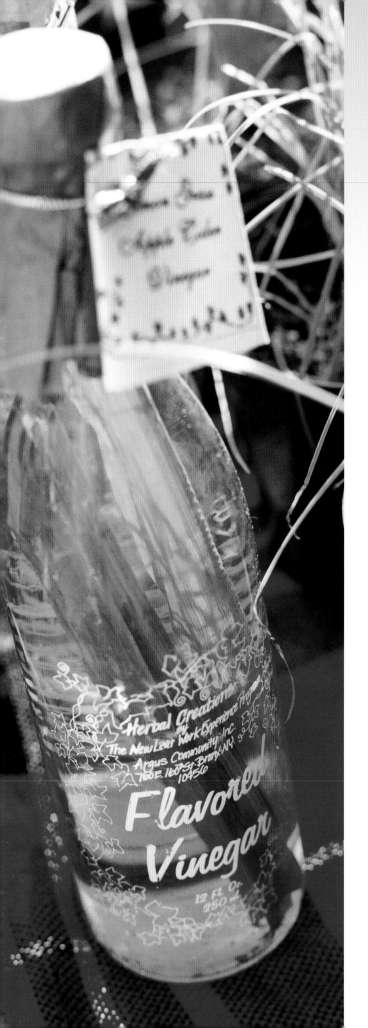

Special Ingredients List

Amaranth: Amaranth dates back eight thousand years. It was used in religious tributes and as a dietary staple of the Aztecs. The Spanish conquistador Cortés outlawed the cultivation of amaranth, which effectively starved the Aztecs and destroyed their culture.

Amaranth is not a true grain, although it is touted as a supergrain. It is related to pigweed, a common pest. Amaranth has a chewy texture and a nutty, slightly peppery flavor. It contains high amounts of calcium, folic acid, magnesium, and iron.

Anaheim chile: A long, tapered chile with a pale to medium bright green color, relatively thick flesh, and a mild flavor. Available fresh, canned, or roasted, but not dried. Also known as the California chile and long green chile. Available in most grocery stores, natural food stores, and Hispanic grocery stores.

Anchovy paste: Pounded anchovies mixed with vinegar and spices and usually sold in a tube. Available in most grocery stores and specialty food stores.

Arame: Dried, shredded seaweed with a greenish-brown color and a mild, delicate flavor. Used as a flavoring in Japanese cuisine. Available in natural food stores and Asian grocery stores.

Azuki beans (also **adzuki**): A favorite in Asia, these small, sweet red beans are processed into red-bean paste to prepare desserts. Excellent with rice or barley, they are available dry and as bean paste.

Barley: The most popular type of barley available in markets today is pearl barley, which has been processed to remove the outer hull and bran. This process removes many of its nutrients. Hulled barley is the densest type of barley, from which only the inedible outer hull has been removed. This barley has a pleasant chewy texture and does not become sticky during cooking like pearl barley. Hulled barley contains two or three times the protein of an equal portion of rice. When cooked, hulled barley is similar to brown rice in appearance, but it is chewier and darker in color. It has a rich, wonderful, whole-grain flavor with slightly nutty tones.

Bean curd sheets: These sheets are made by lifting and drying the thin layer that forms on the surface of hot soymilk as it cools. They are high in protein. They are sold fresh, semi-dried, and dried in Asian grocery stores.

Black beans (turtle beans): These black, oval beans have an earthy flavor and are used widely in Latin, Japanese, and Chinese cookery. They provide dramatic color and flavor in black bean soup and black bean cakes. They are available dried and canned.

Buckwheat: Buckwheat is not a true grain. Buckwheat belongs to the sorrel and rhubarb family. Buckwheat groats have a triangular shape and assertive flavor. Buckwheat is high in amino acids and magnesium. Buckwheat is available in several forms: groats, whole buckwheat, and kasha. Whole buckwheat is white when raw and brown when roasted. Kasha is roasted, hulled buckwheat kernels that are cracked into coarse, medium, and fine granules.

Cannellini beans: These are large white kidney beans often used in Italian dishes such as minestrone soup. They are available dried and canned.

Chickpea flour: Ground dried chickpeas. This flour is used in Middle Eastern cooking and to make chickpea crêpes. Available in some natural food stores and Indian food stores.

Chickpeas (Garbanzo beans): Acorn-shaped beans that are a tan to brown color, chickpeas are key to Middle Eastern and Mediterranean dishes. They are available dried and canned. (See **chickpea flour**, page xv.)

Chinese five-spice powder: A spice blend used in Asian cooking, generally consisting of ground cloves, fennel seeds, star anise, cinnamon, and Szechwan pepper. Available in some grocery stores, natural food stores, and Asian grocery stores.

Chipotle: A dried, smoked jalepeño, this medium-sized chile has a dull tan to dark brown color with a wrinkled skin and a smoky, slightly sweet, relatively mild flavor with undertones of tobacco and chocolate. Available dry or canned in sauce in most grocery stores, natural food stores, and Hispanic grocery stores.

Cranberry beans: These are beige-colored, oval-shaped beans with pink spots. They have a nutty flavor and are used in stews and casseroles. They are available fresh and dried.

Curry paste: A blend of spices that have been combined with a little fat or oil, there are a variety of pastes available such as red, green, or yellow depending on the spices used. Curry paste is used primarily in Indian and Pakistani dishes. The paste is available at most natural foods stores and Asian grocery stores.

Fava beans (broad beans): A personal favorite, they are large, flat beans, pale green when fresh and brown in their dried form. They are time-consuming to shell, and have two pods, an outer shell and another shell around each bean. Both shells should be removed before eating. Their pleasant, nutty flavor combines well with aromatic Italian dishes. They are available fresh, dried, canned, and frozen.

Fish sauce: Made from the liquid of salted, fermented fish and optional seasoning, fish sauce is used as a flavoring in Thai, Vietnamese, and other Asian cuisine. Fish sauce has a very strong odor and a distinctive flavor, which mellows as it cooks. It is available in Asian grocery stores, natural food stores, and grocery stores.

Flageolets: These are actually immature kidney beans; they are pale green in color, smooth, flat, and oval-shaped. They are used in traditional French cassoulet dishes, as well as in soups and cold salads. They are available dried.

Flax seeds: Flax seeds provide a good source of omega-3 fatty acids, fiber, and ligan (plant estrogen). They can be ground and added to salads, soups, and cereal. Flax seeds are available in natural food stores and most grocery stores.

Garam masala: A blend of spices used in Indian cooking, usually containing peppercorns, cardamom, cinnamon, cloves, coriander, nutmeg, turmeric, and/or fennel seeds. Available in specialty food stores, natural food stores, and Indian food stores.

Great Northern beans: These are oval-shaped, large white beans with a mild flavor. A perfect addition to soups, stews, and casseroles, they are available dried and canned.

Hulled hemp seeds: Hemp seeds are high in protein, B vitamins, and dietary fiber. Available in natural food stores and some specialty grocery stores.

Jícama: A legume that grows underground as a tuber, jícama is a large, brown-skinned, white-fleshed, root vegetable. The texture is crispy, and it has a sweet, nutty flavor. Jícama is eaten raw or cooked and tastes wonderful grated in salads. Jícama is available in some grocery stores and Hispanic grocery stores.

Kalamata olives: These are ripe Greek olives that are usually packed in olive oil. These olives have a strong, salty flavor and are a great addition to Greek and Middle Eastern dishes. Toss a few in a salad for added flavor. Kalamata olives are available in Middle Eastern grocery stores, most natural food stores, and some grocery stores.

Kidney beans: Known for their kidney shape, they range in color from pink to brown and are a favorite in chilies and Mexican dishes. They are available dried and canned.

Kombu: A dark-brown kelp that is cut, dried, and folded. It is used as a flavoring in Japanese cooking, in Asian stocks, and soaked and cut into strips and added to soups and stews. Kombu is available in most natural food stores and Asian grocery stores.

Lemongrass: A tropical grass with a citrus flavor, it is used in Asian cooking. The grass is a long stalk that is one to two feet long with a greenish outside color and white interior. Use just the bottom six inches for the best flavor. Lemongrass is available in Asian grocery stores, some natural food stores, and grocery stores.

Lentils: Lentils are small, disk-shaped legumes found in green, brown, yellow, and orange. They cook quickly and boast a slight peppery flavor. They are great in soups, mixed with other vegetables, or in salads. They are available dried.

Lima beans: Medium-sized, flat beans that are white to pale green, they are used extensively in stews and succotash. They are available canned, dried, fresh, and frozen.

Menlo wrappers: These wrappers are made from cornstarch and/or wheat flour and come in rounds or squares. They are used in Filipino cuisine to wrap meat, fish, and vegetables. They can be deep-fried or baked. Menlo wrappers are available in Asian grocery stores.

Millet: These grains are tiny, spherical, pale yellow to reddish-orange in color, and have a delicate, nut-like flavor. Nutritionally powerful, millet equals or surpasses wheat in protein content and is higher in B vitamins, copper, and iron than whole wheat and brown rice. When fresh, this crunchy seed tastes mildly sweet with a very subtle alkaline aftertaste. It is gluten-free and very rich in amino acids and phosphorus.

Miso paste: Miso is a fermented paste made with soybeans that have generally been mixed with grains such as rice or barley. It is very rich in protein and, according to Asian tradition, is used as an aid in digestion. Light yellow miso has a delicate flavor and is about 6 percent salt. Red miso has a stronger flavor and is about 9 percent salt. Miso paste is available in some grocery stores, natural food stores, and Asian grocery stores.

Mung beans: Used frequently in Asian dishes, these small, round legumes are green, yellow, or black. They cook quickly and become soft and sweet tasting. They are available fresh, dried, and sprouted.

Navy beans (pea beans): A smaller version of the Great Northern beans, but less mealy with a milder flavor. They are available dried and canned.

Nopales: The young pads of the prickly pear cactus, they have an oval, flat shape with little spines. To remove the spines, hold the base of pad, and using a sharp knife, run it over the spines. Repeat this on the other side to ensure all the spines have been removed before cutting into strips and cooking. Nopales are available in Hispanic grocery stores and some grocery stores. They are also available canned.

Nori: Dark green to black, these are thin sheets of dried seaweed used to make sushi. They can be sliced into thin strips and added to salads or as a garnish. They are available in most natural food stores and Asian grocery stores.

Oats: The numerous forms in which oats are available are whole kernels, rolled oats, steel-cut oats, and oat bran. One of the most common forms to eat oats is oatmeal, a good source of protein, B vitamins, calcium, unsaturated fats, and fiber. Chewy but moist, oats are sweeter and nuttier than other grains because of their higher lipid profile. Science has found that oats help regulate blood sugar. Oats contain compounds that prevent cancer in animals and act as a laxative.

Pasteurized egg whites: These egg whites have been heated to 140°–180°F (60°–82°C) for a short period of time to kill any bacteria. Pasteurized egg whites are great for making mousses, cheesecakes, and fillings that are not going to be cooked. They are available in the refrigerator or frozen sections of most grocery stores.

Peas (split pea, garden pea): These small green or yellow peas cook quickly and have a nutty flavor. Ideal for soups, stews, purees, and casseroles, they are available fresh, dried, canned, and frozen.

Pinto beans: A medium-sized and reddish-tan bean with brown specks, it is the most popular bean in the United States. Its earthy flavor is a favorite in Mexican dishes. They are available dried and canned.

Poblano chile: Large and fairly mild, the dark green, fresh poblano is about five inches long. This chile has a nutty flavor and is often stuffed for chile rellenos. They are usually roasted and peeled. Substitute Anaheims for poblanos if necessary. When dried, these are called ancho chiles. Available in most grocery stores, natural food stores, and Hispanic grocery stores.

Potato starch (flour): The pure starch remaining from soaking grated potatoes in water, potato starch can be used as a thickener or in baking.

Quinoa: Quinoa is not a true grain; it is related to a leafy vegetable similar to Swiss chard. Because it has a grainlike appearance and uses, it is considered a super-grain for its high levels of iron, potassium, and riboflavin and amounts of protein. This grain has a subtly sweet yet nutty flavor, delivering an almost piquant aftertaste. Ranging in color from light brown, amber, or black, quinoa seeds are flat, pointed, and oval. When cooked, their texture becomes light, springy, and crunchy.

Raw cane sugar: This sugar, also called **Turbinado sugar,** is made from evaporated sugarcane juice. The sugar still has the molasses intact and has a slight nutty flavor similar to brown sugar. It can be substituted one-to-one for white granulated sugar. It is available in most natural foods stores and many grocery stores.

Red beans: Medium-sized, brick-red oval beans, these rich, savory flavored beans are a favorite in soul food and southern cooking. They are available dried or canned.

Rice: A versatile grain, rice has many forms, colors, and flavors. Rice is a good source of B vitamins, such as thiamin and niacin, and provides iron, phosphorus, and magnesium. Rice is usually eaten in its least nourishing form—white rice that has been milled and polished to remove the bran and germ, which contain valuable nutrients. Brown rice is a great complement to almost any meal; it serves well as a base for desserts or drinks.

Rye: Rye is similar nutritionally to wheat. Compared to all the common grains, it has the highest percentage of the amino acid lysine. It contains B vitamins, vitamin E, protein, and iron, including minerals. Rye bread's tangy flavor has more to do with lactic acid fermentation than with the actual taste of rye, which is quite sweet.

Sea salt: A natural salt that has more minerals than table salt and is derived from evaporated sea water. Sea salt is available in fine or coarse crystals and has a full flavor, enabling cooks to use less salt when preparing dishes.

Seasoned rice wine vinegar: Made from rice wine and seasoned with salt and sugar, it has a delicate flavor and is great for salad dressings, salads, and in marinades. It is available both seasoned and plain in Asian grocery stores, natural food stores, and most grocery stores.

Seitan: A great high-protein meat substitute, it is made by extracting the wheat gluten from a whole-wheat flour and water mixture. Seitan has a firm, chewy texture and can be chopped up and substituted for ground meat or sliced and grilled and used in vegetarian steak sandwiches.

Semolina flour: A grainy, pale yellow flour made from ground durum wheat, semolina is used for making pasta dough. It is available in specialty markets.

Soybeans: The most versatile and widely used legume crop of the world, soybeans are available in many forms. Soy oil is used for dressings, soy protein as a meat or milk substitute, and soy flour for pasta and cereals. Soybean paste (**miso**) is used in Asian dishes. **Tofu** (see page xix) and **tempeh** (see page xviii) are made from soybeans.

Sriracha sauce: A Thai hot sauce made from hot peppers, vinegar, salt, and sugar, this chile sauce has a unique flavor and is great added to any Asian-inspired dishes such as marinades, sauces, and stir-fries. Sriracha is available in Asian grocery stores, natural foods stores, and some grocery stores.

Tahini (sesame seed paste): A paste made from ground, hulled, and toasted sesame seeds, tahini is creamy and light beige in color. It is used in Middle Eastern dishes, such as hummus and falafel. It is available in Middle Eastern stores, natural food stores, and some grocery stores.

Teff: This tiny cereal grain tastes almost like hazelnut. The seed can be white, red-purple, or brown. It is a good source of calcium and iron.

Tempeh: Tempeh is a soybean cake made from whole soybeans, which have been fermented to make them easier to digest. Some tempeh is made with added seeds, grains, and other beans. Tempeh has a nutty flavor, which will take on the flavors of marinades and sauces. You can slice and sauté it for use in sandwiches, stir-fries, and casseroles. It can also be crumbled and sautéed and used with tomato sauce to make chili or other favorite meat dishes that use ground meat. Tempeh is available in natural food stores, Asian grocery stores, and some grocery stores.

Tofu: A firm, custard-like substance made from curdled soymilk, tofu is high in protein. It is very versatile and has a bland flavor, which will pick up other flavors added to it. Tofu comes in different degrees of firmness, depending on how much water has been pressed out of the tofu. Extra-firm tofu is good for stir-frying. Silken tofu is ideal for smoothies, pudding, and baking. Tofu is available in natural food stores, Asian grocery stores, and grocery stores.

Tomatillos: Small, pale-green fruits with outer husks, tomatillos resemble green tomatoes. Tomatillos are light to yellowish green, and have a crisp texture and a lemony flavor. Remove the outer husk before using. They are used in southwestern and Mexican cooking and can be cooked or eaten raw. Chopped, they add a refreshing crispness to salsa. Tomatillos are available in most grocery stores and Hispanic grocery stores.

Vanilla bean pod: The dried and cured pod-like fruit of the orchid plant. Inside the pods are tiny black seeds that add great flavor in baking. **To make vanilla sugar**: split the vanilla bean pod in half lengthwise and scrape out the seeds per 2 cups of sugar. Store in an airtight container for 48 hours before using.

Wax Orchards Fruit Sweet Syrup: A rich, very concentrated, natural blend of peach, pear, and pineapple juices, this syrup is sweeter than sugar or honey. It is available in most natural food stores and online.

Wheat: Wheat is one of the most important cereal crops, nourishing much of the world's population. The most common form of wheat is wheat flour, of which there are many varieties (see **whole-wheat pastry flour**, page xix). Wheat contains B vitamins, vitamin E, protein, essential fatty acids, and important trace minerals. Wheat is also available cracked as **bulgur** and as **wheat berries**.

Whole-wheat pastry flour: Made from ground, soft, spring wheat, whole-wheat pastry flour contains the wheat germ and some bran. When combined with unbleached all-purpose flour, it helps produce a tender baking product with a higher nutritional content.

Wild rice: Not a true grain, wild rice is an aquatic grass seed. Wild rice has been part of the Native American diet for over ten thousand years. Boasting a pleasant chewiness, the nutty and rich flavor lends itself to a host of complementary ingredients and dishes. This grain provides twice the amount of protein as brown rice and higher levels of B vitamins.

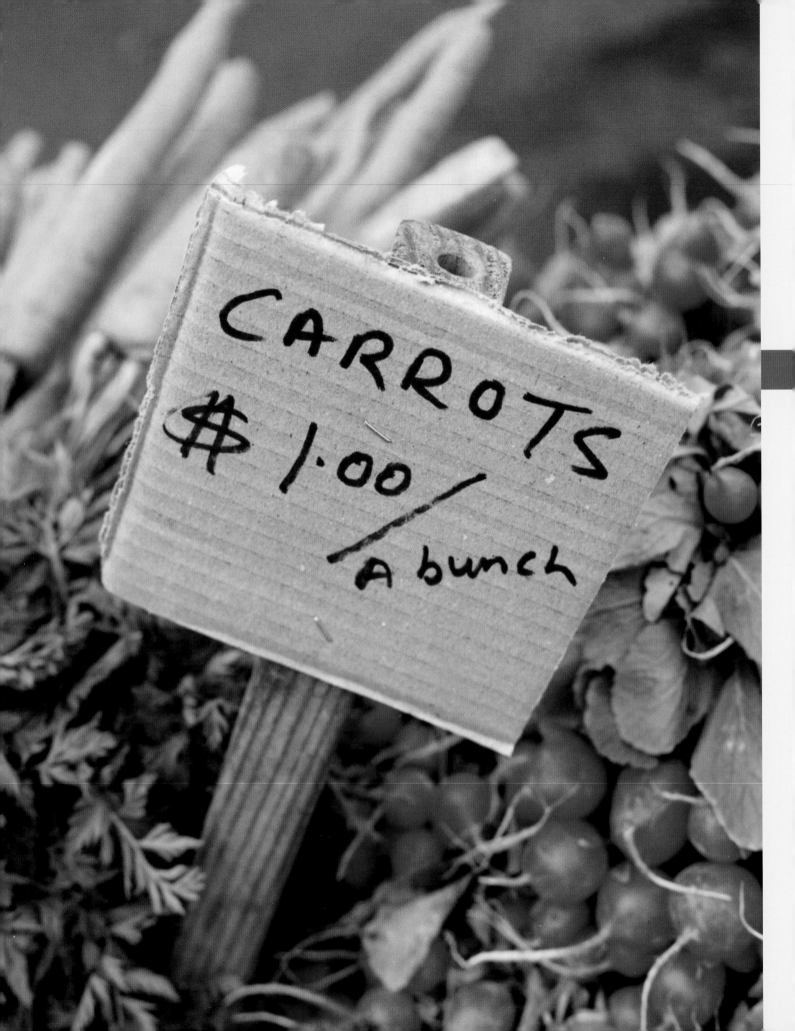

Let's Go Shopping

chapter 1

A healthful and balanced diet calls for you to eat foods that are rich with flavor and provide nutritional benefits. Conscious decisions regarding the quality of the food you purchase, the use of flavor components, and satisfying portions served will help you create a lifestyle of wellness and vitality.

Conscious Cuisine uses fresh seasonal produce as a cornerstone in producing a nutritious and balanced diet. Vegetables supply nearly all the nutrients required for good health. A balanced diet will decrease the need for vitamin supplements and reactive medicines taken to create wellness. Whole-grain products also contain a wealth of vital minerals and vitamins. Many whole grains such as quinoa, barley, and amaranth contain an abundance of protein and iron. All whole grains are complex carbohydrates, which turn into fuel quickly, especially for individuals with an active lifestyle.

When grocery shopping, refocus your meal planning. Select produce items that are in season and build your menus around them. Use high-quality, lean animal proteins to complement your meals rather than as the basis of the meal. They should not dominate the meal in portion size or importance. The USDA recommends five servings of vegetables daily, but the average American eats less than two servings of vegetables a day. Select whole-grain products instead of processed foods as much as possible. You will immediately notice their full flavor and heartiness, but most of all, you will enjoy food that is sustainable and not filled with empty calories.

When time is limited by the demands of your daily schedule, what are some methods to make grocery shopping less of a burden, and what type of foods should you purchase to prepare healthful and nutritious foods? The following guidelines will make shopping a pleasant experience and show you how to make the right decisions.

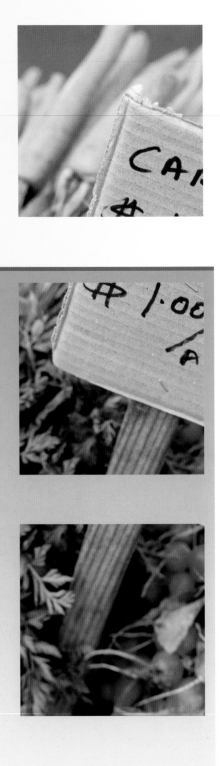

How to Grocery Shop

To make shopping less of a chore, shop monthly or bimonthly at one or more warehouse-type grocers and stock up on all of your essentials. You will save money by buying in bulk and save time from repetitive shopping for the same items weekly. Look for deals on paper products, cleaning products, toiletries, and nonfood items.

Seek out farmers' markets, whole-food markets, and specialty food stores in your area. Even if you have to drive an extra twenty minutes, please invest the time; your body will thank you for it. Choose reputable markets that carry a variety of organic produce as well as whole-grain products.

Before you go shopping, ask yourself these two questions. When do I have time to cook? Which meals will we be eating at home? By first realistically planning when you will have the time to cook and eat at home, you eliminate wasting foods that are purchased and never prepared. Purchase only enough food for the meals that you have planned to prepare and only enough for the people you are responsible for feeding. Don't cook large amounts of food just in case family and friends stop by. This eliminates leftovers and enables you to spend your food dollars on better quality ingredients that are enjoyable to cook and eat.

Reconsider the place of meat in your meal planning. Most Americans were taught to create meals around meat (beef, poultry, and seafood). This has convinced us that a meal is not complete unless it's centered with a large portion of animal protein. This method has produced a culture which consumes massive amounts of protein; the U.S. consumes more red meat than any other country in the world. Animal proteins should complement the other dishes, but they should not dominate the meal in portion size or importance. Eating Conscious Cuisine, you'll be consuming less meat protein and more grains and vegetables, so shop accordingly.

Add fun and variety to shopping by visiting the produce aisle first. Use the freshest produce often and lavishly as the centerpiece of your meals. Purchase only what's in season. Consider how the most beautiful fruits and vegetables might taste in various recipes and, finally, how other foods will complement them. Conscious Cuisine means allowing the seasons to dictate and create your meals. The meat, poultry, and seafood available today are consistent in quality and availability year round, but great produce comes and goes with the seasons. Savor the abundant variety of flavors that nature has awarded us—don't take it for granted.

Remember, good health and longevity are achievable with good, clean food. The main purpose of food is to fuel your body by providing energy, vitamins, minerals, and other nutrients. A conscious selection of nutritious foods can provide great tasting meals, and also ones that can combat illnesses and reduce the occurrence of food-related diseases.

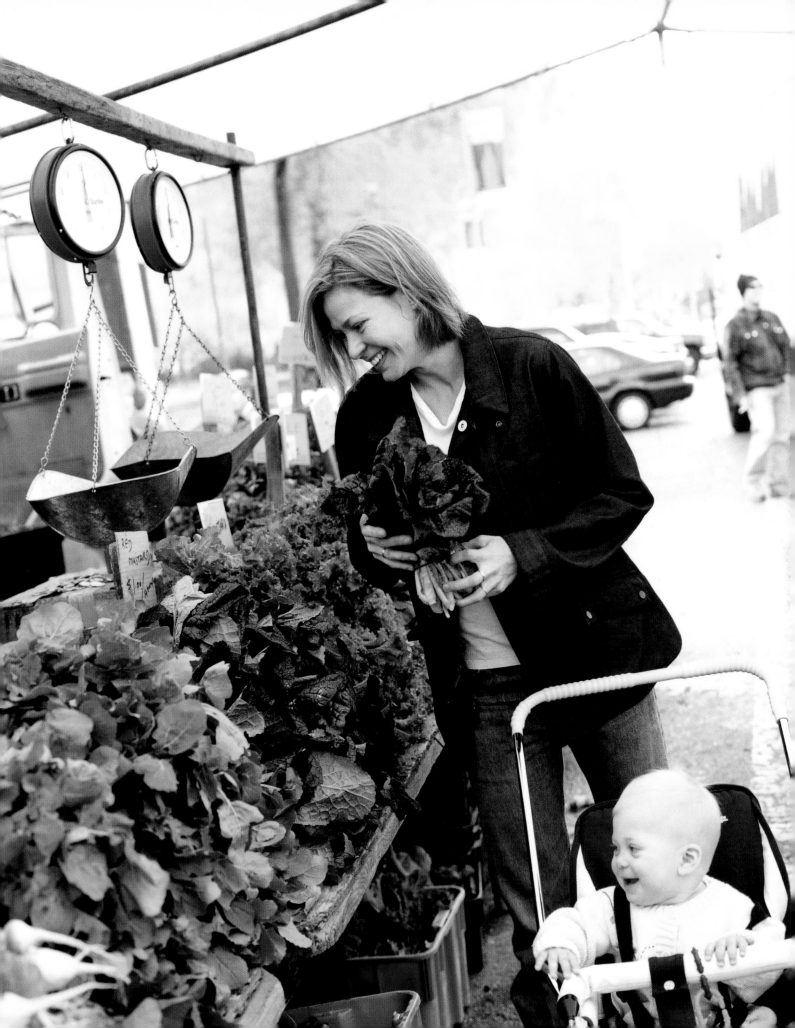

Produce

When shopping for produce, think about what season you are in and where you live. Produce is more flavorful, abundant, and less expensive when it is purchased in season. Buying regionally grown foods creates the opportunity to acquire food that has traveled less, since it is more easily available from local farm stands and markets. These foods are usually allowed to ripen longer in the field, gaining optimum flavor.

Organic Produce

Certified organic produce is grown in fields that have not been treated with any pesticides and chemicals.

As a chef, father, mentor, and member of Chefs Collaborative 2000, I choose organically farmed produce as much as feasibly possible for my family and the guests of Miraval Life in Balance Resort and Spa. Many Americans have forgotten or have never tasted the rich, luscious flavors of vine-ripened tomatoes, peaches, melons, and squash. This produce is given nutrient-rich soil, water, and sunshine, and is harvested only when it has ripened fully and is bursting with succulent juices and flavors.

When choosing a lifestyle focusing on balance, good health, and vitality, certified organic foods provide you with a sustainable option. Organic produce offers a wealth of vital nutrients and cancer-fighting antioxidants, without the addition of harmful or potentially harmful chemicals. Organic produce is harvested fully ripened, allowing its flavors to develop naturally. Conventional produce is routinely packaged and allowed to ripen during shipping, and is often chemically treated to help it ripen faster "off the vine." Besides the noticeable difference in flavor, I cherish the opportunity to support the family and small independent farmers whose efforts and expertise produce delicious crops in a healthful and sustainable manner.

For all of these reasons, I highly recommend that you choose to purchase organic produce whenever possible.

Dairy Products and Eggs

Milk and eggs are two of nature's most nutritious foods. Americans receive most of their calcium from milk products, and eggs are excellent sources of protein and vitamins. From a culinary standpoint, milk and eggs are almost indispensable. Remarkably versatile, these foods lend themselves to use in a vast number of dishes. Milk and eggs can lighten cakes, bind vegetables, or be part of the main dish.

Dairy products also boast a high amount of saturated fat and cholesterol, and one egg contains two-thirds of the total suggested daily maximum intake of cholesterol. Many physicians suggest that dairy products contribute to sinus difficulties and allergies. What are we to do?

If you choose to include dairy products in your diet—and I do include them in *Conscious Cuisine*—make conscious decisions about the type and quality of those products. When using eggs, try to use more egg whites than

Rules of Thumb: Produce

- Bask in the season's best. When in season, produce should be abundant and more flavorful and affordable than when out of season.
- Remember, your produce is going to be the main attraction in your meal.
- Buy the best produce that is available and be flexible. If the broccoli you planned to buy is not at its best, perhaps the crisp green beans are a better choice.
- Make a conscious decision concerning the type of produce you choose to purchase—organic, conventional, or genetically modified.

yolks. Egg whites are free of cholesterol and fat and are almost pure protein. You can reduce your whole egg consumption by using egg whites instead of whole eggs in your breakfast and baking recipes.

I personally enjoy the richness and flavor of organic milk. I also appreciate knowing that it comes from cows that have not been fed steroids or growth hormones to help them produce more milk. It is inevitable that remnants of the chemicals are contained in the milk that the cows produce. I'm a chef, not a scientist, so I do not know if the addition of steroids in dairy cows creates a potential health hazard or not. But, I do know that certified organic milk is different in color, thickness, and, most importantly, flavor. For my family, I purchase organic dairy products. Whatever your choice for milk products may be, use fat-free or reduced-fat milk. Use fat-free yogurt for smoothies and dressings. I have found that reduced-fat sour cream, cottage cheese, ricotta, and cream cheeses are acceptable alternatives to their high-fat counterparts. Very little flavor is lost in these products. There are some good soy cheeses for vegans who want cheese flavor in their recipes.

For other types of cheese, such as blue cheese or cheddar, I do not recommend the low-fat versions. Cheese is a decadent food that has been crafted with skill and love for hundreds of years. Cultures were formed and celebrations held in honor of the delicious cheeses of Europe and America. Conscious Cuisine embraces the luscious flavor of well-made, aromatic, and tantalizing cheeses. When using cheese in recipes, I have taught my staff and guests to choose the highest quality available. Freshly grated Parmesan Reggiano is so superior in flavor to the powdered stuff in the can that you will need at least 1/2 cup of the powdered to mimic the flavor of 1 tablespoon of good quality Parmesan. So buying inexpensively does not necessarily translate into savings, while buying quality does translate into enjoyment.

Rules of Thumb: Dairy and Eggs

- Buy small amounts of good quality cheeses.
- Purchase organic or free-range eggs whenever possible.
- Buy butter instead of margarine. The trans fats in margarine may be far worse for you than the saturated fat in butter.
- Select high-quality dairy products. The rich flavor of quality products will allow you to use less, making them less expensive to use.
- When possible, choose fat-free organic milk, which contains no antibiotics, steroids, or growth hormones.
- Purchase whole milk for infants and young children up to two years of age because it contains essential fatty acids necessary for brain development.
- Choose fat-free and low-fat milk for older children and adults.

Types of Milk

Acidophilus milk has had *Lactobacillus acidophilus* added to help strengthen the intestines.

Buttermilk is cultured milk made with lactic acid and fat-free or low-fat milk.

Dry milk powder is usually made from fat-free milk. One tablespoon of dry milk contains twenty-seven calories, no fat, and has vitamins A and D added to it.

Evaporated milk is made by removing half of the water in the milk. Evaporated fat-free milk contains less than one gram of fat per cup. It's great for low-fat cooking and will even whip when well chilled.

Fat-free milk, the best choice for most adults, has half the calories of whole milk and gets only 5 percent of its calories from fat.

Low-fat or 1 percent milk has 23 percent of its calories from fat.

Reduced-fat or 2 percent milk has 35 percent of its calories from fat.

Grains

We have become a society that worships convenience. However, when cooking for enjoyment, nourishment, and wellness, reducing cooking time by fifteen minutes is a big sacrifice to make in nutritional value and flavor. The grains we eat tend to be heavily refined, a process which removes the outer layers, making the grains easier to chew and quicker to cook. The outer layers of the grain contain most of the fiber, B vitamins, trace minerals, and some of the protein. Most refined grains are "enriched" with nutrients, but this process does not completely replace what has been lost. Grain-based convenience foods not only have fewer nutrients, but they also tend to contain high amounts of sugar, fat, and sodium.

Whole grains are one of the best sources of complex carbohydrates—a nutrition powerhouse! They are rich in soluble fiber (the type of fiber that helps to decrease blood cholesterol) and insoluble fiber (the type of fiber that prevents constipation and protects us from some types of cancer). There is evidence proving that people living in areas where unrefined grains are a significant part of their diet have a lower incidence of intestinal and bowel problems, such as colon cancer, diverticulosis, and hemorrhoids.

Legumes

Legumes (dried beans and peas) paired with grains are the least expensive and most nutritious food sources available. Legumes are low in fat and loaded with high-energy complex carbohydrates, B vitamins, zinc, potassium, magnesium, calcium, and iron. Legumes have more protein than any other vegetable food. The protein is incomplete because of a deficiency in one or more amino acids. Once complemented with grains or a small amount of an animal product, the added food completes the protein by providing complementary amino acids.

Legumes come in a variety of shapes and colors. Many legumes are available canned and are higher in sodium with a softer texture. Otherwise, their nutritional value is the same.

Fish and Shellfish

Fish and shellfish present enthusiastic cooks with the opportunity to create hundreds of delicious dishes that are great sources of protein, while being low in calories, fat, and cholesterol. Fish and shellfish, when prepared mindfully, provide delicate and flavorful dishes that are not only appetizing, but also promote good health.

Fish and shellfish are low in saturated fat and are a good source of vitamin B-12, iodine, phosphorus, and zinc. Fish fat, which takes the form of oil, contains certain types of polyunsaturated fatty acids known as omega-3s. They have anticlotting properties and thus protect against heart attack and high blood pressure. Fish oils also lower our blood cholesterol.

Rules of Thumb: Grains

- Choose whole-grain products as often as possible for their higher nutrient value and flavor.
- Purchase whole grains from a busy, reputable grocer who is dependable for stocking quality products which are rotated often.
- Vary the types of grains that you purchase, and try new ones that are unfamiliar to you such as millet or quinoa.
- Select grains that have been cracked or ground, in addition to whole kernels, to make meals more interesting.
- Store grains, legumes, cereals, and pastas in airtight containers.

Purchasing Fish and Shellfish

Seek out a purveyor or market that emphasizes quality. This establishment should be willing and able to provide information regarding the fish's origin and quality. Your chosen fish market should not only be able to tell you if your choice of fish is lean or oily, firm or flaky in texture, or has heavy or delicate flavor, it should also tell you which methods of cooking provide the most flavorful product.

Smell the fish. It should have a clean sea smell.

When pressed with your finger, the fish should be firm and elastic.

The fish eyes should be clear and full, not milky and sunken.

The gills should be bright red, not gray.

The skin should feel slick and moist. The scales should be firmly attached.

No liquid should be surrounding packaged fillets or steaks.

Frozen fish should not have white frost or cotton-like patches present. These are sure signs of freezer burn.

Shellfish, when purchased live (i.e., crab, lobster), should show noticeable movement. Live clams, mussels, and oyster shells should be tightly closed. Any shells that do not close when tapped should be discarded.

Storing Fish and Shellfish

Purchase only the amount needed for one to two days at the most.

Transport fish and shellfish in a cooler to maintain a consistent cold temperature.

Rinse and rewrap fish immediately. Wrap it in a paper towel, place in a container, and cover the container with a bag of ice.

Fish should not sit in a pool of water at any time. This causes bruising and loss of flavor.

Keep frozen products frozen; place them in the freezer immediately in their original containers.

Freeze fresh fish as quickly as possible. If it is whole, cut it into smaller pieces. Rinse and pat it dry. Wrap it tightly with plastic wrap. Cover the wrap with foil. Label, date, and freeze, preferably at 0°F or below (-20°C or below). Refrigerator freezer compartments do not generally reach this cold temperature. Individual deep freezer units are your best source.

Clams, mussels, and oysters should be stored in their original delivery bags and never iced. Store them around 40°F (5°C).

Live shellfish should be packed with seaweed or damp paper and refrigerated at 40°F (5°C), but not too cold. Avoid contact with fresh water. This will surely kill your crustacean.

Thaw frozen seafood slowly under refrigeration. Remove it from the freezer one to two days before use. Refrain from defrosting it in water, which will dilute the flavor and nutrients.

Rules of Thumb: Legumes

- Purchase legumes that are brightly colored and free from cracks or broken beans. Also check for insect damage (pinhole-sized marks).
- Purchase beans from a busy, reputable grocer who is dependable for stocking quality products which are rotated often.
- Store legumes in a sealed container at a cool room temperature. They should keep for up to a year.

Rules of Thumb: Fish and Shellfish

- Because seafood is one of the most perishable food products, I have detailed guidelines for both purchasing and storing it.

Meats and Poultry

Americans have always had a love affair with meat and poultry. Americans, who make up only 7 percent of the world's population, eat one-third of the world's meat supply.

Despite their wonderful flavor and high protein content, meats and poultry are high in saturated fat and cholesterol. However, meat protein does have some advantages. Meat contains heme iron, the type of iron that is best absorbed by the body. Plant foods also contain iron, but it is nonheme, which does not absorb as well in our bodies. The protein found in meat and poultry is complete with all the amino acids needed by the body.

Conscious Cuisine uses fresh meats and poultry as a complement to meals, relying on the many different types, various cuts, and high-protein content to consciously create delicious and nutritionally balanced meals. *Conscious Cuisine* instills new habits with regard to reducing portion sizes and increasing the quality of the meats and poultry products used to create healthful and delicious meals. By selecting lean, high-quality meats and poultry, we embrace their delicate flavors. When you reduce the portion size of your protein, you must depend more on the flavor and the nutritional benefits of the other components to make the meal balanced and complete. When the protein found in meats and poultry is reduced or eliminated from our diet, the body must replace the nutrients they supply with those from legumes, produce, and a variety of whole grains. In *Conscious Cuisine* there are no bad foods. We must simply make good choices concerning portion sizes and how often we eat higher fat and calorie-denser foods.

So, have your steak and eat it, too!

Purchasing, Handling, and Storing Meats and Poultry

Choose meats and poultry with the latest sell-by date.

Look for marbled, lean meats and moist, plump poultry.

The color of the skin on poultry has nothing to do with quality; it is a result of the type of feed.

Frozen meat or poultry should be rock hard, with no sign of defrosting.

Wash your hands thoroughly and often when handling raw meat and poultry.

Use clean towels to wipe work surface.

Store fresh products in a refrigerator below 40°F (5°C) or freeze them at or below 0°F (-20°C).

Never put cooked foods back into uncooked marinade.

Never use the same utensils for raw and cooked food.

Never defrost foods at room temperature. Plan ahead. Defrost slowly in the refrigerator.

Keep meats and poultry at room temperature for no more than one hour before or after cooking. Refrigerate leftovers promptly.

Cook all meats and poultry to recommended internal temperatures.

Rules of Thumb: Meats and Poultry

- Buy smaller portions (3 1/2 to 4 ounces) per serving.
- Choose extremely lean cuts.
- Remove all excess fat.
- Purchase high-quality, flavorful meats (i.e., organic beef and lamb).
- Substitute chicken or turkey for red meats in your favorite recipes (i.e., smoked turkey legs for ham hocks or chicken sausage for pork sausage).

Shopping Summary

Reduce repetitive trips to the grocer by stocking up on toiletries, paper, and nonfood supplies.

Seek a reputable, busy grocer who receives produce frequently.

Visit the produce area first and design your meals around fresh, seasonal fruits and vegetables.

Choose foods based on quality, freshness, and flavor. It will prove more cost effective, providing better food and less waste.

Limit your consumption of processed foods. Purchase whole grain and organic products as much as possible. You will be able to taste and tell the difference.

Enjoy lean, high-quality meats and poultry. Purchase 3 1/2 to 4 ounces per serving.

Select fresh or frozen seafood that is not heavily breaded. Even though seafood is a healthy choice, 4 to 5 ounces is an ample portion to serve.

Make conscious decisions when choosing dairy products. Certified organic dairy products are available and free of chemicals and steroids. The intense flavor of high-quality cheeses is a more effective choice than using more cheese of lesser quality.

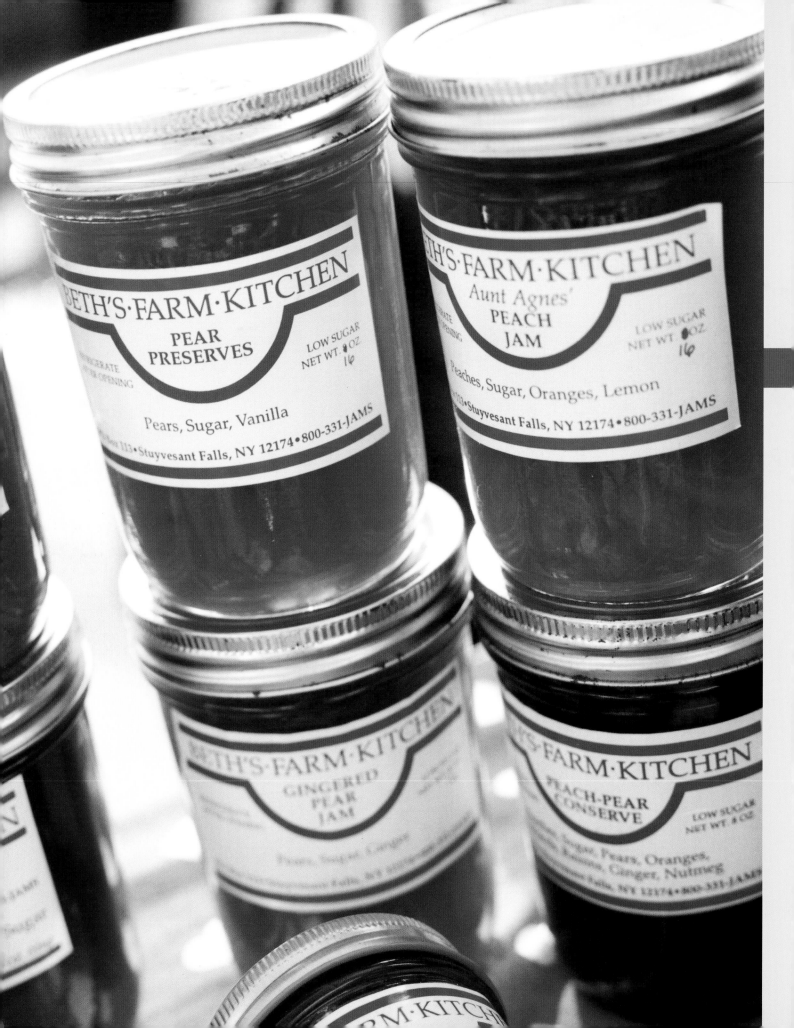

Kitchen Wisdom: Stocking the Pantry and Kitchen

Today's culture of convenience with fast-food restaurants and microwave ovens has created a society of consumers who are ill-equipped to cook foods in the home. The average American eats away from the home four times per week, helping to turn fast food into a multibillion dollar industry. Choosing to invest the time in eating healthfully and making conscious decisions regarding your food's sustainability, portion size, and nutritional content is a life-altering process. I believe this decision will create wellness for you and for those for whom you cook. Eliminating the mystery around food preparation and understanding helpful cooking terminology and methods will bring ease and enjoyment into the kitchen. Listed below are helpful tips for stocking the pantry and understanding recipes and menus with confidence.

Basic Food Products and Utensils

There are countless food, utensil, and equipment options available. These are the basic food products you should have in your pantry and the utensils you should outfit your kitchen with for creating Conscious Cuisine.

I have listed some tasty and nutritious food products that are great to keep on hand in your kitchen to help you make wonderfully delicious meals.

Stocking the Pantry

Condiments and Canned Goods

artichoke hearts

cocoa powder

Dijon mustard

dried beans (canned)

dried fruits

dried herbs

dried vegetables such as dried mushrooms, sun-dried tomatoes, sea vegetables

kombu

light coconut milk

nori

nuts

olives

sea salt

Sriracha (chile) sauce (see page 326)

tahini (sesame seed paste) (see page 327)

tamari (soy) sauce

tomato products

water-packed tuna

whole spices

Grains

Asian noodles

polenta

semolina flour (see page 326)

unbleached all-purpose flour

variety of grains

whole-wheat pasta

whole-wheat pastry flour

Oils

cold-pressed, extra-virgin olive oil

cold-pressed canola oil

toasted sesame oil

Stocks and Glacés

Either purchase or make; keep the following on hand in the freezer or pantry:

high-quality soup and stock bases, such as More Than Gourmet (see page 326)

vegetable stock/glacé

chicken stock/glacé

fish stock/glacé

veal stock/glacé

Sweeteners

corn syrup

honey

pure maple syrup

raw cane sugar (Turbinado)

Wax Orchards Fruit Sweet (see page 326)

(Avoid artificial sweeteners such as saccharin or NutraSweet.)

Vinegars

balsamic vinegar

red wine vinegar

rice wine vinegar

sherry vinegar

white wine vinegar

Stocking the Kitchen

Choosing the right pots, pans, and utensils for your kitchen can be a daunting task, but it does not have to be overwhelming or expensive. Instead of recommending one type or brand over another, I have suggested some helpful utensils and defined the benefits and disadvantages of various types of cookware so you can make educated decisions about which pieces best fit your needs and budget and when and how to use them.

Cookware Types

First consider quality and the expected use and life span of the items you are purchasing. Consider that lower-quality, thin cookware tends to distribute heat unevenly, giving you poor control over your cooking results.

Whether you choose one brand of cookware to outfit your entire kitchen or you choose various brands, keep in mind what foods you wish to prepare.

Aluminum: Heats quickly and evenly and is durable and inexpensive. It can react with acidic food and leave a metallic aftertaste. Usually, this only occurs after long use and multiple, deep scratches to the cooking surface. Aluminum is the most common cookware sold and used in professional kitchens.

Cast iron: Good for frying and searing because it retains heat well. Holds the heat at a uniform temperature, even on high heat. When using cast iron, a little iron from the pan is added to the food, adding some nutrient value. It does react with acidic food and can leave a metallic aftertaste. Needs to be seasoned before the first use to prevent sticking and thoroughly dried after each use to prevent rusting.

Copper: Heats and cools rapidly and evenly. The pans should be lined with stainless steel or alloyed aluminum to avoid foods' reaction to the copper. It is the most impressive cookware of all, but it will need to be polished to maintain its luster.

Glass: Holds heat well and is noncorrosive; can be used on the stovetop and in the oven. Heat conduction is not as uniform as with metal, and glass cookware may chip or break.

Nonstick: Good for reducing the amount of fat used in cooking, durable and easy to clean, but they are not the best pans for browning meats.

Stainless steel: Will not corrode or react with acidic foods. Does not absorb heat well. Purchasing a stainless steel pan with a carbon core produces rapid and evenly distributed heat.

Essential Equipment

Baking pans and baking sheets: Available in nonstick and aluminum, also helpful to place under casseroles that may drip in the oven.

Cutting board: Hardwood (disinfect regularly with a solution of bleach to water, ratio 1 to 8).

Instant-read thermometer: Eliminates guesswork when working with poultry, pork, or other foods where internal temperatures are critical.

Peppermill: Essential for grinding whole peppercorns; the difference in flavor will be noticed by all.

Rolling pins: Available in wooden, marble, plastic, and stenciled.

Knives and Cutters

Chef's knife, eight or ten inches: Used for dicing and chopping.

Fillet or boning knife: Used to remove bones and skin from meat.

Mandoline: Style of cutter used to cut vegetables into thin slices, julienne, jardiniere, and wafer or crinkle-cut.

Paring knife: Small, hand-held knife for cutting and peeling.

Serrated knife: Used to cut breads and crusts.

Slicer: Used to carve roasts.

Vegetable peeler: Used to peel vegetables and fruit.

Bakeware

Muffin pans: Available in nonstick, ceramic, aluminum, and fun-shaped pans for creating breakfast treats.

Measuring cups and spoons: A set each of dry and wet measuring cups ensures more accuracy in baking. Measuring spoons are available ranging from 1/8 teaspoon to 1 tablespoon.

Pastry bag and tips: Used for decorating cakes, etc. Good for getting children involved in the kitchen.

Cookware

Rondo (brassiere): Two-handled shallow pot with lid used for braising.

Saucepans: Selection of aluminum and nonstick pans, ranging in size from one to four quarts.

Sauté pans:
- Aluminum, ranging in size from eight-, ten-, to fourteen-inch diameter, great for cooking on high heat.
- Cast-iron, twelve-inch pan for browning meat, frying, or sautéing; can provide additional iron in your diet.
- Nonstick eight- or ten-inch pan for making omelets and quick sautés. Uses very little oil.

Steamer insert or bamboo steamer: Used to create nutritious entrées and vegetables, the bamboo steamer is available in various sizes.

Stock pot: A must-have to produce chilies, soups, and stocks, great for entertaining a large crowd.

Wooden spoon: Perfect for nonstick pans and starchy foods—one of my favorite utensils.

Favorite Tools for Cooking Fun

These items are not necessities, but I enjoy using them because they allow me to be more creative when making healthful foods.

Chinois: Cone-shaped, fine mesh sieve used for straining soups and sauces to a velvety consistency.

Coffee mill: Used for grinding coffee beans, dry spices, and flours.

Food processor with attachments: A great machine to help with shredding, chopping, pureeing, and whipping.

Food mill: Makes great mashed potatoes, vegetable purees, or creamy soups.

Heavy-duty electric blender: Great for pureeing soups, sauces, and smoothies.

Heavy-duty electric mixer: Speeds up the process when mixing dough and making batters.

Microwave oven: Helpful for reheating, melting chocolate, and making popcorn.

Salad spinner: Gently removes excess water from lettuce.

Spray bottles: An easy way to bottle and control the amount of oil and vinegar used on a dish.

Squeeze bottles: Used to decorate plates with infused oils, vinegars, and sauces.

Vegetable juicer: Produces healthy breakfast drinks, vinaigrettes, sauces, and flavored oils.

Cooking Methods and Terminology

I'm often reminded by guests, friends, and young cooks of the difficulties of understanding new recipes and dinner menus. Once I explain what is meant by a word or method, the recipe and menu instantly becomes more inviting and "user friendly." I'm convinced that the basic knowledge of common cooking methods and terminology will help you to create flavorful and nutritious meals, and understand menus with ease and confidence.

Al dente: Cooked until tender, but still firm (such as pasta and vegetables).

Bisque: Soup based on crustaceans or pureed vegetables.

Blanch: To partially cook an item in water or fat.

Boning: Method used to remove bones from meats, poultry, and fish.

Braise: To cook by searing, then simmering in liquid.

Broth: Flavorful, aromatic liquid.

Brunoise: Small square dice (1/8-inch cubes).

Chiffonade: Leafy vegetables or herbs cut into fine shreds.

Chowder: Thick soup containing potatoes.

Compote: Fruit cooked in syrup with spices or liquor.

Concassée: Tomatoes that have been peeled, seeded, and chopped.

Coulis: Thick puree of fruits or vegetables.

Danger zone: The temperature range for optimum bacteria growth; 45° to 140°F (7° to 60°C). Foods kept within this temperature are at risk for growth of dangerous bacteria.

Deglaze: To use liquid to release flavorful food particles from a pan after roasting or sautéing.

Emulsion: Fat or oil mixed with liquid until well dispersed, either on a permanent or temporary basis.

Essence: Concentrated flavoring extracted from foods.

Fines herbes: A mixture of finely chopped herbs.

Julienne: Vegetables cut into thin strips, 1/8-inch square x 2 inches long.

Mince: To chop into fine pieces.

Mirepoix: Classic seasoning combination of two parts onion, one part carrot, and one part celery, roughly chopped.

Mise en place (put in place): The preparation and organization of ingredients, utensils, and/or serviceware for a particular dish or service.

Mousse: Dish prepared with beaten egg whites and/or whipped cream.

Nouvelle cuisine: New cooking style emphasizing innovative combinations of fresh and light ingredients through classical preparations.

Paillarde: A fillet of chicken, meat, or fish that has been flattened by pounding it out with a mallet. It may be used for a dramatic presentation that will cover the plate entirely, or rolled around a filling to form a roulade.

Pan-sear: To sear food in a hot pan with the least amount of added fat.

Papillote, en: Food cooked enclosed in parchment or foil (moist heat cookery).

Pesto: Thick puree of herbs and oil.

Phyllo (filo) dough: Ultra-thin pastry sheets.

Poach: To cook gently in simmering liquid.

Puree: To process food into a smooth paste.

Raft: Mixture of ingredients used to clarify a consommé.

Reduce: To decrease volume of liquid to gain a thicker consistency and/or concentrate flavors.

Roulade: Meat, poultry, or fish rolled around a filling.

Roux: Thickener of equal parts flour and butter cooked together.

Sauté: To cook quickly in a hot pan with a small amount of fat.

Simmer: To maintain the temperature of a liquid just below the boiling point.

Slurry: Starch combined with a cold liquid, used to prevent lumps when added to hot liquids as a thickener.

Stock: Flavorful liquid of extracted meat, poultry, seafood, and/or vegetables.

Temper: To heat gently and gradually.

Vinaigrette: Cold sauce of oil and vinegar.

Zest: Colored outer part of citrus rind.

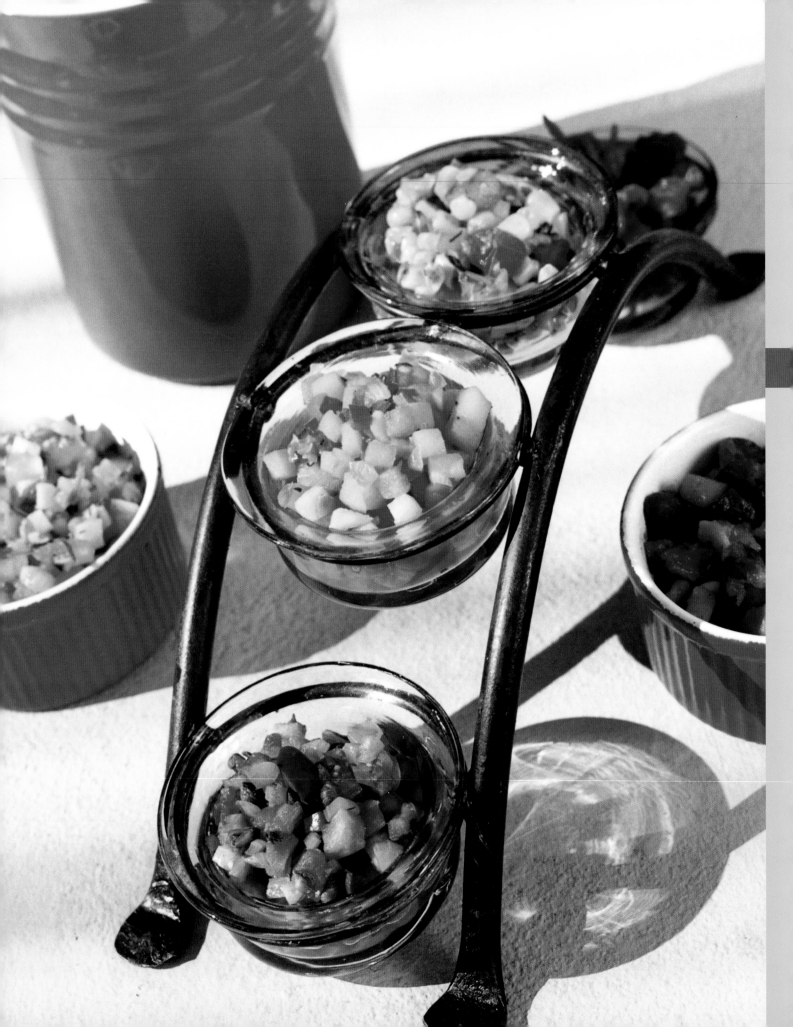

Sauces & Seasonings

Pictured at left: (back to front) Beet, Cranberry, and Jícama Relish, Nopale-Corn Salsa, Pear Chutney, Italian Eggplant Relish, (left and right) Cucumber-Mint Relish, Cranberry Chutney

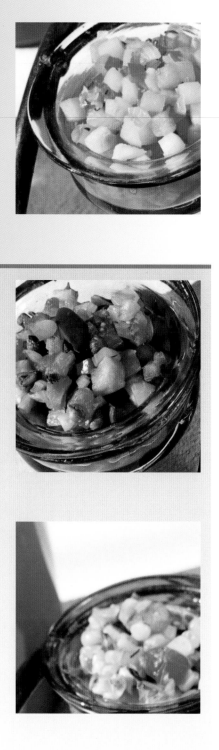

Creative cooks have utilized stocks, infused vinegars, oils, and sauces as dynamic flavor sources for years. Whether it's consciously cooking healthful meals or preparing sinfully delicious family favorites, understanding and using our abundant flavor sources contributes to the creation of inspiring meals.

Unfortunately, foods that are high in fat are usually delicious because fat carries the flavors and adds mouth-feel and texture. Therefore, when you begin to reduce the amount of fat and calories in your favorite recipes, it's very important that you add aromatic ingredients to replace those being removed. Understanding the dynamics of the vast array of flavor sources available to you will unleash new ideas for creating delicious foods. This chapter will help introduce you to the natural flavors of food and teach basic recipes for sauce and condiment preparations to arm you with the tools needed to prepare delicious meals that are balanced in flavor and nutrients.

You may well ask, as a professional chef or home cook, how can I continue to make delicious sauces, but with less fat and fewer calories? This is easily achieved by becoming more consciously aware of two key components.

First, you can increase your use of flavor-packed fruits and vegetables when making sauces, broths, coulis, and chutneys.

Second, you can utilize the wonderful properties of starchy foods rather than thickening agents. Cooking potatoes and grains as part of sauces and soups will thicken them when they are pureed. This method will lighten the sauces and soups, eliminating the use of creams, butter, and roux, and will add extra nutrients and flavor.

Red Wine Reduction

Per 1 tablespoon:
Calories 60; Protein 0g; Total Fat 0g; Saturated Fat 0g; Carbohydrates 5g; Dietary Fiber 0g; Cholesterol 0mg; Sodium 10mg

Do you have some inexpensive wine or opened bottles you have no use for? Reduce them down to make this wonderful glacé. Store at room temperature for two to three months and serve on almost anything. I love to drizzle this reduction on seafood or poultry dishes, steaks, and even cheeses.

You need to stay near the stove when making this because once it starts to thicken, it is done. The syrup will thicken further as it cools.

Ingredients
Makes 1/2 cup.

2 cups (16 ounces) red wine
2 tablespoons corn syrup

Preparation
Combine the wine and corn syrup in a small saucepan. Bring to a boil over medium-high heat. Boil until reduced to a syrupy consistency, about 10 minutes.

Variation
Balsamic Reduction: Substitute 2 cups balsamic vinegar for the wine.

Roasted Yellow Pepper Sauce

Per 1/4 cup:
Calories 40; Protein 1g; Total Fat 1.5g;
Saturated Fat 0g; Carbohydrates 6g; Dietary
Fiber 1g; Cholesterol 0mg; Sodium 135mg

Roasting bell peppers over an open flame brings out their natural sugars and gives them a wonderful smoky flavor and aroma. This is a delightful sauce to be used on virtually any dish or as a dip for vegetables and appetizers. Cut the roasted peppers in broad strips and mix with slivered garlic, basil, and olive oil for a quick and awesome relish.

Ingredients

Makes 2 1/4 cups.

1 teaspoon extra-virgin olive oil
3 large Roasted Yellow Peppers (see page 38), peeled and chopped
1 medium yellow onion, chopped
1 tablespoon plus 2 teaspoons minced garlic
1 tablespoon plus 1 teaspoon chopped fresh oregano
3 tablespoons chopped fresh cilantro
3 cups Vegetable Stock (see page 152)
1 tablespoon cornstarch mixed with 1 tablespoon water
1/2 teaspoon sea salt
1/4 teaspoon freshly ground black pepper

Preparation

Heat a medium saucepan over medium heat and add the olive oil to lightly coat the bottom of the pan. Stir in the roasted peppers, onion, garlic, oregano, and cilantro and cook until the onion has softened, about 2 minutes. Add the stock and simmer for 15 minutes.

Carefully ladle the pepper mixture into a blender and process until smooth.

Strain the pepper mixture through a colander lined with cheesecloth or through a fine mesh strainer.

Pour the strained sauce back into the saucepan and bring to a low boil. Mix in the cornstarch mixture and cook, stirring constantly, until the sauce thickens and coats the back of a spoon, about 5 minutes. Season with salt and pepper.

Use the sauce immediately, or cool quickly by setting in a bowl of ice and water. Store in an airtight container for up to 1 week in the refrigerator or freeze for about 1 month.

English Pea Sauce

Per 1/4 cup:
Calories 90; Protein 4g; Total Fat 1g; Saturated Fat 0g; Carbohydrates 16g; Dietary Fiber 5g; Cholesterol 0mg; Sodium 10mg

I love this sauce for its immediately sweet flavor, beautiful pastel green color, and ability to complement vegetarian and fish courses masterfully, while sneaking in some extra iron, potassium, and beta-carotene.

Ingredients
Makes 2 cups.

1 teaspoon extra-virgin olive oil
1 cup chopped yellow onion (about 1 large)
1 teaspoon minced fresh ginger
1/2 teaspoon minced garlic
4 cups shelled fresh English peas (or frozen peas)
2 cups Vegetable Stock (see page 152)
2 tablespoons cornstarch mixed with 2 tablespoons water
1/4 teaspoon sea salt
1/4 teaspoon freshly ground black pepper

Preparation
Heat a medium saucepan over medium heat and add the olive oil to lightly coat the bottom of the pan. Stir in the onion, ginger, and garlic and cook until the onion has softened, about 2 minutes. Add the peas and cook 2 minutes more. Stir in the stock and simmer until the peas have softened, but are still a bright green, about 5 minutes.

Carefully ladle the pea mixture into a blender and process until smooth.

Strain the pea mixture through a colander lined with cheesecloth or a fine mesh strainer.

Pour the strained sauce back into the saucepan and bring to a low boil. Mix in the cornstarch mixture and cook, stirring constantly, until the sauce thickens and coats the back of a spoon, about 5 minutes. Season with salt and pepper.

Use the sauce immediately, or cool quickly by setting in a bowl of ice and water. Store in an airtight container for up to 1 week in the refrigerator or freeze for about 1 month.

Yellow Tomato Sauce

Yellow tomatoes have less acid than red tomatoes and can create a sauce that is light, vibrantly fresh, and a glorious golden-yellow hue. The addition of fresh basil makes this sauce come alive.

Ingredients
Makes 4 cups.

1/4 teaspoon extra-virgin olive oil
1/2 cup chopped yellow onion (about 1 medium)
2 tablespoons minced garlic
6 yellow tomatoes, chopped
1/2 cup white wine
1 tablespoon finely shredded fresh basil
1/2 teaspoon raw cane sugar (Turbinado)
1/4 teaspoon sea salt
1/8 teaspoon freshly ground black pepper

Preparation

Heat a medium saucepan over medium-high heat and add the olive oil to lightly coat the bottom of the pan. Stir in the onion and garlic and cook until the onion has softened, about 2 minutes. Add the tomatoes and wine and simmer until the tomatoes are cooked, about 15 minutes.

Carefully ladle the tomato sauce into a blender and process until smooth.

Pour the sauce back into the saucepan and bring to a low boil. Stir in the basil, sugar, salt, and pepper.

Use the sauce immediately, or cool quickly by setting in a bowl of ice and water. Store in an airtight container for up to 1 week in the refrigerator or freeze for about 1 month.

Shiitake Mushroom Sauce

Rehydrated shiitake mushrooms add a meaty, smoky flavor that makes this sauce an ideal accompaniment to Asian entrées such as Curried Tofu and Napa Cabbage Roulade (see page 257).

Per 1/4 cup:
Calories 45; Protein 3g; Total Fat 0.5g; Saturated Fat 0g; Carbohydrates 7g; Dietary Fiber 2g; Cholesterol 0mg; Sodium 180mg

Ingredients

Makes 3 cups.

1 cup dried shiitake mushrooms (about 14 medium), rinsed
3 cups filtered water
1 teaspoon toasted sesame oil
1/4 cup chopped green onions (about 2)
1/2 cup finely chopped carrot (about 1 medium)
1/2 teaspoon minced fresh ginger
1/4 teaspoon minced garlic
1 tablespoon sake or white wine
2 tablespoons tamari (soy) sauce
1 tablespoon seasoned rice wine vinegar
1 tablespoon cornstarch mixed with 2 tablespoons water

Preparation

In a bowl, soak the mushrooms in the 3 cups of water for about 20 minutes. Strain the mushrooms through a colander lined with a cheesecloth or a fine mesh strainer and reserve soaking liquid for the sauce. Remove and discard the stems from the mushrooms and julienne the caps.

Heat a medium saucepan over medium-high heat and add the toasted sesame oil to lightly coat the bottom of the pan. Stir in the mushrooms, green onions, carrots, ginger, and garlic and cook quickly to brown the vegetables, 2 to 3 minutes. Add the sake into the pan. Stir in the tamari, rice wine vinegar, and mushroom water. Bring to a boil, reduce heat, and simmer for 10 minutes.

Mix in the cornstarch mixture and cook, stirring constantly, until the sauce thickens and coats the back of a spoon, about 5 minutes.

Use the sauce immediately, or cool quickly by setting in a bowl of ice and water. Store in an airtight container for up to 1 week in the refrigerator or freeze for about 1 month.

Lemon-Garlic Sauce

This light lemon sauce is great for pasta, chicken, or any seafood. Quick and easy to make, it has subtle fresh flavors. For an extra burst of flavor, add a teaspoon of grated lemon zest.

Ingredients

Makes 3 1/2 cups.

1 teaspoon extra-virgin olive oil
3/4 cup minced garlic
1 cup finely chopped green onions (about
   1 bunch)
1/2 cup fresh lemon juice (juice of about 4
   lemons)
1/4 cup white wine
1/4 cup chopped fresh thyme
1/4 teaspoon freshly ground black pepper
4 cups Vegetable Stock (see page 152)
1/4 teaspoon sea salt
1/4 teaspoon honey
3 tablespoons cornstarch mixed with 4
   tablespoons Vegetable Stock

Preparation

Heat a medium saucepan over medium heat and add the olive oil to lightly coat the bottom of the pan. Stir in the garlic and green onions and cook until the onions have softened, about 2 minutes. Stir in the lemon juice, wine, thyme, and pepper. Cook until reduced and the pan is almost dry, about 3 to 5 minutes, to concentrate the flavors in the sauce. Add the stock and bring to a boil. Reduce heat and simmer for 15 minutes. Season with salt and honey.

Strain the onion mixture through a colander lined with cheesecloth or through a fine mesh strainer.

Pour the strained sauce back into the saucepan and bring to a low boil. Mix in the cornstarch mixture and cook, stirring constantly, until the sauce thickens and coats the back of a spoon, about 5 minutes.

Use the sauce immediately, or cool quickly by setting in a bowl of ice and water. Store in an airtight container for up to 1 week in the refrigerator or freeze for about 1 month.

Tarragon Aïoli

Aïoli is a classic, French-style mayonnaise in which an emulsion is made with garlic, egg yolks, and olive oil. American-style mayonnaise is made in the same manner, with a more neutral-flavored oil, and without the garlic. An aïoli is a wonderful accompaniment to vegetables, seafood, or sandwiches. All the delicious flavors of a classic aïoli are available to you, without the fat and calories, by starting with Mayonnaise Nouvelle (see page 120). This recipe provides you with the tastes of Provence, without the guilt.

Ingredients
Makes 1 cup.

1 tablespoon Roasted Garlic (see page 38)
1/2 teaspoon minced fresh garlic
1 cup Mayonnaise Nouvelle (see page 120), low-fat mayonnaise, or soy-based mayonnaise
1 tablespoon minced fresh tarragon
1/8 teaspoon freshly ground black pepper
1/4 teaspoon sea salt
1/2 teaspoon extra-virgin olive oil

Preparation
Place the roasted garlic, fresh garlic, mayonnaise, and tarragon in a blender and process until smooth. Add the pepper, salt, and olive oil. Pulse to combine. Refrigerate until ready to use. The aïoli can be made 1 day ahead; it will keep for 5 days in the refrigerator.

Tamari-Ginger Sauce

Per 1/4 cup:
Calories 50; Protein 2g; Total Fat 0g; Saturated Fat 0g; Carbohydrates 9g; Dietary Fiber 0g; Cholesterol 0mg; Sodium 810 mg

I promise that you will love this Asian-style sauce. It complements a host of entrées from vegetable stir-fries to tofu dishes, shrimp, chicken, or duck. Sriracha sauce is a wonderful Asian chile sauce that's frequently used at sushi restaurants. It is available in Asian markets and some specialty grocery stores. Other chile sauces will work, but this sauce is far superior and is a great condiment to keep on hand.

Ingredients
Makes 2 1/2 cups.

1/2 teaspoon extra-virgin olive oil
1/2 cup chopped green onions (about 4)
2 tablespoons minced garlic
1/4 cup minced fresh ginger
1/4 cup white wine
2 1/2 cups unsweetened orange juice
1/2 cup tamari (soy) sauce
1 tablespoon cornstarch mixed with 2
    tablespoons orange juice
1 teaspoon Sriracha (chile) sauce
1/2 teaspoon fresh lime juice

Preparation
Heat a medium saucepan over medium-high heat and add the olive oil to lightly coat the bottom of the pan. Stir in the green onions, garlic, and ginger and cook until the onions have softened, about 2 minutes. Add the wine and cook until reduced and the pan is almost dry, about 3 to 5 minutes, to concentrate the flavors of the sauce. Mix in the orange juice and tamari and bring to a low boil.

Mix in the cornstarch mixture and cook, stirring constantly, until the sauce thickens and coats the back of a spoon, about 5 minutes. Season with Sriracha sauce and lime juice.

Use the sauce immediately, or cool quickly by setting in a bowl of ice and water. Store in an airtight container for up to 1 week in the refrigerator or freeze for about 1 month.

Carrot-Cardamom Sauce

Per 1/4 cup:
Calories 25; Protein 1g; Total Fat 0g; Saturated Fat 0g; Carbohydrates 6g; Dietary Fiber 0g; Cholesterol 0mg; Sodium 40mg

This is one of my favorite sauces. The bright orange color is so attractive, and the fragrance and taste of the cardamom are magnificent with the sweetness of the carrots.

Ingredients

Makes 4 1/2 cups.

6 cups fresh carrot juice
1 teaspoon ground cardamom
5 tablespoons cornstarch mixed with 6
   tablespoons Vegetable Stock
   (see page 152)

Preparation

Heat the carrot juice and cardamom in a medium saucepan over medium-high heat. Bring to a boil, reduce heat, and simmer for 15 minutes. (The carrot juice will separate; this is okay.) Mix in the cornstarch mixture and cook, stirring constantly, until the sauce thickens and coats the back of a spoon, about 5 minutes.

Pour the sauce into a blender and process to incorporate the carrot juice.

Use the sauce immediately, or cool quickly by setting in a bowl of ice and water. Store in an airtight container for up to 1 week in the refrigerator or freeze for about 1 month.

Asparagus Sauce

This sauce is a great way to use the asparagus stems left over from prepping spears for dinner. The addition of ginger does not dominate the flavor, but adds dimension to the asparagus flavor.

Ingredients
Makes 3 cups.

1/2 teaspoon extra-virgin olive oil
1 cup chopped onion (about 1 large)
2 teaspoons minced garlic
4 cups chopped asparagus stems (about 2 bunches)
1 teaspoon minced fresh ginger
3 cups Vegetable Stock (see page 152)
2 cups fresh spinach, stems removed, washed, and drained
1/4 cup cornstarch mixed with 1/4 cup Vegetable Stock
1/4 teaspoon sea salt
1/4 teaspoon freshly ground black pepper
1/4 teaspoon ground nutmeg

Preparation

Heat a medium saucepan over medium-high heat and add the olive oil to lightly coat the bottom of the pan. Stir in the onion, garlic, asparagus, and ginger and cook until the onion has softened, about 5 minutes. Pour in the stock and simmer for 3 minutes. (Do not overcook asparagus; you want it to be bright green.) Add the spinach and simmer for 2 minutes.

Carefully ladle the asparagus mixture into a blender and process until smooth.

Strain the blended mixture through a colander lined with cheesecloth or through a fine mesh sieve.

Pour the strained mixture back into the saucepan and bring to a low boil. Mix in the cornstarch mixture and cook, stirring constantly, until the sauce thickens and coats the back of a spoon, about 5 minutes. Season with salt, pepper, and nutmeg.

Use the sauce immediately, or cool quickly by setting in a bowl of ice and water. Store in an airtight container for up to 1 week in the refrigerator or freeze for about 1 month.

Basil Sauce

This sauce has a beautiful light green color with a delicious basil flavor. It works well with fresh pasta or seafood. The sauce will keep for about two days, but the vibrant color and flavor of the basil will have to be refreshed with new basil each time it is reheated.

Ingredients
Makes 2 cups.

1 teaspoon extra-virgin olive oil
1/2 cup minced shallots (about 3 medium)
2 teaspoons minced garlic
4 cups finely chopped fresh basil
1/2 cup white wine
2 cups Vegetable Stock (see page 152)
3 tablespoons cornstarch mixed with 2
    tablespoons water
1/4 teaspoon sea salt
Pinch of white pepper

Preparation

Heat a medium saucepan over medium-high heat and add the olive oil to lightly coat the bottom of the pan. Stir in the shallots and garlic and cook until the shallots have softened, about 5 minutes. Quickly add the basil and cook for 1 minute. Pour in the wine and cook until reduced and the pan is almost dry, about 3 to 5 minutes, to concentrate the flavors of the sauce. Add the stock and bring to a boil. Reduce heat and simmer for about 15 minutes.

Carefully ladle the basil mixture into a blender and process until smooth.

Strain the blended mixture through a colander lined with cheesecloth or through a fine mesh strainer.

Pour the strained sauce back into the saucepan and bring to a low boil. Mix in the cornstarch mixture and cook, stirring constantly, until the sauce thickens and coats the back of a spoon, about 5 minutes. Season with salt and pepper.

Use the sauce immediately, or cool quickly by setting in a bowl of ice and water. Store in an airtight container for up to 1 week in the refrigerator or freeze for about 1 month.

Roasted Shallot Sauce

Per 1/4 cup:
Calories 45; Protein 1g; Total Fat 0g; Saturated
Fat 0g; Carbohydrates 9g; Dietary Fiber 0g;
Cholesterol 0mg; Sodium 60mg

You will say WOW! about this underutilized vegetable with its sweet, complex onion flavor, which is great on hearty winter foods, meats, and game. Roast some extra shallots—you can slice them and sprinkle them on top of flat breads and sandwiches, or puree them for a wonderful spread.

Ingredients
Makes 3 cups.

1/2 teaspoon extra-virgin olive oil
3 cups halved Roasted Shallots (see page 38) (about 25 medium)
2 teaspoons minced garlic
1/2 cup chopped mushrooms (1/4 pound)
1 tablespoon fresh thyme
1/2 cup white wine
3 cups Vegetable Stock (see page 152)
1 bay leaf
1/4 teaspoon sea salt
1/8 teaspoon freshly ground black pepper

Preparation

Heat a medium saucepan over medium-high heat and add olive oil to lightly coat the bottom of the pan. Stir in the shallots, garlic, mushrooms, and thyme and cook until the shallots turn golden brown, about 5 minutes. Pour in the wine and cook until reduced and the pan is almost dry, about 3 to 5 minutes, to concentrate the flavors of the sauce. Add the stock and bay leaf and simmer about 15 minutes.

Carefully ladle the shallot mixture into a blender and process until smooth.

Strain the blended mixture through a colander lined with cheesecloth or through a fine mesh strainer. Pour the strained sauce back into the saucepan and bring to a low boil. Season with salt and pepper.

Use the sauce immediately, or cool quickly by setting in a bowl of ice and water. Store in an airtight container for up to 1 week in the refrigerator or freeze for about 1 month.

Saffron-Chive Sauce

Ingredients
Makes 2 1/2 cups.

1/2 teaspoon extra-virgin olive oil
1 cup diced yellow onion (about 1 large)
1 teaspoon minced garlic
1 tablespoon saffron threads
1 cup white wine
3 cups Vegetable Stock (see page 152)
1 cup diced, peeled potatoes (about 2 medium)
1/2 teaspoon sea salt
1/8 teaspoon freshly ground black pepper
2 tablespoons chopped fresh chives

Saffron is made from the stigmas of a beautiful purple crocus found in Spain and the Middle East. Each flower has only three stigmas, and each stigma is hand-picked, which makes saffron very expensive. Its pungent smell, bitter flavor, and yellow color have been used throughout the ages in magic, medicine, and cooking.

This recipe creates all of the pleasures of a wonderful saffron cream sauce without the use of cream or butter. Pureed potatoes thicken the sauce and provide a creamy mouth feel. The flavor is as good as its counterpart without the extra calories and fat—Conscious Cuisine at its best!

Preparation
Heat a medium saucepan over medium-high heat and add the olive oil to lightly coat the bottom of the pan. Stir in the onion, garlic, and saffron and cook until the onion has softened and the saffron has released its color, about 2 minutes. Pour in the wine and cook until reduced and the pan is almost dry, about 3 to 5 minutes, to concentrate the flavors of the sauce. Add the stock and potatoes and bring to a boil. Reduce heat and simmer until the potatoes are soft, about 15 minutes.

Carefully ladle the potato mixture into a blender and process until smooth.

Strain the blended mixture through a colander lined with cheesecloth or a fine mesh strainer. Pour the strained sauce back into the saucepan and bring to a low boil. Adjust the seasonings with salt and pepper. Stir in the chives.

Use the sauce immediately, or cool quickly by setting in a bowl of ice and water. Store in an airtight container for up to 1 week in the refrigerator or freeze for about 1 month.

Beet and Ginger Sauce

Per 1/4 cup:
Calories 30; Protein 1g; Total Fat 0g; Saturated Fat 0g; Carbohydrates 6g; Dietary Fiber 1g; Cholesterol 0mg; Sodium 230mg

The brilliant color, pleasing aroma, and lusciously sweet taste of this sauce have made me a fan of beets forever. This is a great way to introduce beets to kids and to those adults who have negative opinions about beets.

Ingredients
Makes 3 1/2 cups.

1/2 teaspoon extra-virgin olive oil
1 cup chopped yellow onion (about 1 large)
2 cups chopped, peeled beets (about 1 pound)
4 cups Vegetable Stock (see page 152)
1 teaspoon minced fresh ginger
2 tablespoons cornstarch mixed with 2 tablespoons Vegetable Stock
1/2 teaspoon sea salt
1/2 teaspoon white pepper

Preparation

Heat a medium saucepan over medium-high heat and add the olive oil to lightly coat the bottom of the pan. Stir in the onion and beets and cook until onion has softened, about 5 minutes. Add the stock and ginger and bring to a boil. Reduce heat and simmer until the beets are soft, about 20 minutes.

Carefully ladle the beet mixture into a blender and process until smooth.

Strain the blended mixture through a colander lined with cheesecloth or a fine mesh strainer. Pour the strained sauce back into the saucepan and bring to a low boil. Mix in the cornstarch mixture and cook, stirring constantly, until the sauce thickens and coats the back of a spoon, about 5 minutes. Season with salt and pepper.

Use the sauce immediately, or cool quickly by setting in a bowl of ice and water. Store in an airtight container for up to 1 week in the refrigerator or freeze for about 1 month.

Marinara Sauce

Per 1/2 cup:
Calories 40; Protein 1g; Total Fat 0g; Saturated Fat 0g; Carbohydrates 6g; Dietary Fiber 1g; Cholesterol 0mg; Sodium 470mg

This quick and easy marinara sauce will inspire you to create many wonderful dishes. The nutty flavor of the browned garlic and the brightness of fresh basil provide a wonderful overtone of freshness.

Ingredients
Makes 3 cups.

1 32-ounce can of diced tomatoes
1/2 teaspoon extra-virgin olive oil
2 tablespoons minced garlic
2 tablespoons finely shredded fresh basil
1/2 teaspoon sea salt
1/2 teaspoon freshly ground black pepper
1/2 teaspoon raw cane sugar (Turbinado)

Preparation

Add the tomatoes with their juices to a medium saucepan. Bring to a boil over medium-high heat. Reduce heat and simmer for about 20 minutes, stirring frequently and skimming off the foam as it rises to the top.

Heat a small sauté pan over medium heat and add the olive oil to lightly coat the bottom of the pan. Stir in the garlic and cook until golden, about 2 minutes, watching carefully.

Add the garlic to the tomatoes. Season the tomato mixture with the basil, salt, pepper, and sugar.

Carefully ladle the tomato mixture into a blender and process until smooth.

Use the sauce immediately, or cool quickly by setting in a bowl of ice and water. Store in an airtight container for up to 1 week in the refrigerator or freeze for about 1 month.

Roasted Garlic-Ricotta Sauce

I created this sauce to rival the classic Alfredo sauce. Try this and you will agree that great-tasting food does not necessarily mean high fat and calories. Enjoy the rich, comforting flavors of my version at 60 calories and 1.5 grams of fat, compared to the heavy traditional taste of butter, cream, and cheese that weighs in at 240 calories and 26 grams of fat.

Per 1/4 cup:
Calories 60; Protein 2g; Total Fat 1.5g; Saturated Fat 0.5g; Carbohydrates 7g; Dietary Fiber 0g; Cholesterol 5mg; Sodium 140mg

Ingredients
Makes 3 cups.

1/2 teaspoon extra-virgin olive oil
1/3 cup chopped Roasted Garlic (see page 38)
1/4 cup chopped Roasted Shallots (see page 38)
1/2 cup white wine
3 cups Vegetable Stock (see page 152)
3 tablespoons cornstarch mixed with 3 tablespoons water
1/2 cup fat-free ricotta cheese
1 tablespoon plus 1 teaspoon chopped fresh basil
1 tablespoon chopped fresh oregano
1/2 teaspoon sea salt
1/4 teaspoon freshly ground black pepper

Preparation

Heat a medium saucepan over medium-high heat and add the olive oil to lightly coat the bottom of the pan. Stir in the roasted garlic and shallots and cook until lightly browned, about 3 minutes. Pour in the wine and cook until reduced and the pan is almost dry, about 3 to 5 minutes, to concentrate the flavors of the sauce. Add the stock and bring to a boil. Reduce heat and simmer for 15 minutes.

Mix in the cornstarch mixture and cook, stirring constantly, until the sauce thickens and coats the back of a spoon, about 5 minutes.

Place the ricotta cheese and about 1/3 cup of the garlic mixture into a blender. With the blender on, slowly pour in the remaining sauce through the opening in the blender lid; the sauce will thicken.

Transfer the sauce back into the saucepan and stir in the basil, oregano, salt, and pepper.

Use the sauce immediately, or cool quickly by setting in a bowl of ice and water. Store in an airtight container for up to 1 week in the refrigerator or freeze for about 1 month.

Toasted Fennel and Tomato Sauce

Per 1/4 cup:
Calories 35; Protein 1g; Total Fat 0g; Saturated Fat 0g; Carbohydrates 5g; Dietary Fiber 1g; Cholesterol 0mg; Sodium 160mg

Toasting fennel seeds releases oils from the seeds to develop a wonderfully complex flavor and aroma. This sauce makes a beautiful base for your favorite Manhattan-style clam chowder or seafood cioppino.

Ingredients
Makes 2 cups.

2 tablespoons whole fennel seeds
1/4 teaspoon extra-virgin olive oil
1/4 cup chopped yellow onion (about 1 small)
1/2 cup white wine
2 cups canned tomato juice
1/8 teaspoon sea salt
1/4 teaspoon freshly ground black pepper
2 tablespoons balsamic vinegar

Preparation

In a dry sauté pan, toast the fennel seeds over medium heat until they are golden brown and release a nutty aroma, about 2 minutes. Shake the pan constantly so the seeds do not burn. Cool seeds and grind with a mortar and pestle or a spice grinder.

Heat a medium saucepan over medium-high heat and add the olive oil to lightly coat the bottom of the pan. Stir in the onion and ground fennel seeds and cook until the onion has softened, about 5 minutes. Pour in the wine and cook until reduced and the pan is almost dry, about 3 to 5 minutes, to concentrate the flavors of the sauce. Stir in the tomato juice; reduce heat and simmer for 5 to 7 minutes. Season with salt, pepper, and balsamic vinegar.

Use the sauce immediately, or cool quickly by setting in a bowl of ice and water. Store in an airtight container for up to 1 week in the refrigerator or freeze for about 1 month.

Red Pepper Puree

Per 1 tablespoon:
Calories 5; Protein 0g; Total Fat 0g; Saturated Fat 0g; Carbohydrates 1g; Dietary Fiber 0g; Cholesterol 0mg; Sodium 30mg

This red pepper puree (coulis) offers a delicious and visually satisfying complement to poultry, seafood, and vegetables. It is used to represent the sun in the critically acclaimed Eclipse Soup (see page 164), a combination of Black Bean Soup and Butternut Squash Soup.

Ingredients

Makes 3/4 cup.

1/2 teaspoon extra-virgin olive oil
1 1/2 cups diced red bell pepper (1 1/2 medium)
2 Roasted Red Peppers (see page 38), peeled, seeded, and diced
1/2 cup diced yellow onion (about 1 medium)
1/2 cup diced celery (1 medium rib)
1 teaspoon minced garlic
1 tablespoon finely shredded fresh basil
1/2 teaspoon sea salt
1/2 teaspoon freshly ground black pepper

Preparation

Heat a small sauté pan over medium-high heat and add the olive oil to lightly coat the bottom of the pan. Stir in the peppers, roasted peppers, onion, celery, garlic, basil, salt, and pepper. Cook until the vegetables are soft and tender, about 3 minutes.

Carefully ladle the ingredients into a blender and puree until smooth.

Use the puree immediately or store in an airtight container in the refrigerator for up to 3 days.

Basil Pesto

Pesto is a traditional Italian pasta sauce made by grinding together fresh garlic, basil, pine nuts, Parmesan cheese, and olive oil. Traditional pesto has remarkable flavor, but is extremely high in fat and calories. This version delivers flavor and reduces the fat and calories dramatically by using Thickened Vegetable Stock to replace an equal volume of oil and substituting pumpkin seeds for pine nuts to provide a nutty flavor without as much fat. I add olive oil at the end to provide flavor, not volume.

Ingredients
Makes 2 1/2 cups.

2 cups packed fresh basil
1 cup Thickened Vegetable Stock (see page 153)
1/4 cup fresh oregano
1/4 cup toasted, shelled pumpkin seeds
2 tablespoons Roasted Garlic (see page 38)
1/4 teaspoon sea salt
1/4 teaspoon freshly ground black pepper
1/4 cup extra-virgin olive oil

Preparation
In a blender, combine the basil, vegetable stock, oregano, pumpkin seeds, roasted garlic, salt, and pepper. Process until finely chopped, then slowly drizzle the olive oil into the blender through the hole in the lid. Blend until the mixture is smooth and thick. Adjust seasoning with additional salt and pepper as needed.

Store in an airtight container in the refrigerator for up to 1 week.

Roasted Peppers

Ingredients

Red or yellow bell peppers,
   or Anaheim or poblano chiles

When bell peppers and chiles are roasted, they develop a sweet and smoky flavor that complements cheeses, meats, and other vegetables—a simple and beautiful way to add complex flavors to a dish.

Preparation

Preheat the broiler. Arrange the peppers on a roasting pan and place under the broiler. Broil on each side until the skin has blistered and turned black, about 10 minutes total, using tongs to turn the peppers as they blacken. Carefully remove the peppers from the oven, place in a bowl, and cover with plastic wrap. (This will make removing the skins easier.) Cool for 20 minutes, peel off the skins, and remove the stems and seeds. Gently rinse off any remaining charred skin.

Variations

If you have a gas stove, you can roast the peppers directly on the stovetop. Arrange the peppers on the burner rack. Cook until all the sides are blackened and blistered, turning with tongs.

You also can roast peppers on a grill following the same directions as above.

Roasted Garlic

Ingredients

Whole garlic bulbs
Olive oil
Sea salt
Freshly ground black pepper

Roasted garlic cloves and shallots are a quintessential flavor source that I rely on for a number of recipes. When they are pureed, they provide thickening and a deep, earthy flavor in salad dressings and sauces. They also create an uplifting flavor in vegetable spreads and flatbreads. Try to keep these little flavor treats on hand.

Preparation

Preheat the oven to 350°F (175°C). Trim off the top of each garlic bulb to expose the garlic cloves. Peel excess skin off the sides of the garlic bulbs. Place in a baking pan. Lightly drizzle the tops of the garlic bulbs with olive oil and sprinkle with salt and pepper.

Cover the pan with foil. Bake for 40 minutes or until the garlic cloves are soft and lightly brown on top.

Variation

Roasted Shallots: Substitute whole shallots for the garlic bulbs; increase baking time by about 10 minutes, depending on their size.

Fresh Herb Mix

Ingredients
Makes 1 1/4 cups.

1/4 cup finely chopped fresh basil
1/4 cup finely chopped fresh oregano
1/2 cup finely chopped fresh parsley
1/4 cup finely chopped fresh thyme

This herb mixture is great for general seasoning. Use it to season meats, vegetables, and grains. It appears in various recipes used throughout the book. The absence of one of the four herbs is okay; use what you have on hand and have fun!

Preparation
Combine all the herbs in a small bowl and mix well.
Store in an airtight container in the refrigerator for up to 1 week.

Herb Crust

Ingredients
Makes 1 1/2 cups.

1/2 cup finely chopped fresh parsley
1/4 cup finely chopped fresh basil
1/4 cup finely chopped fresh oregano
1/4 cup finely chopped fresh thyme
1 tablespoon chopped fresh chives
1 teaspoon finely chopped fresh rosemary
1/2 teaspoon sea salt
1/2 teaspoon freshly ground black pepper

I use this herb crust to create dishes such as herb-crusted baked halibut or chicken. It has an attractive appearance plus provides the delicate flavor of fresh herbs.

Preparation
Combine all the ingredients in a small bowl and mix well.
Store in an airtight container in the refrigerator for up to 1 week.

Blackening Spice Mix

Ingredients
Makes 1/2 cup.

1/4 cup chile powder
1 tablespoon paprika
1 teaspoon cayenne pepper
1 teaspoon dried basil, crumbled
1 teaspoon dried thyme, crumbled
1 teaspoon dried oregano, crumbled
1 teaspoon granulated garlic
1 teaspoon granulated onion
1 teaspoon ground cumin
1 teaspoon curry powder
1 teaspoon raw cane sugar (Turbinado)
1 teaspoon freshly ground black pepper
1/4 teaspoon sea salt

Use this spice mixture for blackening poultry, meats, or seafood or use as a grill seasoning. Keep this great mix on hand to add a personal touch to many dishes.

Preparation
Combine all the ingredients in a small bowl and mix well.
Store in an airtight container in the refrigerator for up to 1 month.

Jerry's Prime Rib Rub

Ingredients
Makes 2 cups.

1/4 cup dried thyme
1/4 cup dried oregano
2 tablespoons dried basil
1 tablespoon dried tarragon
1 tablespoon dried rosemary
5 bay leaves, crushed
2 tablespoons minced garlic
2 tablespoons paprika
4 teaspoons sea salt
4 teaspoons freshly ground black pepper
1 cup extra-virgin olive oil

I receive a call every holiday season for the best way to season a prime rib of beef. I developed this quick rub for my brother-in-law, Jerry, who cooks an awesome prime rib for our family celebrations.

Preparation
Crumble the herbs into a medium bowl. Combine with remaining ingredients and mix well.
    Spread mixture on beef before using.

Asian Dry Rub

Ingredients
Makes 1 cup.

1/2 cup packed light brown sugar
1/4 cup finely chopped cilantro
2 tablespoons finely chopped green onions
2 tablespoons seasoned rice wine vinegar
2 tablespoons toasted sesame oil
2 tablespoons water
2 teaspoons minced garlic
2 teaspoons minced fresh ginger
2 teaspoons grated lemon zest
2 teaspoons tamari (soy) sauce
1/2 teaspoon crushed red chiles

Try this on sautéed or baked tofu, ribs, duck, or shrimp. The flavor is intensely Asian.

Preparation
Combine all the ingredients in a medium bowl and mix well.
Store in an airtight container in the refrigerator for up to 1 week.

Asian Marinade

Ingredients
Makes 2 cups.

1/2 cup packed light brown sugar
1/2 cup unsweetened orange juice
1/4 cup finely chopped fresh cilantro
2 tablespoons finely chopped green onion
2 tablespoons seasoned rice wine vinegar
2 tablespoons toasted sesame oil
2 tablespoons water
2 teaspoons minced garlic
2 teaspoons minced fresh ginger
2 teaspoons grated lemon zest
2 teaspoons tamari (soy) sauce
1 teaspoon Chinese five spice powder
1/2 teaspoon crushed red chiles

Zip up your Asian rub by also using this quick marinade. It makes a fantastic sauce or Asian barbecue with duck, chicken, or pork.

Preparation
Combine all the ingredients in a medium bowl and mix well.
Store in an airtight container in the refrigerator for up to 1 week.

Tomato-Rosemary Chutney

Per 2 tablespoons:
Calories 20; Protein 1g; Total Fat 0g; Saturated Fat 0g; Carbohydrates 4g; Dietary Fiber 0g; Cholesterol 0mg; Sodium 45mg

Chutneys are a fantastic flavor source and a convenient way to add to the enjoyment of your favorite dishes. Because of the acid in the vinegar or wine found in chutneys, they will keep up to one week refrigerated. Chutneys can be served hot or cold and will soon become staple condiments you keep on hand to enhance a host of meals. Try this tomato-herb mixture on lamb, chicken, shrimp, or pasta.

Ingredients
Makes 2 cups.

1/2 teaspoon extra-virgin olive oil
1 cup finely chopped red onion (about 1 large)
2 teaspoons minced garlic
4 cups diced, peeled tomatoes (about 4 medium)
2 tablespoons balsamic vinegar
1 tablespoon finely chopped fresh rosemary
1/4 teaspoon sea salt

Preparation
Heat a sauté pan over medium-high heat and add the olive oil to lightly coat the bottom of the pan. Stir in the onion and cook until the onion has softened, about 2 minutes. Add the garlic and cook for 2 minutes. Mix in the tomatoes, vinegar, and rosemary.

Simmer until the tomatoes start to cook down, about 15 minutes. Season with salt.

Store in an airtight container in the refrigerator for 4 or 5 days.

Pear Chutney

The combination of sweet pears with red onion and apple cider vinegar creates a perfect accompaniment to grilled pork tenderloin. Photo on page 16.

Per 1/4 cup:
Calories 60; Protein 0g; Total Fat 0g; Saturated Fat 0g; Carbohydrates 12g; Dietary Fiber 2g; Cholesterol 0mg; Sodium 95 mg

Ingredients
Makes 3 cups.

1 teaspoon extra-virgin olive oil
1/2 cup finely chopped red onion (about 1 medium)
6 medium Bosc pears, peeled, cored, and diced
1/4 cup brandy
1/2 teaspoon finely chopped fresh rosemary
1/2 cup apple cider vinegar
1 teaspoon finely chopped jalapeño chile
1/4 cup finely chopped red bell pepper
1 cup unsweetened apple juice
1/2 teaspoon sea salt

Preparation
Heat a large sauté pan over medium-high heat and add the olive oil to lightly coat the bottom of the pan. Stir in the onion and cook until the onion has softened, about 2 minutes. Stir in the pears.

Carefully pour the brandy into the sauté pan and ignite to burn off the alcohol. (Be very careful, the flame may burn high. Never pour alcohol directly from the bottle into a hot pan.) Cook 2 minutes, then add the remaining ingredients.

Reduce the heat and simmer the mixture until the pears are soft, about 15 minutes.

Transfer to a bowl, cover, and refrigerate for 1 hour before serving.

Store in an airtight container in the refrigerator for 4 or 5 days.

Cranberry Chutney

Don't wait until Thanksgiving to enjoy this chutney on sandwiches or on breakfast breads. Photo on page 16.

Per 1/4 cup:
Calories 40; Protein 0g; Total Fat 0g; Saturated Fat 0g; Carbohydrates 9g; Dietary Fiber 2g; Cholesterol 0mg; Sodium 0mg

Ingredients
Makes 3 1/2 cups.

1 12-ounce bag fresh cranberries (about 3 cups)
2 Granny Smith apples, peeled and diced
1 cup unsweetened orange juice
1 cup diced, dried (about 25) or fresh (about 12) apricots
1/2 teaspoon minced fresh ginger
1 tablespoon honey
1 teaspoon ground cinnamon
1/4 teaspoon ground cloves

Preparation
Heat a medium saucepan over medium-high heat. Add the cranberries and apples and cook until the cranberries begin to pop, about 3 minutes. Add the remaining ingredients and simmer until cranberries have broken down and chutney is thick, about 10 to 15 minutes.

Transfer chutney to a bowl, cover, and refrigerate for 1 hour before serving.

Store in an airtight container in the refrigerator for 4 or 5 days.

Papaya Chutney

Papaya is an ideal fruit to use in making chutney. By adding jalapeños, we create a sweet but spicy condiment that is delicious with poultry, fish, pastas, and canapés.

Ingredients

Makes 3 cups.

2 cups diced, peeled papaya (about 2
   medium)
1/2 cup unsweetened orange juice
1/4 cup finely chopped green onion
1/4 cup chopped jícama
1/4 cup unsweetened pineapple juice
2 tablespoons finely chopped red bell
   pepper
1 teaspoon finely shredded fresh mint
1/2 teaspoon minced fresh cilantro
1/2 teaspoon finely chopped jalapeño chile
1/2 teaspoon minced fresh ginger
1/8 teaspoon sea salt

Preparation

Combine all the ingredients in a medium bowl and mix well. Cover and refrigerate the chutney for 1 hour before serving.

Store in an airtight container in the refrigerator for 4 or 5 days.

Beet, Cranberry, and Jícama Relish

Per 2 tablespoons:
Calories 40; Protein 1g; Total Fat 1.5g;
Saturated Fat 0.5g; Carbohydrates 6g; Dietary
Fiber 1g; Cholesterol 0mg; Sodium 10mg

Thanksgiving will not be the same once you complement your turkey with this relish. Photo on page 16.

Ingredients

Makes 3 cups.

2 cups unsweetened apple juice
2 cups 1/2-inch cubes, peeled beets
1 cup diced jícama
1/2 cup dried cranberries
1/2 cup chopped walnuts
Grated zest of 1 orange
1 cinnamon stick

Preparation

In a medium saucepan, combine all the ingredients and mix well. Bring to a boil over medium-high heat. Reduce heat to low and simmer uncovered until the beets are soft, about 45 minutes.

Transfer to a bowl, cover, and refrigerate for 1 hour before serving.

Store in an airtight container in the refrigerator for 4 or 5 days.

Cucumber-Mint Relish

Per 2 tablespoons:
Calories 5; Protein 0g; Total Fat 0g; Saturated
Fat 0g; Carbohydrates 1g; Dietary Fiber 0g;
Cholesterol 0mg; Sodium 75mg

I love this cool relish on chilled shrimp cocktail or grilled sea scallops. You'll love the ease of preparation and the fresh, lively flavor. Photo on page 16.

Ingredients

Makes 2 1/2 cups.

2 cups diced, peeled cucumber (1 medium)
1/4 cup minced red onion
1/4 cup seasoned rice wine vinegar
1 tablespoon chopped fresh mint
1 teaspoon minced garlic
1/2 teaspoon raw cane sugar (Turbinado)
1/4 teaspoon toasted sesame oil
1/8 teaspoon sea salt
1/8 teaspoon freshly ground black pepper

Preparation

Combine all the ingredients in a medium bowl and mix well. Cover the bowl with plastic wrap and refrigerate the relish for 1 hour before serving.

Store in an airtight container in the refrigerator for 4 or 5 days.

Asian Eggplant Relish

This relish is a great accompaniment to Asian-style poultry, lamb, and pork dishes. It is also makes a wonderful vegetarian canapé.

Ingredients

Makes 6 cups.

1 teaspoon extra-virgin olive oil
2 cups diced yellow onion (about 2 large)
1/2 cup diced red bell pepper (about 1 small)
1/2 cup diced yellow bell pepper (about 1 small)
1/2 cup diced green bell pepper (about 1 small)
4 cups chopped tomatoes (about 5 medium)
4 cups 1/4-inch cubes, peeled eggplant (about 1 medium)
1 tablespoon chopped Roasted Garlic (see page 38)
1 1/4 cups unsweetened pineapple juice
1/2 cup fresh lime juice
5 teaspoons curry powder
5 teaspoons ground cumin
1 teaspoon chile powder
2 teaspoons garam masala
1 tablespoon tomato paste
1/8 teaspoon ground cardamom
2 teaspoons grated lemon zest

Preparation

Heat a sauté pan over medium-high heat and add the olive oil to lightly coat the bottom of the pan. Stir in the onions, peppers, tomatoes, eggplant, and garlic and cook until eggplant has softened, about 5 minutes. Stir in the remaining ingredients and simmer for 5 minutes.

Remove from the heat and cool. Store in an airtight container in the refrigerator for up to 1 week.

Italian Eggplant Relish

Per 2 tablespoons:
Calories 15; Protein 0g; Total Fat 0g; Saturated
Fat 0g; Carbohydrates 3g; Dietary Fiber 0g;
Cholesterol 0mg; Sodium 55mg

Serve this savory mixture on toast points with fresh mozzarella cheese for a
crowd-pleasing appetizer. Heat with white wine and stir in a little butter to
create an inspiring sauce for shrimp or scallops. Photo on page 16.

Ingredients

Makes 4 cups.

1/4 teaspoon extra-virgin olive oil
6 cups diced, peeled eggplant (about
    1 large)
2 cups diced yellow onion (about 2 large)
1 cup diced celery (3 medium ribs)
2 teaspoons minced garlic
1/4 cup finely chopped kalamata olives
2 cups diced, peeled tomatoes (about 3
    medium, see Chef's Tip, page 186)
1/4 cup balsamic vinegar
2 tablespoons Fresh Herb Mix (see
    page 39)
1/2 cup tomato juice
2 tablespoons capers

Preparation

Heat a large sauté pan over medium-high heat and add the olive oil to
lightly coat the bottom of the pan. Stir in the eggplant, onion, celery, and
garlic and cook until the onion has softened, about 5 minutes. Add the
remaining ingredients and simmer until the eggplant is soft and the tomato
juice is reduced by half, 10 to 20 minutes.

Remove from heat and cool.

Store in an airtight container in the refrigerator for 4 or 5 days.

Tomatillo Salsa

Per 1/4 cup:
Calories 45; Protein 1g; Total Fat 2g; Saturated Fat 0g; Carbohydrates 6g; Dietary Fiber 2g; Cholesterol 0mg; Sodium 0mg

Though their popularity originated in the southwestern United States, tomatillos can now be found in the produce aisles of many well-stocked supermarkets. This small, green, papery-skinned fruit provides the tart, sweet flavor in *salsa verde*. Tomatillo salsa is extremely versatile; it can accompany poultry, seafood, and even meats and makes for a cool dip with any Mexican-style dinner.

Ingredients
Makes 1 1/2 cups.

2 cups tomatillos, papery skin removed, cut in quarters (about 8 ounces)
1/4 cup chopped red onion
1 teaspoon minced garlic
1/4 jalapeño chile, finely chopped
1/2 cup water
1/2 teaspoon raw cane sugar (Turbinado)
4 tablespoons chopped fresh cilantro
1/2 cup tomatillos, papery skin removed, chopped (about 2 ounces)
1/4 cup chopped red bell pepper
1/3 cup chopped avocado

Preparation

Heat a dry medium saucepan over medium-high heat and add the quartered tomatillos. Cook, stirring constantly, until the tomatillos have started to brown, about 3 minutes. Add the onion, garlic, jalapeño, water, sugar, and 3 tablespoons of the cilantro. Bring to a boil, reduce heat, and simmer until the tomatillos are soft, about 5 minutes.

Remove from heat, pour the mixture into a blender, and process until smooth.

Pour the pureed salsa into a mixing bowl and stir in the remaining 1 tablespoon cilantro, chopped tomatillos, red bell pepper, and avocado.

Cover with plastic wrap and refrigerate the salsa for 1 hour before serving.

Store in an airtight container in the refrigerator for 4 or 5 days.

Nopale-Corn Salsa

Nopales are the paddle-shaped pads of the prickly pear cactus indigenous to the Southwest. The pads are cleaned of the prickly spines and grilled, sautéed, or simmered to make a delicious and interesting addition to salads or beef entrées. This is an authentic and satisfying salsa with true southwestern flavors. Photo on page 16.

Ingredients
Makes 4 cups.

2 1/2 cups diced nopales (2 medium cactus pads), spines removed
3/4 cup fresh or frozen corn kernels
2 teaspoons finely chopped Roasted Garlic (see page 38)
1/2 cup finely chopped green onion
1 cup chopped, peeled tomato (1 medium)
1 cup chopped jícama
1/4 cup chopped fresh cilantro
2 teaspoons finely chopped, seeded jalapeño chile
1/2 teaspoon sea salt
1/4 teaspoon freshly ground black pepper

Preparation
Heat the nopales in a large sauté pan over medium-high heat and cook until they are lightly browned, about 2 minutes. Add the corn, garlic, and green onions and cook, stirring constantly, for about 5 minutes. Remove from the heat and stir in the remaining ingredients.

Transfer to a bowl, cover, and refrigerate for 1 hour before serving.

Store in an airtight container in the refrigerator for 4 or 5 days.

Fruit Salsa

Per 2 tablespoons:
Calories 10; Protein 0g; Total Fat 0g; Saturated Fat 0g; Carbohydrates 2g; Dietary Fiber 0g; Cholesterol 0mg; Sodium 0mg

This delicious and light accompaniment uplifts the flavors in sea scallops, shrimp, and mild fish. The addition of jalapeños and onions makes this suitable for grilled meats. The key ingredient is the marriage of the cool mint with the fresh fruit.

Ingredients
Makes 4 cups.

1 cup diced strawberries
1 1/2 cups diced pineapple
1 cup diced papaya
1/4 cup diced kiwifruit (about 1)
1 teaspoon finely shredded fresh mint
1/2 teaspoon finely chopped fresh cilantro
1/2 cup unsweetened orange juice
1 tablespoon finely chopped green onion
1/2 teaspoon finely chopped jalapeño chile

Preparation
Combine all the ingredients in a large bowl and mix well. Cover and refrigerate for about 1 hour before serving.

Variation
Omit onions and jalapeño and serve with ice cream.

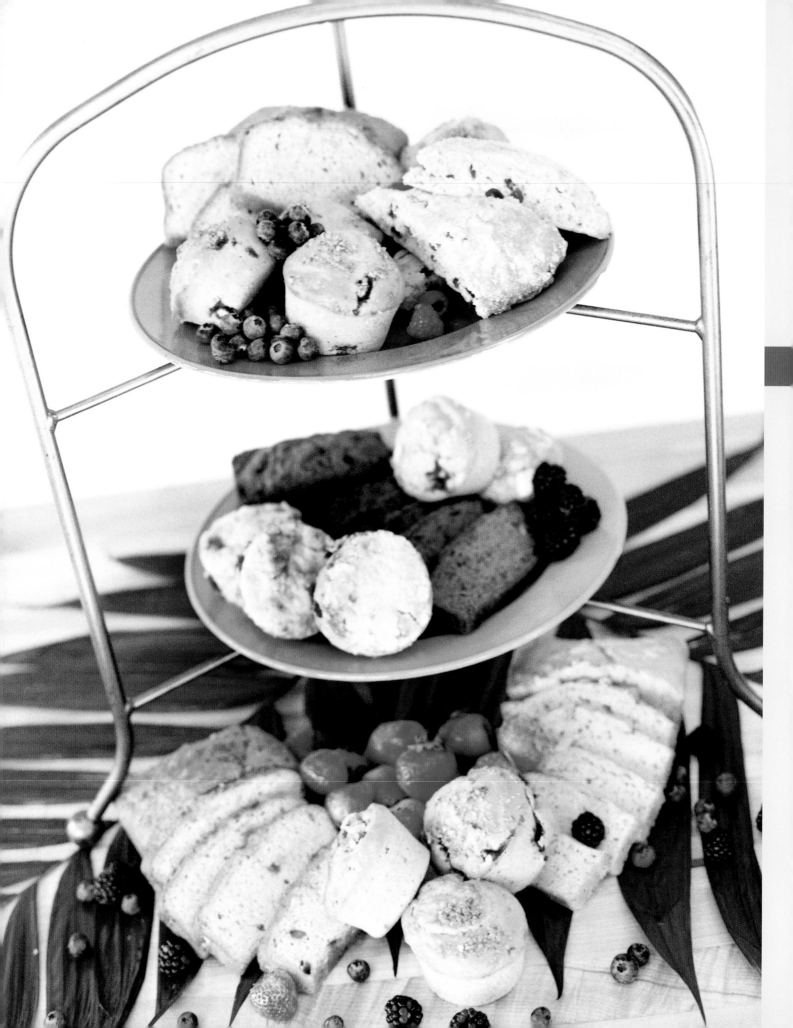

Breakfast:
Breaking the Fast

Pictured at left: (top) Almond-Poppy Seed Bread, Blueberry Muffins, Cranberry-Orange Scones, (middle) Dried Cherry Crumb Cakes, Zucchini Bread, Raspberry Muffins, (bottom) Banana Bread, Raspberry/Blackberry Muffins, Almond-Poppy Seed Bread

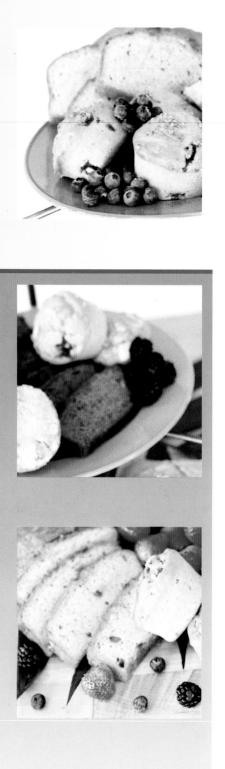

Beginning each morning by eating a balanced breakfast sets the stage for a day filled with healthful and nutritious food. Breakfast is a very important meal when you are seeking to achieve a healthful lifestyle and control weight. A balanced breakfast, consisting of carbohydrates, proteins, moderate amounts of fats, vitamins, minerals, and fiber, is essential to refuel your body with the vital nutrients you need to be mentally focused, and to provide you with the energy needed to be at your best in today's demanding world.

In creating a balanced and healthful lifestyle, you may find it necessary to retrain yourself to practice better eating habits. A balanced meal to start your day does not have to consist of three whole eggs, three strips of bacon, hash brown potatoes, juice, and toast. This typical American breakfast accounts for 1,284 calories and 93 grams of fat. This is overwhelming, considering that the average woman should consume about 2,000 calories and 67 grams of fat per day (based on no more than 30 percent of calories from fat). It's not surprising that after eating the typical American breakfast we feel more tired and bloated than energized and renewed.

I often hear from friends and guests how difficult it is to find the time to eat breakfast because morning schedules are so busy. Others tell me that breakfast doesn't appeal to them—the standard breakfast fare seems too boring or heavy.

Breakfast is worth making time for, especially when you'll be eating these rich-tasting, satisfying, and energy-boosting foods. All will help you start your day being more conscious of the types of foods and portion sizes that you consume.

On some days you'll find time to prepare an enjoyable full meal for breakfast, on others your fast-paced life will demand something quick. The recipes included in this chapter will help you create sensational morning starters, from quick and easy juice drinks to luscious brunch-style entrées.

Juices and Smoothies

We have all heard and read that we should eat more fresh fruits and vegetables. Including energy-boosting, delicious fresh fruit and vegetable beverages can be a fun, convenient, and easy way to get the recommended four to five servings of fresh fruits and vegetables daily. Juice and smoothies provide antioxidants, vitamin C, beta-carotene, minerals, and fiber.

Cereals

An easy way to have a healthy breakfast is to keep a supply of Miraval Granola on hand. Add your choice of fresh fruit and milk, and you have a breakfast that is ready in minutes and supplies many of the B vitamins, vitamin E, iron, and fiber that you need each day. Cooked cereals, full of whole-grain goodness, take a little more time, but you can combine the dry ingredients the night before and add the liquid just before cooking.

Entrées

In this section you will find recipes that go beyond just bacon and eggs. Many, such as Warm Fruit and Berry Strudel, are elegant enough for a weekend brunch with guests. For those mornings when you want a hearty meal, try Breakfast Scramble made with egg whites, or Tofu Scramble. Both are good sources of high-quality, low-fat protein.

Breads

Who doesn't enjoy the smell of baking bread? To save time on busy mornings, bake your muffins the evening before using one of the delicious low-fat muffin variations. The muffins can be frozen for up to a month and reheated just before eating. Bread is an important source of nutrients, providing complex carbohydrates which include the majority of each day's intake of calories, B vitamins, and fiber.

55

Liquid Sunshine

This is one of my favorite juice drinks. It's extremely easy to make—just toss the washed, unpeeled chunks into a juicer—and its flavors are as luscious as a ray of sunshine. The use of ginger not only provides an interesting burst of flavor, it also aids in digestion and alleviates motion sickness. To turn this drink into a sensational Dreamsicle float, add a scoop of frozen vanilla yogurt or ice cream.

Ingredients
Makes 1 serving.

5 carrots
1/2 apple
1-inch piece fresh ginger
Pinch of nutmeg

Preparation
Place all the ingredients into a juicer and process according to manufacturer's directions. Serve in a tall glass.

Beet Sensation

Even if you have never been a fan of beets, this drink, with its vibrant color and sweetness, will make you love the old root veggie. The carrots, apples, and beets provide you with a natural dose of vitamins A and C and beta-carotene. Its refreshing flavors, including a hint of tartness from the lemon, make this drink an ideal cooler any time of the day.

Ingredients
Makes 1 serving.

5 carrots
1/2 apple
1/2 beet, scrubbed
1/2 lemon
Lemon wedge or slice, for garnish

Preparation
Place the carrots, apple, beet and lemon into a juicer and process according to manufacturer's directions. Serve in a tall glass garnished with a lemon wedge.

Mudslide

Per serving:
Calories 260; Protein 5g; Total Fat 5g;
Saturated Fat 0.5g; Carbohydrates 53g; Dietary
Fiber 4g; Cholesterol 0mg; Sodium 80mg

Kids big or small will love the nutty and chocolatey flavors in this drink, which are reminiscent of a candy bar. Just don't tell them that it's packed with stuff that's good for them.

Ingredients
Makes 1 serving.

2 teaspoons carob powder or chocolate
   syrup
3/4 cup soymilk, rice milk, or fat-free milk
1/2 medium banana
1 teaspoon almond, cashew, or peanut butter
1 teaspoon honey
1 1/2 cups ice cubes

Preparation
Combine all the ingredients in a blender and process until smooth. Serve in a tall glass.

Omega-3 Smoothie

Per serving:
Calories 240; Protein 3g; Total Fat 3g;
Saturated Fat 0g; Carbohydrates 55g; Dietary
Fiber 7 g; Cholesterol 0mg; Sodium 10mg

This is Conscious Cuisine at its best. Close your eyes and you can embrace memories of home-cooked apple pie. Plus, Omega-3 fatty acids—which lower blood cholesterol and triglycerides and reduce the chance of blood clot formation—are contained in both the hemp and flax seeds.

Ingredients
Makes 1 serving.

3/4 cup unsweetened apple juice
1/2 medium banana
1 teaspoon ground flax seeds
1 teaspoon ground hemp seeds
1/2 teaspoon ground cardamom
1 teaspoon ground cinnamon
1 1/2 cups ice cubes

Preparation
Combine all the ingredients in a blender and process until smooth. Serve in a tall glass.

Nordine's Power Punch

Per serving:
Calories 260; Protein 16g; Total Fat 1.5g;
Saturated Fat 0g; Carbohydrates 51g; Dietary
Fiber 5g; Cholesterol 5mg; Sodium 190mg

My good friend and two-time Mr. Universe winner, Nordine Zouareg, drinks this strawberry-banana punch regularly. Three of the four food groups are represented in this delicious blend, providing a burst of nutrients to start the day—or begin a Total Body Workout.

Ingredients
Makes 1 serving.

2 tablespoons soy or whey protein powder
1/2 cup fat-free milk
1/2 cup plain fat-free yogurt
1/2 cup strawberries
1/2 medium banana
1 1/2 cups ice cubes

Preparation
Combine all the ingredients in a blender and process until smooth. Serve in a tall glass.

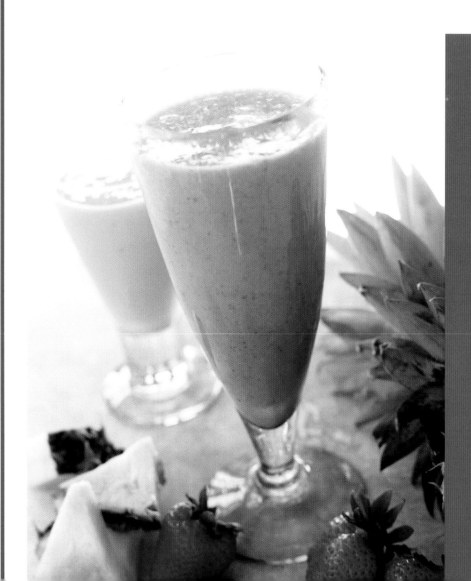

Don Juan

Per serving:
Calories 160; Protein 2g; Total Fat 1g;
Saturated Fat 0g; Carbohydrates 41g; Dietary
Fiber 4g; Cholesterol 0mg; Sodium 30mg

A summertime sensation, this drink blends the cool, tropical flavors of pineapple, mango, and coconut. But beware—this beverage may cause you to dream of the islands!

Ingredients
Makes 1 serving

1/4 cup unsweetened pineapple juice
1/2 medium banana
1/4 cup light coconut milk
1/4 cup chopped mango or mango puree
1 1/2 cups ice cubes

Preparation
Combine all the ingredients in a blender and process until smooth. Serve in a tall glass.

Oat Bran

Per 1/2 cup oats and 2 tablespoons milk:
Calories 140; Protein 4g; Total Fat 1g;
Saturated Fat 0g; Carbohydrates 32g; Dietary
Fiber 3g; Cholesterol 0mg; Sodium 20mg

Cereals are a quick and convenient way to start the day with essential nutrients. While eating hot cereals, we are forced to slow down to enjoy their textures and flavors. Bran cereals can help lower your cholesterol and reduce the risk of cancer. Sometimes oat bran has a lackluster flavor, but this recipe adds sweetness and character to the nutritious whole grain.

Ingredients
Makes 8 servings.

2 cups water
2 cups unsweetened apple juice
1 1/3 cups oat bran
1 Granny Smith apple, cored, finely
    chopped
1/2 cup raisins
2 tablespoons pure maple syrup
1/2 teaspoon ground cinnamon
1/2 teaspoon ground caraway seed
1 cup fat-free milk

Preparation
Combine the water and apple juice in a medium saucepan and bring to a boil over medium heat. Add the oat bran, apple, raisins, maple syrup, cinnamon, and caraway. Reduce heat to low and simmer, stirring frequently with a whisk until the mixture begins to thicken, about 4 to 6 minutes. Remove from heat and let stand uncovered 5 minutes. Serve with the milk.

Oat Bran and Carrot Cereal

Per 1/2 cup:
Calories 90; Protein 3g; Total Fat 1.5g;
Saturated Fat 0g; Carbohydrates 23g; Dietary
Fiber 3g; Cholesterol 0mg; Sodium 5mg

You'll love this satisfying hot cereal—the apple juice and carrot provide sweetness and the oat bran provides substance and fiber. The delicious punch of freshly grated nutmeg lifts the cereal to the next level of flavor.

Ingredients
Makes 4 cups.

3 cups unsweetened apple juice
1 cup water
1/2 teaspoon freshly grated nutmeg
1 1/2 cups oat bran
1/2 cup shredded carrot (about 1 medium)
Vanilla soymilk, optional

Preparation
In a medium saucepan, combine the apple juice, water, and nutmeg. Bring to a boil over medium heat. Stir in the oat bran and reduce heat to low. Simmer, whisking vigorously to prevent clumping, until thickened, 2 to 3 minutes. Remove from heat and stir in the carrot.

Serve with vanilla soymilk, if desired.

Quinoa-Couscous Breakfast Cereal

Per 1/2 cup:
Calories 180; Protein 4g; Total Fat 1.5g;
Saturated Fat 0g; Carbohydrates 40g; Dietary
Fiber 3g; Cholesterol 0mg; Sodium 10mg

This is a great way to make a balanced, nutritious breakfast for children. Serve it as is, or create a fantastic breakfast cake by preparing the cereal the night before, pressing it into an 8-inch-square pan, refrigerating it, and cutting it into bars the next morning. The sweetness and tartness of the dried fruit blend well with the nutty flavor of the quinoa to make a quick and delicious morning meal.

Ingredients
Makes 6 cups.

3 cups unsweetened apple juice
2 cups water
1 cup quinoa
1/4 cup dried cranberries
1/4 cup dried blueberries
1/4 cup chopped dried apricots
1/4 cup raisins
1 teaspoon ground cinnamon
1/2 teaspoon ground allspice
1 cup uncooked couscous
1/2 cup soymilk, rice milk, or fat-free milk,
  optional

Preparation

In a medium saucepan, combine the apple juice and water. Bring to a simmer over medium heat.

Rinse and drain the quinoa in a fine mesh strainer. Heat a medium sauté pan over medium heat; add the quinoa and toast it. Stir constantly until the grains begin popping, 2 to 3 minutes.

Add the quinoa, dried fruits, and spices to the saucepan. Simmer, stirring occasionally, until the quinoa is clear and soft, 12 to 15 minutes. Stir in the couscous. Remove pan from heat and cover. Let stand until the couscous has absorbed the liquid and is fluffy, 5 to 7 minutes.

Stir in the soymilk, if desired.

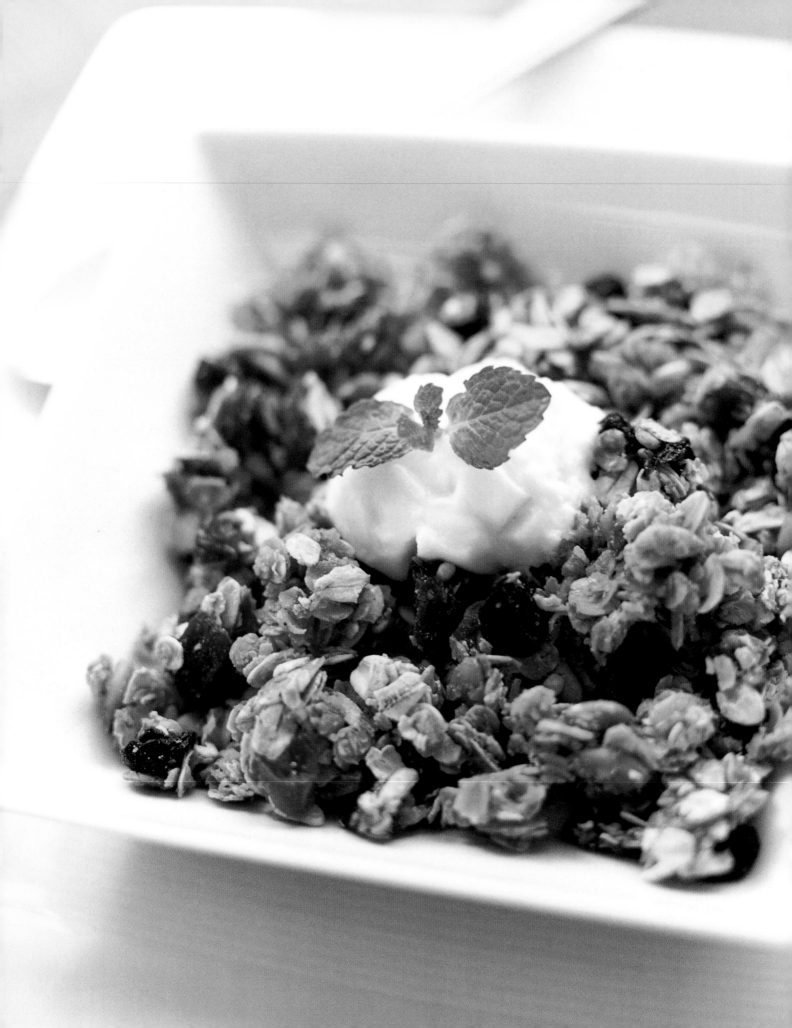

Miraval Granola

Per 1/2 cup:
Calories 230; Protein 7g; Total Fat 4g;
Saturated Fat 4g; Carbohydrates 49g; Dietary
Fiber 6g; Cholesterol 0mg; Sodium 0mg

Believed to be healthful, traditional granola can be high in fat and calories from high-fat nuts, butter, and sugar, typically 1/2 cup at 420 calories and 20 grams of fat. I've created depth of flavor in this delicious low-fat version by toasting the grains rather than caramelizing them. Pumpkin and sunflower seeds replace macadamia nuts, pecans, and walnuts to retain a nutty flavor and a crunchy mouth feel. The natural sweetness of the dried fruits eliminates the need for brown sugar, and the use of honey and a vanilla bean creates rich flavor without using butter. This mindful selection of ingredients and the unique preparation illustrate Conscious Cuisine at its best.

Ingredients
Makes 11 cups.

6 cups rolled oats
3 cups oat bran
1/4 cup shelled pumpkin seeds
1/4 cup shelled sunflower seeds
1 cup honey
1 vanilla bean, split in half lengthwise
3 cups unsweetened apple juice
1/3 cup chopped dried apricots
1/3 cup golden raisins
1/3 cup dried cherries
1/3 cup dried chopped dates
1/3 cup dried blueberries

Preparation
Preheat the oven to 400°F (205°C). Spread out the rolled oats and oat bran evenly on 2 baking sheets. Toast in the oven for 5 to 8 minutes or until golden.

On another baking sheet, spread out the pumpkin and sunflower seeds and toast for 5 minutes or until lightly browned.

Scrape the seeds from the vanilla bean pod and combine with the honey in a small saucepan. (The remaining pod can be put to another use such as flavoring vanilla sugar, see page xix.) Simmer the honey and vanilla seeds over low heat to flavor the honey, 5 to 7 minutes.

In a medium saucepan, combine the apple juice and dried fruits. Simmer until softened, about 5 minutes, and drain the fruit.

In a large bowl, combine the oat mixture, seeds, and fruit mixture. Stir in the warm honey, and stir to coat the mixture as evenly as possible.

Spread the mixture evenly onto 2 baking sheets. Bake 10 to 15 minutes or until golden brown, stirring every 2 minutes to prevent burning.

Cool the granola completely. Can be stored in an airtight container for up to 1 month.

Steel-Cut Oats

Conscious Cuisine means selecting and preparing foods that provide both flavor and health benefits. Steel-cut oats are a great example of this. Oats are a good source of fiber and vital nutrients and have cholesterol-lowering attributes. Steel-cut oats are oat groats that have been cut lengthwise; they are minimally processed and thus retain most of their nutrients. The cooking time is longer than for old-fashioned, quick, or instant oats, but the nutty whole-grain flavor and nutritional superiority are worth the extra 15 minutes.

Ingredients
Makes 3 cups.

3 1/2 cups water
1 cinnamon stick
1 cup steel-cut oats
1/4 teaspoon sea salt

Preparation

Combine the water and cinnamon stick in a small saucepan. Simmer over low heat for 5 minutes.

Heat a dry saucepan over medium heat and toast the oats, stirring constantly, until golden, about 3 minutes. Stir the oats and salt into the hot water and simmer, stirring occasionally, until the oats are soft, about 15 to 20 minutes. Remove the cinnamon stick before serving.

Breakfast Blintz Purses

Per 1 blintz:
Calories 150; Protein 10g; Total Fat 0.5g;
Saturated Fat 0g; Carbohydrates 25g; Dietary
Fiber less than 1 gram; Cholesterol 30mg;
Sodium 280g

It's challenging and fun to remake traditional foods—such as blintzes, a typical brunch item—into lighter and more delicious versions. In this recipe, the richness of fat-free ricotta cheese replaces high-fat Mascarpone. The granola adds sweetness and texture.

Ingredients
Makes 10 blintzes.

10 fresh chives
2 cups fat-free ricotta cheese
1 tablespoon chopped dried cranberries
1 tablespoon chopped dried apricots
1 teaspoon ground cinnamon
1/4 teaspoon ground nutmeg
1 teaspoon pure vanilla extract
1/4 cup Miraval Granola (see page 63)
10 purchased crêpes or Crêpes (see
*   page 67)*

Preparation
Blanch the chives in boiling water for 1 second. Plunge the chives in a bowl of ice water to stop the cooking process. Set aside.

Preheat the oven to 350°F (175°C). In a mixing bowl, combine the ricotta cheese, dried fruits, spices, vanilla, and granola.

Place one crêpe on a clean cutting board and spoon 2 tablespoons of the ricotta-cheese mixture onto the center of the crêpe. Fold up the sides of the crêpe, and tie the crêpe closed with a chive to make a decorative package. Repeat with remaining crêpes, cheese mixture, and chives.

Place blintzes on a nonstick baking sheet. Spray lightly with vegetable oil. Bake for 10 to 15 minutes or until golden brown.

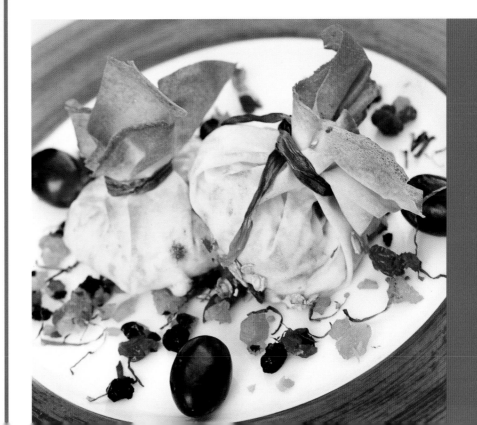

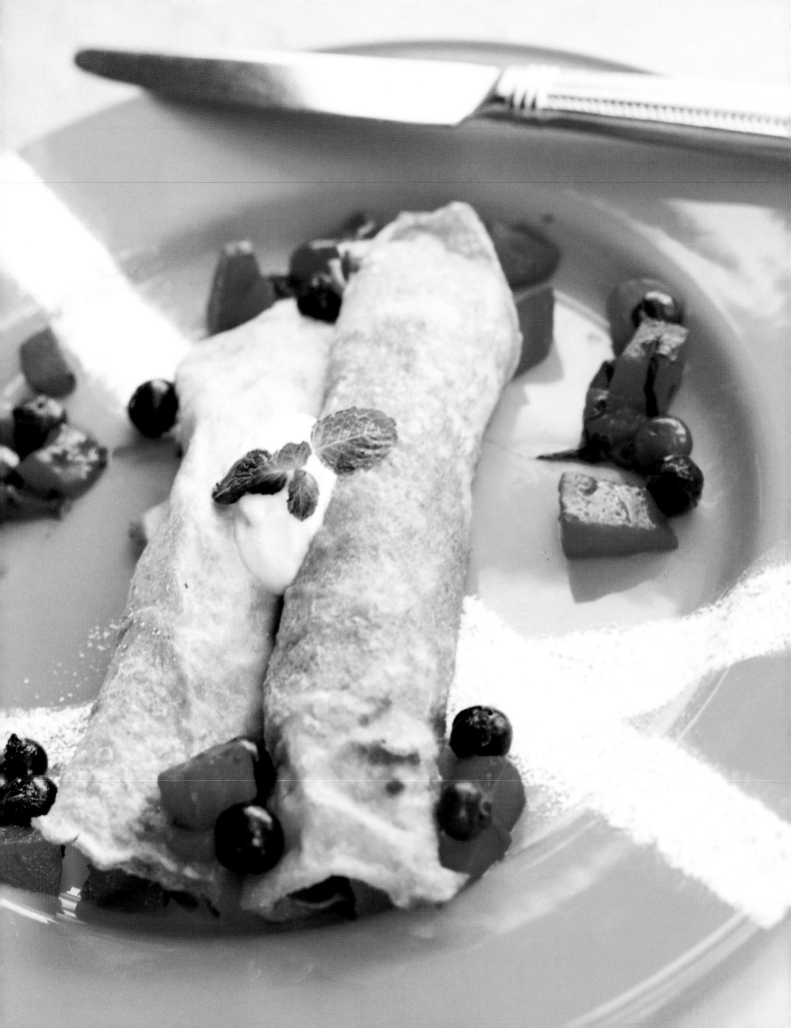

Applesauce Crêpes with Fresh Fruit Compote

Per 2 crepes:
Calories 250; Protein 7g; Total Fat 1g;
Saturated Fat 0g; Carbohydrates 56g; Dietary
Fiber 7g; Cholesterol 0mg; Sodium 110mg

Thin, scrumptious crêpes have been a staple of French cuisine for centuries. This is a revival of an old favorite. Applesauce is used to flavor the crêpes and provide enough body to eliminate the need for oil.

Crêpes are extremely versatile. Try these dusted with powdered sugar for a sensational light dessert, or filled with savory foods for a luscious entrée.

Ingredients
Makes 10 crêpes.

Crêpes
1 1/2 cups unsweetened applesauce
1 cup fat-free milk
2 large egg whites
1/2 cup unbleached all-purpose flour
1/2 cup whole-wheat pastry flour
1/8 teaspoon sea salt

Berry Compote
1 vanilla bean, split in half lengthwise
2 cups chopped, peeled pears (2 medium)
2 cups chopped, peeled apples
  (2 medium)
1 pint (2 cups) fresh blueberries
1/2 cup unsweetened apple juice
1 teaspoon finely shredded fresh mint

Vanilla fat-free yogurt

Preparation

For the Crêpes: Combine the unsweetened applesauce, milk, and egg whites in a small bowl and mix well. Whisk in the flours and salt until the batter is smooth. Let rest for 15 minutes.

Heat a nonstick crêpe pan (or small sauté pan) over medium-high heat. Coat pan with cooking spray and ladle in enough batter to just cover the bottom of the pan. Cook until set and slightly browned, then flip and cook the other side in the same manner. Repeat with remaining batter.

Stack the crêpes on a plate as they are cooked. (Layered between waxed paper or plastic wrap, the crêpes can be stored in the refrigerator for up to 7 days.)

For the Berry Compote: Scrape the seeds from the vanilla bean pod and combine with the pears, apples, blueberries, and apple juice in a small saucepan. (The remaining pod can be put to another use such as flavoring vanilla sugar, see page xix.) Bring to a boil over medium heat; reduce heat and simmer until pears and apples are just soft, 15 to 20 minutes. Drain the liquid into a bowl and reserve for another sauce. Stir shredded mint into fruit mixture.

To serve: Place a crêpe on a clean cutting board; spoon 1 tablespoon of fruit compote onto the crêpe and roll it up. Place 2 crêpes on each plate with a dollop of vanilla yogurt.

Warm Fruit and Berry Strudel

Per slice:
Calories 290; Protein 4g; Total Fat 4g;
Saturated Fat 1.5g; Carbohydrates 21g; Dietary
Fiber 2g; Cholesterol 21mg; Sodium 250mg

For an elegant breakfast entrée or evening dessert, this strudel is both attractive and sinfully delicious. When working with phyllo dough, butter is typically used in between each layer. When creating desserts and strudels, I lighten the recipe by using hazelnut, walnut, pistachio, or olive oil (or cooking spray) between the layers of phyllo to complement the flavors of each dish. Look for phyllo dough in your grocer's freezer.

Ingredients

Makes 2 strudels; 8 slices.

2 medium Granny Smith apples, peeled, cored
2 medium Bosc pears, peeled, cored
2 vanilla beans, split in half lengthwise
1/2 cup honey
2 tablespoons finely chopped pecans
1 tablespoon finely shredded fresh mint
1 cup fresh raspberries
1 cup fresh blueberries
8 sheets phyllo dough (about 1/3 of a 1 lb. box)
1 cup Product 19 cereal or other unsweetened cereal
Hazelnut oil in spray bottle (or cooking spray)
Vanilla fat-free yogurt, optional

Preparation

Preheat the oven to 425°F (205°C).

Cut the apples and pears into wedges, about 8 wedges from each.

Scrape the seeds from the vanilla bean pods and combine with the honey in a medium saucepan. (The remaining pod can be put to another use such as flavoring vanilla sugar, see page xix.) Heat the honey and vanilla seeds over medium heat until warm, about 3 minutes. Stir in the apples and pears, and cook until the fruit starts to soften, about 10 minutes. Remove from heat and cool completely. Fold the pecans, mint, and berries into the honey mixture. Let stand for 10 minutes, then drain off excess liquid.

Using a clean coffee grinder, grind up the cereal, or crumble by hand into small crumbs, and place in bowl.

To assemble: Carefully unfold the phyllo sheets. Place one sheet on a clean cutting board and spray with hazelnut oil, brushing oil in a thin layer across the phyllo sheet. Sprinkle with 1 tablespoon of the cereal crumbs. Place another sheet of phyllo on top of first sheet. Spray with oil and sprinkle with crumbs. Repeat with 2 more layers of phyllo for a total of 4 layers.

Place 1 3/4 cups of the fruit mixture along the bottom long edge of the layered phyllo rectangle. Fold edges in on both sides of the fruit mixture and roll up. Spray the top with hazelnut oil. Place the strudel seam side down on a nonstick baking sheet. Repeat with remaining phyllo, crumbs, hazelnut oil, and fruit mixture.

Bake for 10 to 12 minutes, or until golden brown. Cut each strudel diagonally into 4 pieces.

Serve with a dollop of vanilla fat-free yogurt, if desired.

Variation

Replace the fresh berries with dried fruit, or use any combination of apples, pears, or peaches.

Blue Corn Waffles

This is a southwestern breakfast treat. For an extra special twist, serve these with prickly pear syrup. If you have leftovers, cool them on a wire rack, individually wrap them in plastic wrap, place them in a freezer bag, and freeze. Reheat the waffles in a toaster for a quick and delicious breakfast.

Ingredients
Makes 12 waffles.

2 cups whole-wheat pastry flour
1 cup blue (or yellow) cornmeal
2 teaspoons baking powder
1 teaspoon ground allspice
1 can (8 ounces or 1 cup) cream-style corn
1 cup low-fat buttermilk
1 cup plain, fat-free yogurt
4 large egg whites
1 tablespoon canola oil

Preparation
Sift the flour, cornmeal, baking powder, and allspice into a medium mixing bowl. In a separate bowl, mix all the remaining ingredients. Make a well in the center of the dry ingredients; pour in the corn mixture and stir until smooth.

Heat a waffle iron and coat with vegetable spray. Pour 3/4 cup of batter onto the iron and bake until golden brown. Repeat with remaining batter.

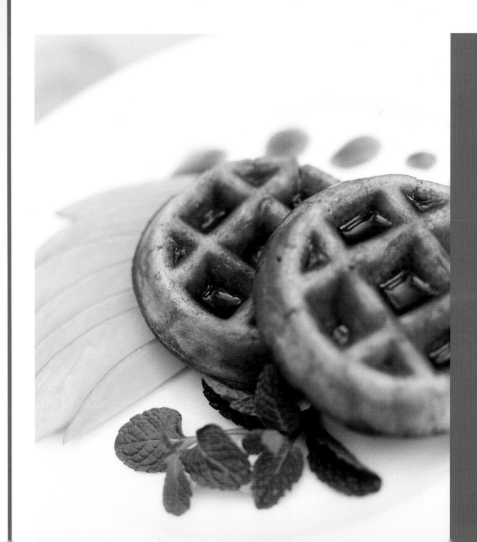

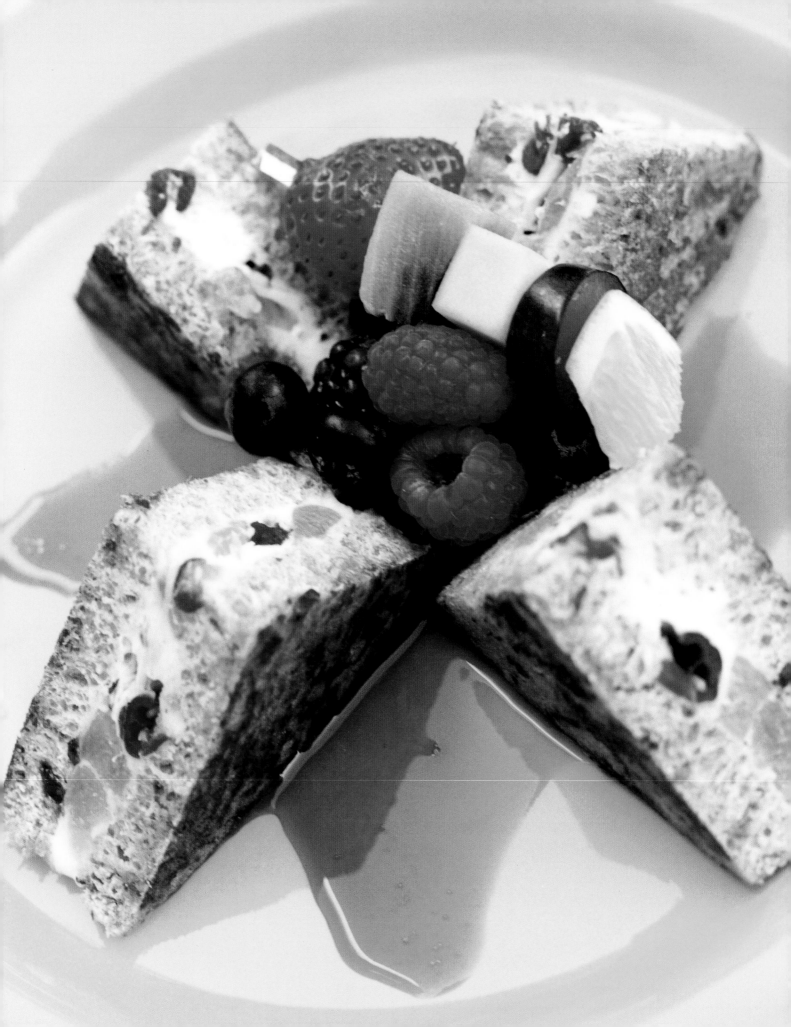

Stuffed French Toast

This is an attractive breakfast treat inspired by two classic French dishes: French toast and the *croque-monsieur* (a grilled ham and cheese sandwich). Serve with fresh fruit and pure maple syrup.

Ingredients
Makes 8 servings.

Filling
1 cup (8 ounces) reduced-fat cream cheese
1 1/2 teaspoons chopped dried cherries
1 1/2 teaspoons chopped dried blueberries
1 1/2 teaspoons chopped dried apricots
1 teaspoon minced fresh mint

French Toast
8 slices cinnamon raisin bread
4 large egg whites
1/2 cup low-fat buttermilk
1 teaspoon ground cinnamon
1/2 teaspoon ground allspice
1 tablespoon pure maple syrup

Garnish
Fresh berries, optional

Preparation

For the Filling: In a mixing bowl, soften the cream cheese by stirring vigorously or by warming slightly over a water bath. Stir in the dried fruits and mint.

For the French Toast: Spread 2 tablespoons of the cheese mixture on a slice of bread and top with another slice of bread. Repeat to make 4 sandwiches.

Heat a griddle over medium-high heat. Lightly coat with cooking spray.

In a mixing bowl, beat the egg whites and buttermilk until just combined. Whisk in the cinnamon, allspice, and maple syrup. Dip both sides of each sandwich into the batter and place on the hot griddle. Cook until browned, about 3 minutes, and flip. Cook until browned on remaining side.

Cut each sandwich into 4 pieces and serve warm. Garnish with fresh berries, if desired.

Apple-Buckwheat Griddle Cakes

Per 2 pancakes:
Calories 90; Protein 4g; Total Fat 3g; Saturated Fat 0g; Carbohydrates 13g; Dietary Fiber 1g; Cholesterol 20mg; Sodium 120mg

Both hearty and elegant, these griddle cakes are a great way to enjoy the flavors and benefits of buckwheat. The sweetness of the apples marries well with this old-fashioned grain's hearty flavor. Serve these with fresh raspberry sauce or pure maple syrup.

Ingredients
Makes 6 servings.

1/2 cup Granny Smith apple, peeled, cored, and diced
1/8 teaspoon ground cinnamon
1/2 teaspoon unsweetened apple juice
1/4 cup buckwheat flour
1/4 cup whole-wheat pastry flour
3/4 teaspoon baking powder
1/8 teaspoon sea salt
1 large egg
1 tablespoon canola oil
1 tablespoon honey
3/4 cup fat-free milk
2 large egg whites

Preparation

Combine the apple, cinnamon, and apple juice in a medium saucepan over medium heat. Cook until the apple is tender, 7 to 10 minutes. (The natural juice from the apple will produce a glaze.) Place the apple mixture in a bowl and refrigerate until cool.

Sift the flours, baking powder, and salt into a medium mixing bowl. In a separate bowl, mix together the egg, oil, honey, and milk. Make a well in the center of the dry ingredients; pour in the egg mixture and stir until just moistened.

With an electric mixer, whip the egg whites until stiff peaks form. Gently fold the egg whites into the batter. Fold in the chilled apple mixture.

Heat a griddle over medium heat and coat with cooking spray. Spoon batter by 1/4 cupfuls onto the griddle. Cook until bubbles appear and edges begin to look dry. The bottoms should be golden brown. Turn the pancakes over—they will rise and the middles will become light and fluffy—and cook until golden brown.

Mango-Strawberry Griddle Cakes

With cool, contrasting flavors and a light, airy texture, this is a wonderful summertime treat when strawberries are at their best. Serve with pure maple syrup, fruit compote, or fruit preserves.

Ingredients
Makes 6 servings.

1 cup unbleached all-purpose flour
1 tablespoon baking powder
1/2 teaspoon baking soda
1/4 teaspoon sea salt
3/4 teaspoon honey
3/4 teaspoon canola oil
1/4 teaspoon pure vanilla extract
1/2 cup fat-free ricotta cheese
1 1/2 cups low-fat buttermilk
1 large egg white
1 teaspoon freshly grated lemon zest
1/3 cup diced mango
1/3 cup sliced strawberries

Preparation
Sift the flour, baking powder, baking soda, and salt into a medium mixing bowl. In a separate bowl, mix the honey, oil, vanilla, ricotta cheese, and buttermilk.

Make a well in the center of the dry ingredients; pour in the ricotta cheese mixture and stir until just moistened.

With an electric mixer, whip the egg white until stiff peaks form. Gently fold the egg white into the batter. Fold in the lemon zest, mango, and strawberries.

Heat a griddle over medium heat and coat with cooking spray. Spoon batter by 1/4 cupfuls onto the griddle. Cook until bubbles appear and edges begin to look dry. The bottoms should be golden brown. Turn the pancakes over—they will rise and the middles will become light and fluffy—and cook until golden brown.

Banana-Buckwheat Griddle Cakes

I've used this recipe for years and improved the quality of the flours and dairy products to make it more nutritious. It's a great recipe to make with children, teaching them to notice the difference in flours and the multiple uses of bananas. Serve with pure maple syrup, fruit compote, or fruit preserves.

Ingredients
Makes 6 servings.

1/4 cup buckwheat flour
1/4 cup whole-wheat pastry flour
3/4 teaspoon baking powder
1/8 teaspoon sea salt
1 large egg
3/4 teaspoon canola oil
3/4 teaspoon honey
3/4 cup fat-free milk
2 large egg whites
1/2 cup diced banana (about 1 medium)
1 pinch ground cinnamon
3/4 teaspoon freshly grated lemon zest
3/4 teaspoon fresh lemon juice

Preparation
Sift the flours, baking powder, and salt into a medium mixing bowl. In a separate bowl, mix together the egg, oil, honey, and milk. Make a well in the center of the dry ingredients; pour in the egg mixture and stir until just moistened.

With an electric mixer, whip the egg whites until stiff peaks form. Gently fold the egg whites into the batter. Fold in the banana, cinnamon, lemon zest, and lemon juice until just combined.

Heat a griddle over medium heat and coat with cooking spray. Spoon batter by 1/4 cupfuls onto the griddle. Cook until bubbles appear and edges begin to look dry. The bottoms should be golden brown. Turn the pancakes over—they will rise and the middles will become light and fluffy—and cook until golden brown.

Potato–Wild Rice Griddle Cakes

Per griddle cake:
Calories 80; Protein 3g; Total Fat 0g; Saturated Fat 0g; Carbohydrates 17g; Dietary Fiber 1g; Cholesterol 0mg; Sodium 290mg

This is a handy way to use up leftover baked potatoes and cooked wild rice. It makes a very substantial potato pancake—perfect with eggs and fruit as a healthy substitute for hash browns.

Ingredients
Makes 8 servings.

3 cups cooked wild rice
1 mashed, peeled, baked potato
1 tablespoon mashed Roasted Garlic (see page 38)
1 teaspoon sea salt
1/4 teaspoon freshly ground black pepper
1/4 teaspoon ground nutmeg
2 tablespoons chopped fresh herbs, such as thyme, chives, basil, oregano, or parsley

Preparation
Combine the rice and potato in a mixing bowl; add the garlic, salt, pepper, nutmeg, and herbs. Stir to combine (this will be a thick mixture). Taste and adjust the seasoning, if necessary, with additional herbs, salt, and pepper.

Scoop up about 1/3 cup of the potato mixture; mold with your hands to form a round, flat cake. Repeat with remaining mixture to make 8 cakes.

Heat a griddle over medium-high heat and lightly spray with olive oil. Cook cakes on griddle, turning once, until browned and heated thoroughly, about 5 minutes on each side.

Pistachio and Potato Cakes

Per 2 potato cakes:
Calories 140; Protein 7g; Total Fat 2.5g;
Saturated Fat 0g; Carbohydrates 23g; Dietary
Fiber 2g; Cholesterol 0mg; Sodium 135mg

These potato cakes are surprisingly light, and the pistachio adds an interesting flavor note. Serve with apple compote or as a substitute for blini with smoked salmon.

Ingredients
Makes 6 servings.

1 cup whole-wheat pastry flour
2 teaspoons baking powder
1/4 teaspoon ground allspice
1 cup fat-free milk
4 large egg whites
2 tablespoon honey
1 tablespoon extra-virgin olive oil
2 cups potatoes, peeled, cooked, and
    mashed (about 1 1/2 pounds)
1/4 cup pistachio nuts, finely chopped

Preparation

Sift the flour, baking powder, and allspice into a medium mixing bowl. In a separate bowl, mix together the milk, egg whites, honey, and oil. Stir in the potatoes and nuts. Make a well in the center of the dry ingredients; pour in the potato mixture and stir until smooth.

Heat a griddle over medium heat and coat with cooking spray. Spoon batter by 1/4 cupfuls onto the griddle. Cook until bubbles appear and edges begin to look dry. The bottoms should be golden brown. Turn the pancakes over—they will rise and the middles will become light and fluffy—and cook until golden brown.

Salmon Patties

This is a lovely alternative to pork sausage on the breakfast table or brunch buffet. The addition of grapes gives the recipe moisture and a touch of sweetness. Photo on page 80.

Per salmon patty:
Calories 80; Protein 8g; Total Fat 2.5g; Saturated Fat 0g; Carbohydrates 5g; Dietary Fiber 0g; Cholesterol 20mg; Sodium 220mg

Ingredients
Makes 6 salmon patties.

1/2 pound fresh salmon fillets (without skin or bones)
1 large egg white
1/2 teaspoon sea salt
3/4 teaspoon freshly ground black pepper
1/4 cup chopped green onion
1 tablespoon chopped fresh chervil, parsley, dill, or cilantro
1/2 cup chopped seedless grapes
1/2 cup potato (about 1 small), diced, blanched, and peeled

Preparation
Preheat the oven to 350°F (175°C).

Place the salmon into a food processor and pulse until roughly chopped, about 3 times. Add the egg white, salt, and pepper. Process until smooth. Transfer mixture to a bowl. Fold in the green onion, herbs, grapes, and potato.

Heat a griddle over medium heat and coat with cooking spray. Using a 1/4-cup measure, form 6 patties and place on the hot griddle. Brown the patties on both sides.

Place the patties on an ungreased baking sheet and bake until cooked through, about 5 minutes.

Chicken Patties

This is a great basic recipe to build upon—try topping these patties with cooked tomatoes and spinach, or add chiles to create a southwestern breakfast sausage. Photo on page 79.

Per chicken patty:
Calories 100; Protein 16g; Total Fat 1.5g; Saturated Fat 0g; Carbohydrates 5g; Dietary Fiber 0g; Cholesterol 40mg; Sodium 280mg

Ingredients
Makes 5 chicken patties.

1/2 pound boneless, skinless chicken breasts
1 large egg white
1/2 teaspoon sea salt
1/4 teaspoon freshly ground black pepper
2 tablespoons finely chopped red bell pepper
1/4 cup minced red onion
1 tablespoon chopped fresh herbs, such as thyme, oregano, basil, and parsley
2 tablespoons fat-free milk
1/2 cup potato (about 1 small), diced, partially cooked, and peeled

Preparation
Preheat the oven to 350°F (175°C).

Place the chicken into a food processor and pulse until roughly chopped, about 3 times. Add the egg white, salt, and pepper. Process until smooth. Transfer to a bowl. Fold in the bell pepper, onion, herbs, milk, and potato.

Heat a griddle over medium heat and coat with cooking spray. Using a 1/4-cup measure, form 5 patties and place on the hot griddle. Brown the patties on both sides.

Place the patties on an ungreased baking sheet and bake until cooked through, about 5 minutes.

Miraval Omelet

Per omelet:
Calories 110; Protein 13g; Total Fat 2.5g;
Saturated Fat 1g; Carbohydrates 10g; Dietary
Fiber 2g; Cholesterol 5mg; Sodium 520mg

This omelet illustrates how versatile and flavorful egg whites are—the possibilities for seasoning and filling combinations are endless. And by eliminating the egg yolks, we decrease the fat and cholesterol by half. Serve with fresh fruit. The photo at the right includes Chicken Patties (see page 77).

Ingredients
Makes 1 omelet.

1/4 teaspoon extra-virgin olive oil
1/4 cup diced fresh shiitake mushrooms
1 tablespoon finely chopped green onion
1/4 cup diced fresh tomato
1/4 cup packed fresh spinach
3 large egg whites, lightly whipped
1/8 teaspoon sea salt
1/8 teaspoon freshly ground black pepper
1 tablespoon low-fat cream cheese

Preparation
Preheat the broiler.

Heat a sauté pan with a flameproof handle over medium heat and add the olive oil. Add the vegetables and sauté until they begin to soften, about 5 minutes. Pour the egg whites over the vegetables and season with salt and pepper. Cook until the bottom is done and the sides are firm, about 4 minutes. Spread the cream cheese on top of the omelet.

Place the pan under the broiler for about 2 minutes to finish cooking the top of the omelet. Remove from heat. Fold over half the omelet and serve.

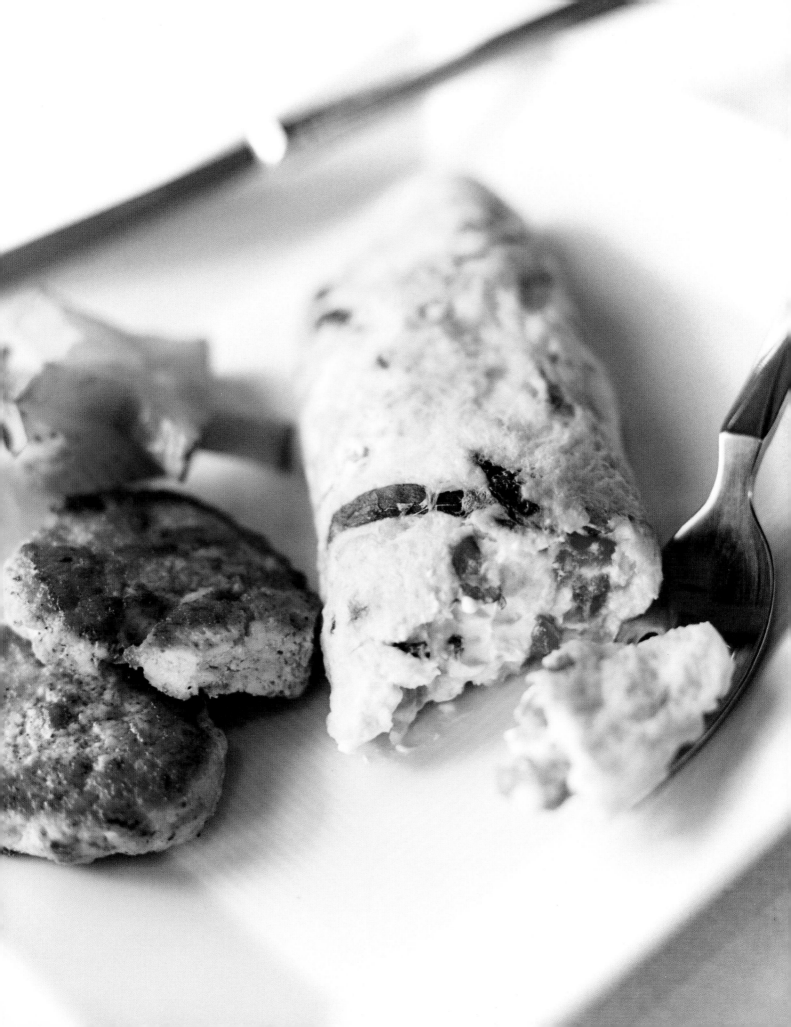

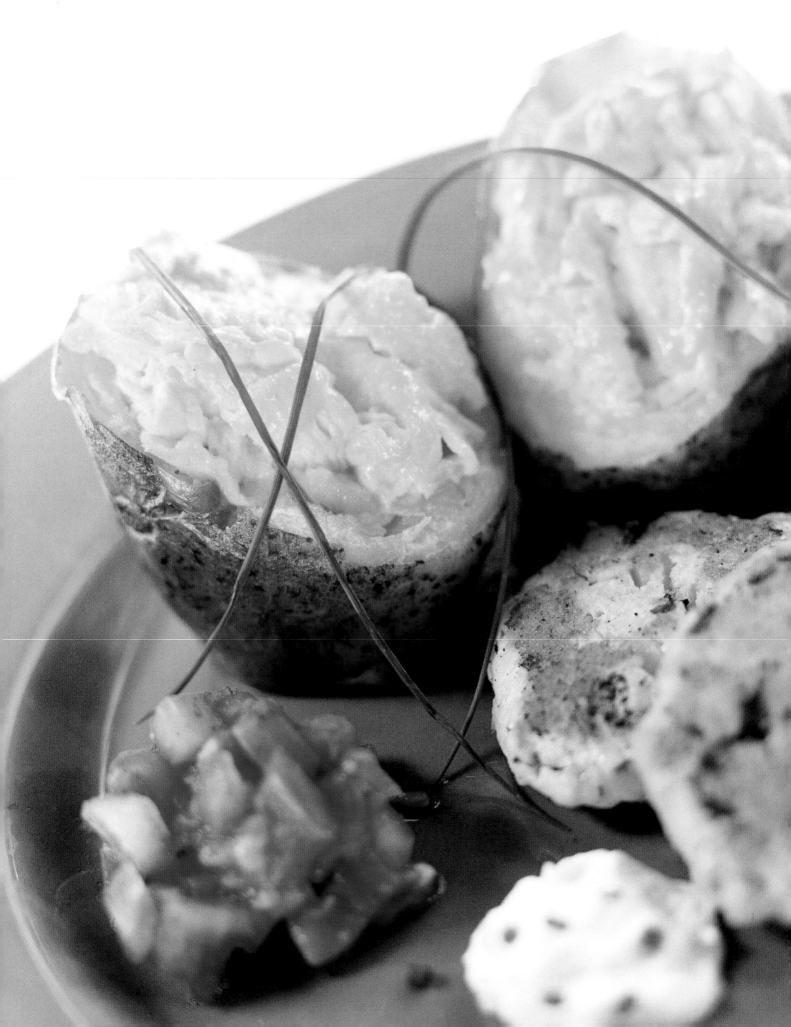

Breakfast Scramble

Per serving:
Calories 300; Protein 14g; Total Fat 4g;
Saturated Fat 1g; Carbohydrates 54g; Dietary
Fiber 5g; Cholesterol 105mg; Sodium 310mg

Bake extra potatoes and refrigerate them to use in this special breakfast recipe. It's full of flavor and low in fat. The photo at the left includes Salmon Patties (see page 77).

Ingredients
Makes 2 servings.

2 medium russet potatoes, baked
1/2 teaspoon extra-virgin olive oil
1 large egg
3 large egg whites
1/8 teaspoon sea salt
1/8 teaspoon freshly ground black pepper

Garnish
1 tablespoon salsa
1 tablespoon fat-free sour cream
1/2 teaspoon chopped fresh chives

Preparation

Make four potato cups by first cutting off both ends (about 1 inch) of the potatoes—this will form a flat base. Reserve the ends. Make a diagonal cut to halve potatoes crosswise. Set the potatoes up on the flat ends and carefully scoop out from the angled ends to form cups, leaving a wall of about 1/2 inch. Scoop out the 4 ends to make little cups for sour cream and salsa.

Heat a sauté pan over medium-high heat and add the olive oil. In a mixing bowl, whip together the egg, egg whites, salt, and pepper. Pour into the sauté pan and cook, stirring until set, about 5 minutes. Remove from heat and stuff into the potato cups.

Serve two potato cups per plate with the salsa and sour cream spooned into the reserved potato ends. Garnish with the chives.

Tofu Scramble

Hey, it took a while for me to try tofu—it wasn't until my assistant, Heidi DeCosmo, spooned this onto my breakfast plate and I thought it was scrambled eggs. I was excited to learn that tofu can really taste great! The photo shows Tofu Scramble in a Menlo cup.

Per serving:
Calories 90; Protein 2.5g; Total Fat 2.5g; Saturated Fat 0g; Carbohydrates 4g; Dietary Fiber: less than 1 gram; Cholesterol 0mg; Sodium 270mg

Ingredients

Makes 3 servings.

1/2 teaspoon extra-virgin olive oil
1/4 cup finely chopped red onion
1 tablespoon finely chopped red bell
  pepper
1 tablespoon finely chopped fresh shiitake
  mushrooms
1 1/2 cups crumbled firm tofu (18 ounces,
  drained)
1/2 teaspoon tahini (sesame seed paste)
1 teaspoon tamari (soy) sauce
1/2 teaspoon curry powder
Fresh fruit

Preparation

Heat a sauté pan over medium-high heat and add the olive oil. Add the onion, bell pepper, and mushroom. Sauté until the onion begins to soften, about 2 minutes. Add the tofu, tahini, tamari, and curry powder. Cook, stirring constantly, until the tofu has begun to dry out and is the consistency of scrambled eggs.

Serve with fresh fruit.

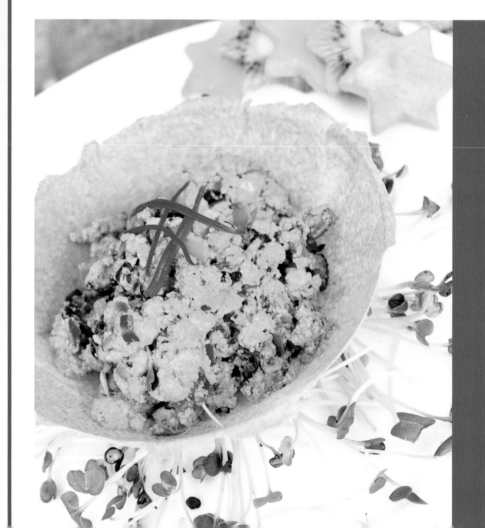

Vegetable Quiche with Rice Crust

Per wedge:
Calories 120; Protein 7g; Total Fat 3g;
Saturated Fat 1g; Carbohydrates 16g; Dietary
Fiber 1g; Cholesterol 55mg; Sodium 230mg

Chef Heidi DeCosmo created this delightful quiche. It's wonderful on a brunch buffet or as a colorful breakfast or luncheon entrée.

Ingredients
Makes 8 servings.

Crust
2 cups cooked brown rice
2 large egg whites
1 tablespoon finely chopped fresh parsley
1 teaspoon finely chopped fresh oregano
1/4 teaspoon sea salt
1/8 teaspoon freshly ground black pepper

Filling
1/2 teaspoon extra-virgin olive oil
1/2 cup finely diced red bell pepper
1/2 cup finely diced mushroom
1/4 cup finely chopped red onion
1 cup chopped, packed fresh spinach
2 large egg whites
2 large eggs
3/4 cup fat-free milk
1/8 teaspoon sea salt
1/8 teaspoon freshly ground black pepper
Pinch of nutmeg
1/4 cup freshly grated Parmesan cheese

Preparation
Preheat the oven to 350°F (175°C).

For the Crust: In a mixing bowl, combine the rice, egg whites, parsley, oregano, salt, and pepper. Coat an 8-inch pie pan with cooking spray. Press the rice mixture over the bottom and up the sides of the pie pan to form a crust. Bake for 15 minutes or until the crust is set and lightly browned.

For the Filling: Heat a sauté pan over medium heat and add the olive oil to lightly coat the bottom of the pan. Add the bell pepper, mushroom, onion, and spinach; sauté until the onion softens, about 5 minutes. Remove from heat and set aside.

In a mixing bowl, whip the egg whites, eggs, and milk until frothy. Add the salt, pepper, nutmeg, and cheese.

To assemble: Place the pie pan with prepared crust on a baking sheet. Spread the vegetables over the bottom of the crust and pour the egg mixture over them.

Bake for 55 minutes or until the eggs have set. Cut into 8 wedges to serve.

Vegetable Quiche Cups

Per serving:
Calories 90; Protein 6g; Total Fat 3g; Saturated Fat 0.5g; Carbohydrates 11g; Dietary Fiber 1g; Cholesterol 70mg; Sodium 150mg

I love this adaptation of the classic quiche. Serve the individual quiches with fresh fruit or a fruit salsa. And yes—real men do eat quiche!

Ingredients
Makes 6 servings.

1/2 teaspoon extra-virgin olive oil
1/2 cup diced fresh shiitake mushrooms
1/4 cup diced red onion
1/4 cup diced red bell pepper
1/2 cup diced zucchini (about 1 small)
1/2 cup diced cauliflower
1/2 cup diced broccoli
1/2 cup diced carrots
1 tablespoon plus 2 teaspoons chopped, mixed fresh herbs
3 sheets phyllo dough
2 large eggs
2 large egg whites
1/2 cup fat-free milk
1/8 teaspoon sea salt
1/8 teaspoon freshly ground black pepper
Pinch of ground nutmeg

Preparation
Preheat oven to 400°F (205°C).

Heat a sauté pan over medium-high heat and add the olive oil to lightly coat the bottom of the pan. Add the vegetables and sauté until soft, about 5 minutes. Mix in 1 tablespoon herbs. Set aside.

On a clean cutting board, lay out one sheet of phyllo dough and lightly coat with cooking spray. Cover with another sheet of phyllo and spray again. Sprinkle with the remaining 2 teaspoons of herbs. Cover with the remaining sheet of phyllo and spray well with cooking spray. Cut the stacked phyllo rectangle crosswise into 6 strips, approximately 2 3/4 inches wide, then cut lengthwise in half. You should have 12 strips approximately 2 3/4 inches wide by 6 inches long.

Coat a 12-cup muffin pan with cooking spray. You will make the quiche in alternating cups, leaving an empty cup between quiches. (The first row will have 2 quiches, the second will have 1 quiche, and so on.) Place a phyllo strip in the bottom of a cup and place another over it at right angles to form a cup. Let the ends hang over or scrunch to make a rim. Repeat to make 6 cups.

In a mixing bowl, beat the eggs, egg whites, milk, and seasonings until combined.

Add 1/4 cup of the vegetable mixture to each muffin cup. Pour 1/3 cup of the egg mixture into each cup. Bake for 25 to 30 minutes or until the eggs have set and are golden on top. Cool in the pan about 5 minutes. Carefully run a knife around the edge of the cups and remove quiches.

Dried Cherry Crumb Cake

Per serving:
Calories 100; Protein 3g; Total Fat 1.5g;
Saturated Fat 0g; Carbohydrates 18g; Dietary
Fiber: less than 1 gram; Cholesterol 0mg;
Sodium 85mg

Your guests will never believe that this coffeecake is low in fat and good for you. They will assume that it's just another fantastic breakfast treat created in your wonderful kitchen.

Ingredients
Makes 16 servings.

Crumb Topping
3 tablespoons unbleached all-purpose flour
3 tablespoons raw cane sugar (Turbinado)
1 1/2 teaspoons butter

Cake
1 1/2 cups unbleached all-purpose flour
2/3 cup raw cane sugar (Turbinado)
1 1/2 teaspoons baking powder
1/4 teaspoon baking soda
1/8 teaspoon sea salt
1/8 teaspoon ground nutmeg
1/2 cup dried, pitted, tart cherries
1 cup fat-free buttermilk
1 teaspoon freshly grated orange zest
1 tablespoon canola oil
*2 tablespoons prune puree or unsweetened
    applesauce*
1 teaspoon pure vanilla extract
2 large egg whites

Preparation

Preheat the oven to 350°F (175°C). Lightly coat a 9-inch cake pan with cooking spray and dust with flour; set aside.

For the Crumb Topping: In a small bowl, combine the flour and sugar. Using a pastry blender or 2 knives, cut in the butter until the mixture resembles coarse meal. Set the crumb mixture aside.

To make the Cake: In a medium mixing bowl, combine the flour, sugar, baking powder, baking soda, salt, nutmeg, and cherries; stir well and set aside.

In a large bowl, combine the buttermilk, orange zest, oil, prune puree, vanilla, and egg whites; whisk until egg whites are well beaten. Gradually add the flour mixture, stirring just until the dry ingredients are moistened.

To assemble: Pour the batter into the prepared cake pan and sprinkle the crumb mixture over the batter.

Bake for 40 to 50 minutes or until a wooden pick inserted in the center comes out clean. Cool in the pan on a wire rack.

Cut into 16 wedges. Serve warm or at room temperature.

Low-Fat Muffin Mix

Per muffin:
Calories 120; Protein 4g; Total Fat 1g;
Saturated Fat 0g; Carbohydrates 23g; Dietary
Fiber 1g; Cholesterol 0mg; Sodium 90mg

This versatile muffin mix can be the foundation for endless variations of muffins. We have included several favorites here, but experiment and create your own original breakfast treats. Please note the quality of the ingredients called for here. The use of unbleached all-purpose flour, whole-wheat pastry flour, and raw cane sugar (also called Turbinado sugar) ensures that we are using the least processed ingredients available, which retain more of their natural goodness. The banana adds flavor, body, and moisture, which reduces the amount of oil needed. These muffins are low in fat, but high in flavor.

Ingredients
Makes 12 muffins.

1 cup whole-wheat pastry flour
1 cup unbleached all-purpose flour
1/2 teaspoon baking soda
Pinch sea salt
1/4 teaspoon ground cinnamon
1/8 teaspoon ground nutmeg
2 large egg whites
2/3 cup fat-free milk
2/3 cup plain, fat-free yogurt
1 1/4 cups raw cane sugar (Turbinado)
1 tablespoon pureed banana
2 teaspoons canola oil
1/4 teaspoon pure vanilla extract

Preparation
Preheat oven to 350°F (175°C). Coat 12 muffin cups with cooking spray.

In a mixing bowl, combine the flours, baking soda, salt, cinnamon, and nutmeg. In a separate bowl, mix together the egg whites, milk, yogurt, sugar, banana puree, oil, and vanilla. Make a well in the center of the dry ingredients; pour in the egg mixture and stir until just moistened. If making a variation, stir the fruit into the batter until just combined.

Scoop 1/3 cup of batter into each prepared muffin cup. If making a variation, sprinkle with the desired topping.

Bake for 30 to 35 minutes or until a wooden pick inserted in centers comes out clean.

Remove muffins from the oven and let cool in the pan on a wire rack for about 5 minutes. Remove from muffin pan and cool completely.

Variations
Banana-Nut Muffins
2 ripe bananas, mashed
1 tablespoon finely chopped walnuts for the topping

Per muffin:
Calories 130; Protein 4g; Total Fat 1.5g; Saturated Fat 0g; Carbohydrates 26g; Dietary Fiber 2g; Cholesterol 0mg; Sodium 90mg

Blueberry Muffins
1 cup fresh or frozen blueberries (1 pint)
1 tablespoon finely chopped pecans for the topping

Per muffin:
Calories 130; Protein 4g; Total Fat 2g; Saturated Fat 0g; Carbohydrates 25g; Dietary Fiber 2g; Cholesterol 0mg; Sodium 90mg

Lemon Raspberry Muffins

Grated zest and juice of 1 lemon (about 1 tablespoon zest and 1/3 cup juice)

1 cup fresh or frozen raspberries (1 pint)

1 tablespoon finely chopped almonds for the topping

Per muffin:
Calories 120; Protein 4g; Total Fat 1g; Saturated Fat 0g; Carbohydrates 24g; Dietary Fiber 2g; Cholesterol 0mg; Sodium 90mg

Orange Cranberry Muffins

Grated zest and juice of 1 orange (about 1 tablespoon orange zest and 1/2 cup juice)

1 cup fresh, frozen, or dried cranberries

1 tablespoon finely chopped almonds for the topping

Per muffin:
Calories 130; Protein 4g; Total Fat 1.5g; Saturated Fat 0g; Carbohydrates 25g; Dietary Fiber 2g; Cholesterol 0mg; Sodium 90mg

Apple Spice Muffins

For spices, use:

1 teaspoon ground cinnamon

1/4 teaspoon ground allspice

1/4 teaspoon ground nutmeg

1/4 teaspoon ground ginger

1 cup chopped, peeled apples (1 large)

1 tablespoon finely chopped walnuts for the topping

Per muffin:
Calories 130; Protein 4g; Total Fat 2g; Saturated Fat 0g; Carbohydrates 25g; Dietary Fiber 2g; Cholesterol 0mg; Sodium 90mg

Cranberry-Orange Scones

Light and tasty, these scones are lower in fat than traditional ones. Add a little orange marmalade, and you have a scrumptious, quick breakfast.

Ingredients

Makes 12 scones.

1 cup unbleached all-purpose flour
1 cup whole-wheat pastry flour
2/3 cup plus 2 teaspoons raw cane sugar
   (Turbinado)
2 teaspoons baking powder
1/2 teaspoon baking soda
1/4 teaspoon sea salt
3 tablespoons butter, chilled, cut into small
   pieces
1/2 cup chopped dried cranberries
2 teaspoons freshly grated orange zest
1 cup plain, fat-free yogurt
1/4 cup fat-free milk

Preparation

Preheat the oven to 400°F (205°C). Coat a baking sheet with cooking spray.

In a mixing bowl, combine the flours, 2/3 cup sugar, baking powder, baking soda, and salt. Using a pastry blender or 2 knives, cut in the butter until mixture resembles coarse meal. Add the cranberries and orange zest; toss well to distribute.

In a separate bowl, mix together the yogurt and milk. Add the yogurt mixture to the flour mixture, stirring until the dry ingredients are just moistened (dough will be sticky).

Turn the dough out onto a lightly floured surface, and with floured hands, knead 4 or 5 times.

Pat the dough into an 8-inch circle on prepared baking sheet. Cut the dough into 12 wedges (do not separate the wedges). Sprinkle the 2 teaspoons sugar over the dough. Bake for 12 minutes or until golden.

Almond–Poppy Seed Bread

Almond extract adds a lot of flavor to this bread without adding the fat of almonds. The bread has a beautiful, light texture and is a real crowd-pleaser.

Ingredients

Makes 1 loaf of 14 slices.

1 cup whole-wheat pastry flour
1/2 cup unbleached all-purpose flour
1 cup raw cane sugar (Turbinado)
1 1/2 teaspoon baking powder
1/4 teaspoon sea salt
3/4 cup fat-free milk
1/3 cup prune puree or unsweetened
   applesauce
3 large egg whites
1 tablespoon canola oil
1/2 teaspoon pure vanilla extract
1 tablespoon pure almond extract
1 tablespoon poppy seeds
1 3/4 teaspoons freshly grated lemon zest
2 tablespoons sliced almonds

Preparation

Preheat oven to 350°F (175°C). Lightly coat a 9 x 5-inch loaf pan with cooking spray and dust with flour; set aside.

Sift the flours, sugar, baking powder, and salt into a medium mixing bowl. In a separate bowl, mix together the milk, prune puree, egg whites, oil, and extracts. Make a well in the center of the dry ingredients; slowly add the milk mixture and stir with a wooden spoon until just moistened. Stir in the poppy seeds and lemon zest.

Pour the batter into the prepared loaf pan. Sprinkle the almonds on top of the batter. Bake for 30 to 40 minutes or until a wooden pick inserted in the center comes out clean. Cool in the pan on a wire rack for 10 minutes; remove from pan and cool completely. Cut into 14 slices to serve.

Banana-Nut Bread

Per slice:
Calories 120; Protein 3g; Total Fat 1.5g;
Saturated Fat 0g; Carbohydrates 24g; Dietary
Fiber 1g; Cholesterol 0mg; Sodium 115mg

This is one of the most requested recipes at Miraval. It's so flavorful and versatile that it can be served at any meal, providing a wonderful bread alternative that's nutritious and delicious.

Ingredients

Makes 1 loaf of 14 slices.

1 cup unbleached all-purpose flour
1 cup whole-wheat pastry flour
1 teaspoon baking powder
1/2 teaspoon baking soda
1/4 teaspoon sea salt
1 cup mashed, very ripe banana (about 3 small)
1 cup raw cane sugar (Turbinado)
1/4 cup plain, fat-free yogurt
1/4 cup prune puree or unsweetened applesauce
2 large egg whites
1 teaspoon pure vanilla extract
1/4 cup chopped pecans, toasted

Preparation

Preheat oven to 350°F (175°C). Lightly coat a 9 x 5-inch loaf pan with cooking spray and dust with flour; set aside.

In a medium mixing bowl, combine the flours, baking powder, baking soda, and salt.

In another mixing bowl, combine the banana, sugar, yogurt, prune puree, egg whites, and vanilla. Whisk until blended, about 2 minutes. Add the dry ingredients to the banana mixture, stirring with a wooden spoon until just moistened. Spoon the batter into the prepared loaf pan. Sprinkle the pecans on top of the batter.

Bake for 1 hour or until a wooden pick inserted in the center comes out clean. Cool in the pan on a wire rack for 10 minutes; remove from pan and cool completely. Cut in 14 slices to serve.

Zucchini Bread

Wow! This bread is good. Compare its flavor to a traditional zucchini bread recipe, and you'll discover that using high-quality ingredients not only reduces fat and calories, it also produces a superior product. For example, I found that using pureed prunes added so much texture, flavor, and sweetness to this bread that I could reduce the sugar content and eliminate the oil. Now, that's a good thing!

Ingredients

Makes 1 loaf of 14 slices.

1 1/4 cups unbleached all-purpose flour
3/4 cup whole-wheat pastry flour
2 1/4 teaspoons baking soda
1/4 teaspoon sea salt
3/4 teaspoon ground nutmeg
1 1/2 teaspoons ground cinnamon
3 large egg whites
3/4 cup raw cane sugar (Turbinado)
3/4 cup prune puree or unsweetened
　applesauce
1 cup grated zucchini

Preparation

Preheat the oven to 350°F (175°C). Lightly coat a 9 x 5-inch loaf pan with cooking spray and dust with flour; set aside.

In a medium mixing bowl, combine the flours, baking soda, salt, nutmeg, and cinnamon.

In a separate mixing bowl, combine the egg whites, sugar, and prune puree. Add the dry ingredients to the egg white mixture, stirring until well combined, but do not overmix. Fold in the zucchini. Pour the batter into the prepared loaf pan.

Bake for 45 minutes to 1 hour or until a wooden pick inserted in the center comes out clean. Cool in the pan on a wire rack for 10 minutes; remove from pan and cool completely. Cut into 14 slices to serve.

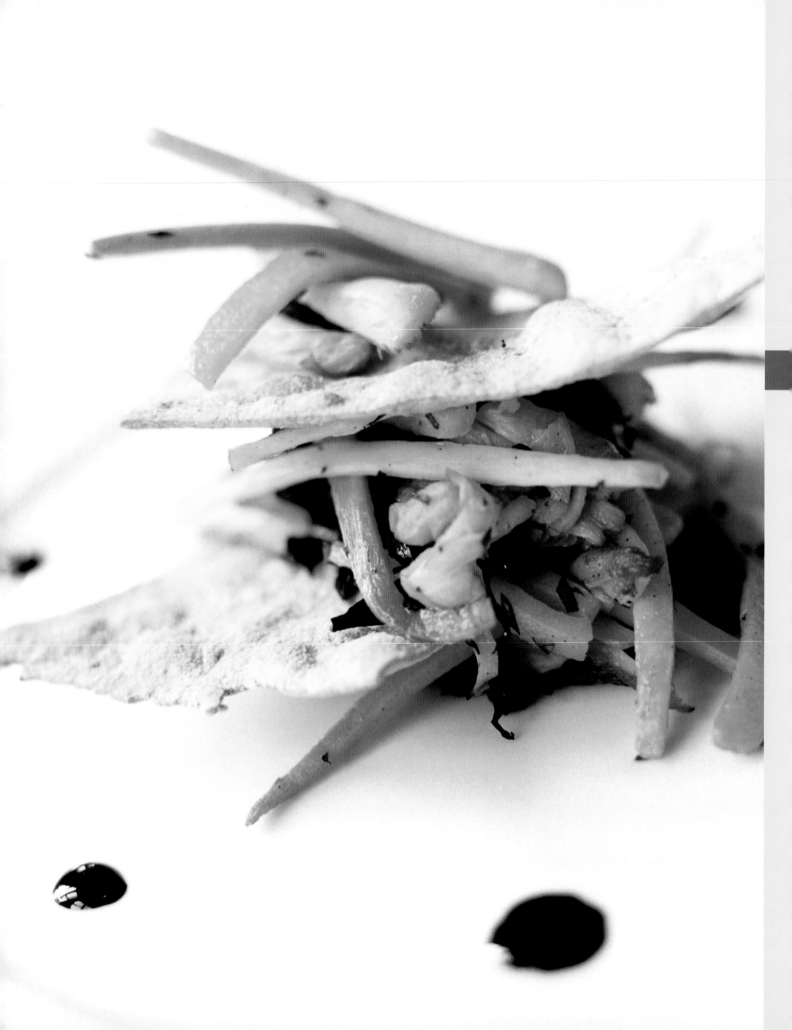

Appealing Appetizers

Pictured at left: Chickpea Napoleons with Pan-Roasted Vegetables

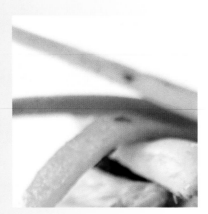

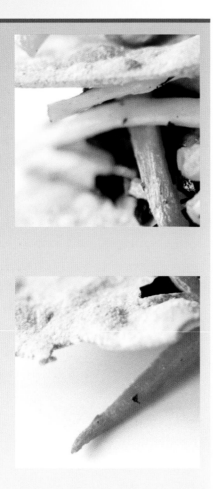

Creating amazing appetizers to serve as starters, hors d'oeuvres, or as a series of small dishes begins with quality ingredients and a conscious approach to cookery. Popular dishes prepared in restaurants are often inundated with excessive fat and calories for two reasons—first, the mammoth portions are designed to make the consumer feel that the restaurant is providing good value for their money, and second, cooking methods such as deep-fat frying increase the fat content to foods. *Conscious Cuisine* illustrates how alternative cooking methods can create satisfying meals without adding excess fats.

As a professional chef and culinary student, I was taught to use high-fat and high-calorie ingredients such as heavy cream, butter, and puff pastry to prepare great-tasting dishes. How are we to achieve the same gastronomic satisfaction without using these ingredients?

In *Conscious Cuisine,* simple and nutritious foods such as garbanzo beans are used to make a delicious Middle Eastern hummus, or dry beans milled into flour to make spectacular crêpes or homemade lavosh crackers. Ultra-thin, light, flaky phyllo pastry is used to make luscious vegetable bundles, Napoleons, and strudels. Reduced-fat cream cheese is used in place of cream sauce to bind the spinach in Baked Oysters Florentine—our version of Oysters Rockefeller. Fresh seasonal vegetables are oven roasted instead of fried to release their natural flavors and sweetness. High-quality, aged cheeses are used sparingly to provide a sensual taste without being heavy and overly rich.

Conscious Cuisine gives you license to prepare appealing appetizers that beg you to notice their artful appearance, interesting textures, and bold flavors. Creative recipes such as Fresh Vegetable Silo, Ahi Tuna Sashimi, and Middle Eastern Crêpes Filled with Roasted Eggplant, Apricots, and Scallops give you appealing appetizers as a flavorful alternative to start a meal.

Chickpea Lavosh

Per 3 crackers:
Calories 100; Protein 4g; Total Fat 1g;
Saturated Fat 0g; Carbohydrates 19g; Dietary
Fiber less than 1 gram; Cholesterol 0mg;
Sodium 130mg

I have used this versatile lavosh cracker recipe in various forms and flavors for about fifteen years. Replacing the ordinary flour with great-tasting equivalents like freshly milled garbanzo beans, mesquite flour, teff flour, or oat flour allows me to develop a host of new dishes and garnishes. This recipe also lends itself to the addition of flavorful herbs and vegetables to produce a wonderful basil, carrot, or tomato cracker with many other possible variations.

Ingredients

Makes 10 servings.

1/2 cup chopped yellow onion (about 1 medium)

1 tablespoon chopped Roasted Garlic (see page 38)

1 1/2 teaspoons seasoned rice wine vinegar

2 tablespoons water

1 plus 1/4 cup chickpea (garbanzo bean) flour

1/2 cup unbleached all-purpose flour

1/2 cup semolina flour

1/2 teaspoon ground cumin

1/2 teaspoon ground coriander

1/2 teaspoon sea salt

1/4 teaspoon white pepper

Preparation

Preheat the oven to 375°F (190°C).

Place the onion, garlic, vinegar, and water into a food processor. Puree until all liquid has been released from the onion and the mixture is smooth, about 3 minutes. (The liquid from the onion is what binds this dough together.) Add 1 cup of the chickpea flour and all remaining ingredients. Process until a dough is formed. Remove the dough from the bowl and knead with remaining 1/4 cup of the chickpea flour until the dough is smooth and firm.

Cut the dough into quarters and roll out each piece on a lightly floured surface. Roll dough out until very thin, and then cut into 3-inch triangles. You should be able to cut about 6 triangles out of each quarter piece of dough. Place the triangles on a baking sheet lined with parchment paper. Prick the triangles with a fork and brush lightly with water. Bake for 5 to 7 minutes or until golden brown.

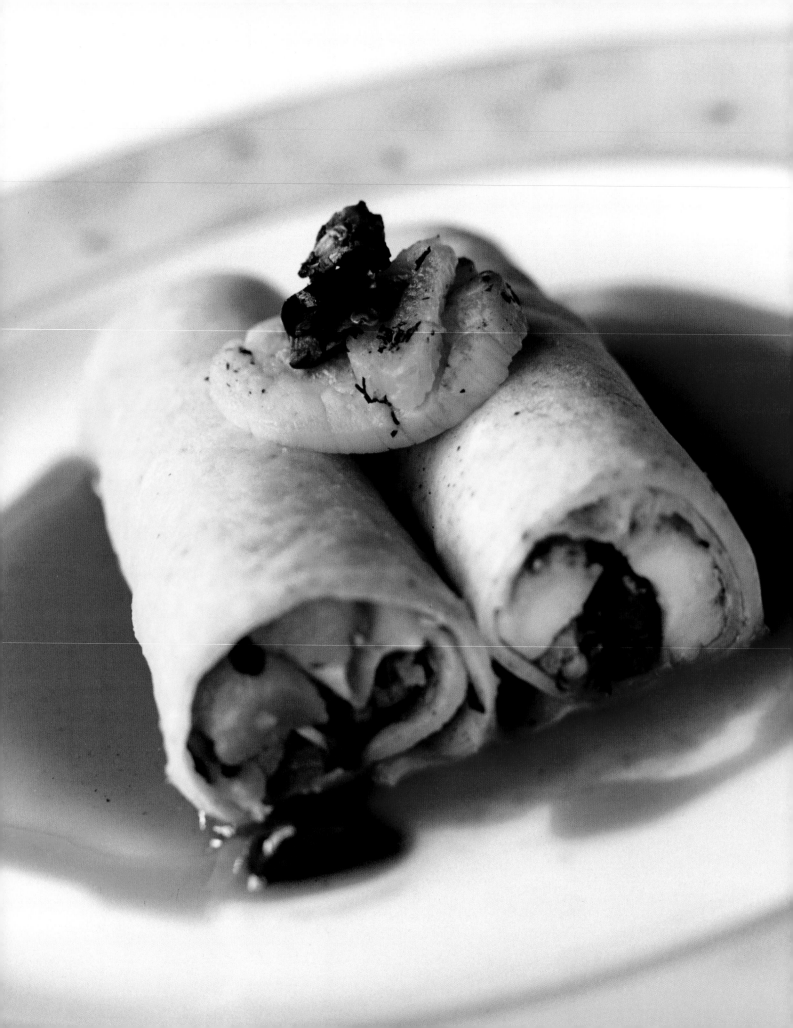

Middle Eastern Crêpes Filled with Roasted Eggplant, Apricots, and Scallops

Per filled crêpe:
Calories 180; Protein 15g; Total Fat 2.5g;
Saturated Fat 0g; Carbohydrates 22g; Dietary
Fiber 2g; Cholesterol 45mg; Sodium 510mg

Crêpe batters have a much thinner consistency than pancake batters, creating a thin, low-calorie delicacy that can be served hot, cold, sweet, or savory. Allow the crêpe batter to stand for at least 30 minutes prior to using to develop the elasticity of the flour. Stir the batter well before pouring into the pan, using only enough batter to lightly coat the pan.

Ingredients
Makes 12 crêpes.

Crêpes
1/2 cup whole-wheat pastry flour
1 cup cornmeal, plus additional for dusting
1 teaspoon raw cane sugar (Turbinado)
1/4 teaspoon baking powder
1/2 teaspoon sea salt
1 teaspoon ground cumin
1/4 teaspoon cayenne pepper
1/4 teaspoon paprika
1 large egg
4 large egg whites
1 cup beer
1 cup fat-free milk
1 teaspoon extra-virgin olive oil

Filling
1 medium eggplant, peeled and chopped
2 teaspoons Fresh Herb Mix (see page 39)
1/2 cup chopped dried apricots
1/4 cup chopped Kalamata olives
1/4 teaspoon sea salt
1/4 teaspoon freshly ground black pepper
1/2 teaspoon extra-virgin olive oil
16 ounces scallops, about 2 cups
1/4 cup sherry

Garnish
Red Pepper Puree (see page 36), optional
Basil Oil (see page 115), optional

Preparation

For the Crêpes: In a medium mixing bowl, stir together the flour, cornmeal, sugar, baking powder, salt, cumin, cayenne, and paprika. Make a well in the center of the dry ingredients. Add the egg, egg whites, beer, milk, and oil to center of the well. Stir to make a thin batter. Strain the batter to remove any lumps. Allow the batter to rest for 30 minutes.

Heat a nonstick crêpe pan (or 10-inch sauté pan) over medium heat and lightly coat with cooking spray. Add about 1/8 cup of the batter, or just enough to coat the bottom of the pan, and cook for about 1 minute. Flip over, and cook other side until dry to the touch, about 1 more minute. Remove the crêpe from the pan. Repeat with remaining batter, coating with cooking spray as needed.

Lightly dust each crêpe with cornmeal to prevent them from sticking together. Stack on a baking sheet until all the batter is used.

For the Filling: Preheat the oven to 425°F (220°C). Place the eggplant on a baking sheet and coat with cooking spray. Bake for 5 to 10 minutes or until the eggplant has just softened. Place in a mixing bowl and stir in the herbs, apricots, olives, salt, and pepper.

Heat a medium sauté pan over medium-high heat and add the olive oil to lightly coat the bottom of the pan. Add the scallops and cook until lightly browned, about 3 minutes. Turn the scallops over and cook another 3 minutes. Add the sherry and stir to remove any browned bits from the bottom of the pan. Cook another minute to reduce the sherry until the pan is almost dry, about 3 to 5 minutes. Remove the scallops from the pan and carefully cut in 3 equal rounds. Mix the scallops with the eggplant mixture.

To assemble: Place one crêpe on a clean cutting board and spoon on 1/2 cup of filling. Fold the end over the filling and roll up to form a log. Repeat with remaining crêpes and filling. Place the assembled crêpes on a baking sheet and keep warm in a 200°F (95°C) oven.

Cut each crêpe in half. To serve, place one crêpe (2 pieces) on each serving plate and drizzle with Red Pepper Puree and Basil Oil.

Chickpea Napoleons with Pan-Roasted Vegetables

Layering Chickpea Lavosh crackers with the hearty flavors of roasted fall vegetables creates a lovely Napoleon. Use any extra crackers as a tasty alternative to bread or to zip up salads and soups. Photo on page 92.

Ingredients
Makes 10 servings.

20 Chickpea Lavosh crackers (see
    page 95)

Pan-Roasted Vegetables
1/2 teaspoon extra-virgin olive oil
*2 cups julienned parsnips (about 4
    medium)*
1 cup julienned butternut squash (1 small)
1 cup julienned carrots (2 medium)
*1 cup julienned oyster mushrooms (about
    3 1/2 ounces)*
*2 cups lightly packed Swiss chard, cleaned
    and roughly chopped*
*2 tablespoons Fresh Herb Mix (see
    page 39)*
1/4 teaspoon sea salt
1/4 freshly ground black pepper

Balsamic Reduction (see page 19)

Preparation

For the Pan-Roasted Vegetables: Heat a large sauté pan over medium-high heat and add the olive oil to lightly coat the bottom of the pan. Add the parsnips, squash, carrots, and mushrooms. Cook until they have softened, about 2 minutes. Stir in the Swiss chard and sauté until wilted, about 1 minute. Season with the mixed herbs, salt, and pepper.

To assemble: Place 2 tablespoons of the vegetable mixture in the center of a plate. Place one lavosh cracker on top of vegetables. Place 2 tablespoons of the vegetables on top of the lavosh. Top with another piece of the lavosh, rotating it slightly clockwise. Drizzle Balsamic Reduction over the Napoleon in thin lines.

Roasted Vegetable Strudel

Per serving:
Calories 130; Protein 5g; Total Fat 3g;
Saturated Fat 0.5g; Carbohydrates 22g; Dietary
Fiber 3g; Cholesterol 0mg; Sodium 250mg

Roasting is a quick and easy way to cook vegetables and release their natural sweetness and flavors. Spinach can be substituted for the arugula, but arugula has a unique peppery flavor. Add the sweet teardrop or cherry tomatoes right before folding up the phyllo dough. The quick cooking time for the strudel will allow the tomatoes to warm throughout, then burst with flavor.

Ingredients
Makes 6 servings.

Filling
1 bunch of medium asparagus (about 24
*   stems), stem ends removed, cut in half*
*   lengthwise and crosswise*
1 medium carrot, peeled, cut into 1/2 x
*   2-inch sticks*
1 medium zucchini, cut into 1/2 x 2-inch
*   sticks*
1 medium portobello mushroom, gills
*   removed, julienned*
1/2 teaspoon extra-virgin olive oil
1/4 teaspoon sea salt
1/8 teaspoon freshly ground black pepper
1 tablespoon Fresh Herb Mix (see
*   page 39)*

Phyllo
9 phyllo dough sheets
Olive oil spray
3 tablespoons Fresh Herb Mix

1 cup teardrop or cherry tomatoes
3/4 cup lightly packed arugula, washed
*   and dried*
Yellow Tomato Sauce (see page 22)

Garnish
Finely chopped vegetables, optional
Parsley, optional

Preparation

For the Filling: Preheat the oven to 450°F (230°C).

Place the asparagus, carrot, zucchini, and portobello mushroom on a baking sheet and toss with the olive oil. Season with the salt, pepper, and herbs. Roast the vegetables for 10 minutes or until they look lightly browned and moist. Remove the vegetables from the oven and transfer to a clean dish.

Reduce the oven temperature to 425°F (220°C).

For the Phyllo: Gently lay one sheet of phyllo dough on a clean cutting board. Lightly mist with olive oil spray. Sprinkle with 1 teaspoon of the mixed herbs. Repeat with phyllo and herbs to make 2 more layers (3 total). Keep remaining phyllo sheets covered with a damp towel.

Cut the rectangle in half lengthwise. On each half, place 1/2 cup of the roasted vegetables. Arrange 3 tomatoes and 2 tablespoons of arugula on top. Fold in the sides and bottom of the dough over the vegetables.

Begin to gently roll up the strudel. You will be making a long tube, like a burrito. Repeat with remaining phyllo and vegetables to make a total of 6 strudel rolls.

Place the strudels on a baking sheet lined with parchment paper. Lightly mist the top and sides of each strudel with olive oil spray. Bake the strudels for 10 to 12 minutes, or until golden brown.

To serve: Trim the ends off each strudel so you can see the colors inside. Ladle 1/4 cup of Yellow Tomato Sauce on each plate. Arrange strudel on top of the sauce. Garnish with vegetables and parsley, if using.

Wild Mushroom Phyllo Stack

Per serving:
Calories 80; Protein 3g; Total Fat 2g; Saturated Fat 0g; Carbohydrates 11g; Dietary Fiber 1g; Cholesterol 0mg; Sodium 180mg

If you are not a fan of blue cheese, perhaps you have only eaten the pre-crumbled domestic kind. Try selecting a higher quality cheese such as Roquefort or Saga Bleu for a true representation of this well-crafted cheese. It complements the earthy flavors of mushrooms so well that you will become a blue cheese–lover instantly. A sensational appetizer or hors d'oeuvre, this is a sure crowd-pleaser.

Ingredients
Makes 6 servings.

Mushroom Filling
1/4 teaspoon extra-virgin olive oil
1 cup julienned fresh shiitake mushrooms (about 3 1/2 ounces)
1 cup julienned fresh oyster mushrooms
1 cup julienned portobello mushrooms, gills removed (about 7 ounces)
1 cup julienned button mushrooms (1/2 pound)
1 teaspoon minced garlic
1 tablespoon minced shallot
1 tablespoon brandy
1 cup lightly packed fresh spinach leaves
1 tablespoon Fresh Herb Mix (see page 39)
1 teaspoon crumbled Roquefort cheese
1/4 teaspoon sea salt
1/8 teaspoon freshly ground black pepper

Phyllo
4 phyllo dough sheets
Olive oil cooking spray
3 tablespoons Fresh Herb Mix

About 6 tablespoons Red Wine Reduction (see page 19)
About 2 teaspoons finely crumbled Roquefort cheese

Preparation
Preheat the oven to 350°F (175°C). Line a baking sheet with parchment paper.

For the Mushroom Filling: Heat a large sauté pan over medium-high heat and add the olive oil to lightly coat the bottom of the pan. Add the shiitake and oyster mushrooms and cook for 1 minute. Add the portobello mushrooms and cook for 1 minute. Add the button mushrooms and cook for 1 minute more. Mix in the garlic and shallot and cook until all the mushrooms have softened, about 2 minutes more. Add the brandy and stir to deglaze the pan. Cook until all the liquid is absorbed, about 3 minutes.

Mix in the spinach, herbs, cheese, salt, and pepper. Set aside.

For the Phyllo: Carefully lay one sheet of phyllo dough on a clean cutting board. Lightly mist the pastry sheet with olive oil spray and sprinkle with 1 tablespoon of the herbs. Layer two more phyllo sheets, misting each layer with olive oil and sprinkling with herbs. Finish with the fourth phyllo sheet. Cut the pastry lengthwise into 6 equal strips. Cut each strip into 6 triangles. You will have a total of 36 triangles.

Place the triangles on the parchment paper-lined baking sheet. Place another piece of parchment on top of the triangles. Cover with another baking sheet. This helps the dough stick together and makes the triangles more stable. Bake for 5 to 10 minutes or until golden brown.

To serve: Drizzle a design on the plate using the Red Wine Reduction. Place one triangle on the plate. Place 1 tablespoon of the mushroom mixture on top of the triangle. Top with another triangle and another 1 tablespoon of the mushroom mixture, ending with a triangle. Arrange the triangles so they each point in a different direction. Sprinkle 1/4 teaspoon of cheese around the plate.

Spanakopita

Per 3 triangles:
Calories 120; Protein 5g; Total Fat 3.5g;
Saturated Fat 0g; Carbohydrates 18g; Dietary
Fiber 0g; Cholesterol 0mg; Sodium 230mg

This is a wonderful vegan rendition of the classic Greek appetizer. Tofu and miso replace the feta cheese. These little pastry pillows are so luscious, you'll find it hard to believe they are nondairy.

Ingredients

Makes 20 servings of 3 triangles per serving.

Filling

1/2 teaspoon extra-virgin olive oil
2 teaspoons minced garlic
1 cup chopped yellow onion (about 1
   large)
2 cups chopped button mushrooms (1
   pound)
1 cup chopped fresh shiitake mushrooms
1/4 cup white wine
5 cups packed, chopped fresh spinach
1 1/4 cups crumbled, extra-firm tofu (about
   7 ounces)
2 tablespoons finely chopped fresh
   oregano
2 tablespoons finely chopped fresh basil
2 tablespoons finely chopped fresh parsley
2 teaspoons miso paste
1 teaspoon tamari (soy) sauce
1/2 teaspoon sea salt
1/2 teaspoon freshly ground black pepper
1/8 teaspoon ground nutmeg

Phyllo

1 16-ounce box phyllo dough (28 sheets)
Olive oil cooking spray

Preparation

Preheat the oven to 350°F (175°C). Line a baking sheet with parchment paper.

For the Filling: Heat a medium sauté pan over medium-high heat and add the olive oil to lightly coat the bottom of the pan. Add the garlic and onion. Cook until the onion has softened, about 2 minutes. Add the mushrooms and cook 1 minute. Pour in the white wine and boil until the pan is almost dry, about 2 minutes. Add the spinach and cook until just wilted, about 2 minutes. Remove to a mixing bowl and cool completely.

Combine the spinach mixture with the tofu, herbs, miso, tamari, salt, pepper, and nutmeg. Mix well and set aside.

For the Phyllo: Unfold the phyllo dough on a baking sheet and cover with a damp cloth to keep it from drying out as you work. On a clean cutting board, lay out one sheet of phyllo. Lightly mist the phyllo with cooking spray. Repeat to make a total of 3 layers.

Cut the layered phyllo sheets crosswise into 6 strips, approximately 2 3/4 inches x 12 inches. Place 1 tablespoon of the spinach mixture on the end of each phyllo strip. Fold the bottom left corner to the right edge over the spinach mixture. You will be forming small triangles. Keep folding, about 4 times (like folding a flag), to seal in the filling. Repeat with each strip. Place the triangles on the prepared baking sheet and mist with cooking spray.

Repeat the process with the remaining sheets of phyllo dough, stacking the sheets, cutting into strips, and folding up around the filling. Lightly mist the triangles with cooking spray and bake for 15 to 20 minutes or until golden brown.

Tyson® Roll

Per serving:
Calories 90; Protein 10g; Total Fat 2.5g;
Saturated Fat 1g; Carbohydrates 8g; Dietary
Fiber 1g; Cholesterol 20mg; Sodium 150mg

Ingredients

Makes 8 servings.

1 medium zucchini
1 medium yellow squash
1 medium eggplant
2 medium portobello mushrooms
1/4 cup Fine Herb Vinaigrette (see
    page 123)
8-ounce boneless, skinless chicken breast
1/4 cup goat cheese
1/2 cup dry-pack sun-dried tomatoes,
    reconstituted in water and julienned
Balsamic Reduction (see page 19)

This is an attractive appetizer that I created for a party for Tyson Foods®—the chicken people. Sun-dried tomatoes and goat cheese pay homage to the tender strips of grilled chicken. Thinly sliced vegetables are grilled quickly over a hot grill. Brushing the vegetables with Fine Herb Vinaigrette instead of oil to prevent sticking adds flavor while reducing the calories.

If you don't have a sushi mat, find one at an Asian grocery store or kitchen supply store. It is inexpensive and indispensable for making a tight, sushi-style roll with ease.

Preparation

Heat a grill to medium heat.

Using a mandoline or thin, sharp knife, slice the zucchini, yellow squash, and eggplant lengthwise. Brush or wipe the portobello mushrooms with a paper towel; remove the dark gills and julienne the caps. Rub all the vegetables with some of the vinaigrette. Grill the vegetables on each side until grill marks form. Lay vegetables out on a baking sheet to cool.

Season the chicken breast with the remaining vinaigrette. Grill on each side for 6 minutes or until it's cooked through. Cool completely and julienne.

Soften the goat cheese by stirring vigorously in the top of a double boiler over low heat.

Place a sushi mat on a worktable and cover with plastic wrap. Lay out 2 pieces of grilled zucchini lengthwise on the plastic wrap. Repeat with 2 pieces of yellow squash strips overlapping the edges of the zucchini slightly. Finally, lay out 2 pieces of eggplant over the squash, again overlapping the edges slightly. Spread 1 teaspoon of the goat cheese across the bottom of the vegetables. On top of the goat cheese, arrange 1 teaspoon of the sun-dried tomatoes. Place 1/4 cup of the chicken on top of the tomatoes, then 2 tablespoons of the mushrooms.

Carefully lift the plastic wrap away from the vegetables while using the sushi mat to roll as tightly as possible. Trim any excess vegetable off the ends. Repeat with remaining vegetables to make 8 rolls.

To serve: Cut each roll into 4 pieces. You can cut 2 of the pieces on an angle so that when you stand them on the flat sides, they make a nice presentation. Arrange 4 pieces on each serving plate and drizzle with Balsamic Reduction.

This roll makes an awesome hors d'oeuvre as well. Slice it into one-inch rounds and skewer them with rosemary stems rather than toothpicks for an attractive presentation.

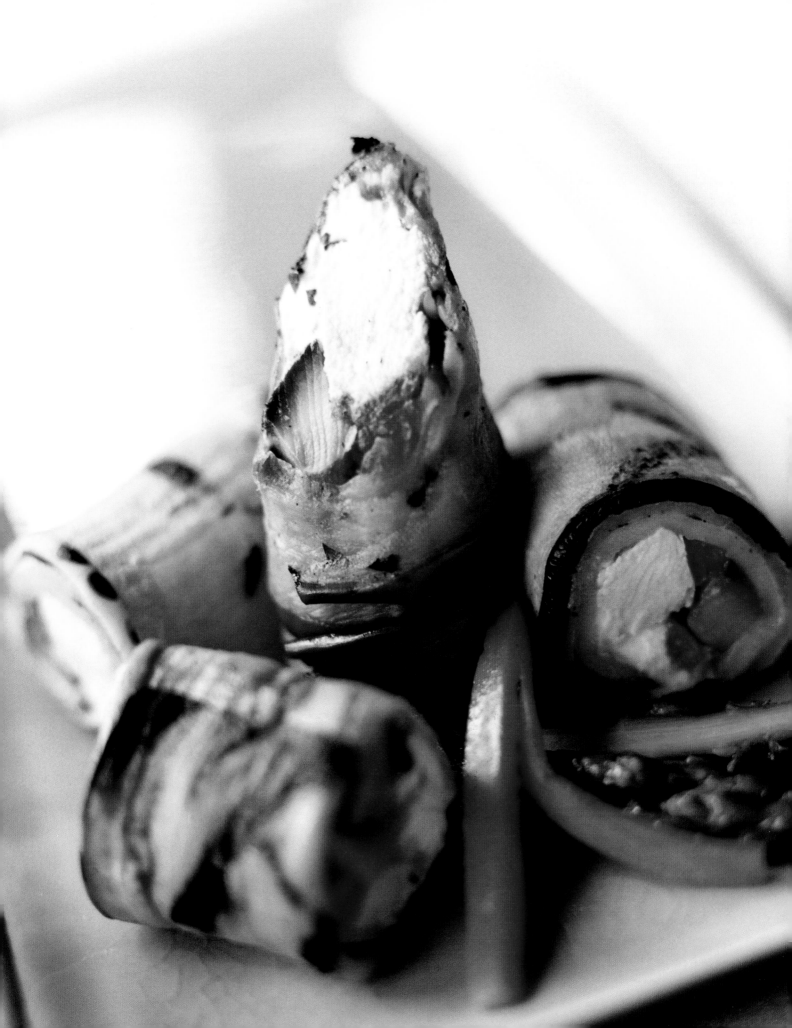

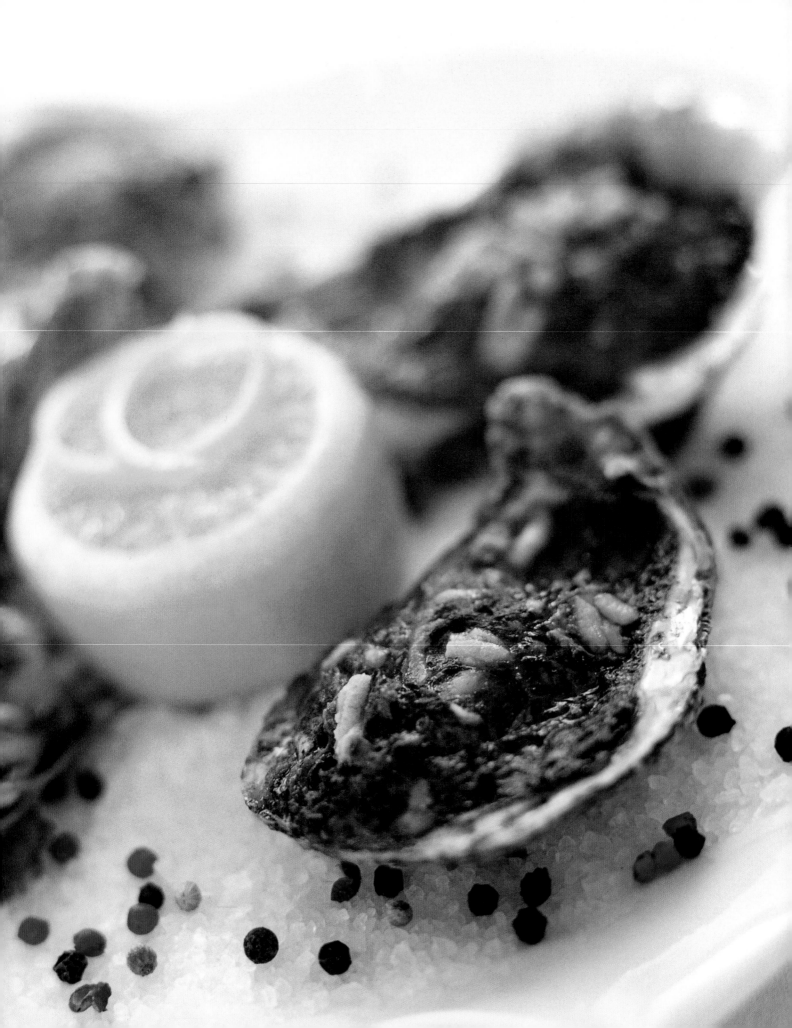

Baked Oysters Florentine

Per serving:
Calories 170; Protein 10g; Total Fat 6g;
Saturated Fat 2g; Carbohydrates 14g; Dietary
Fiber 3g; Cholesterol 45mg; Sodium 660mg

Oysters Rockefeller were first created in New Orleans in 1899 by Jules Alciatore of Antoine's restaurant. It successfully marries spinach, garlic, and cheese with the richness of fresh oysters. Being a great fan of this recipe, I set out to duplicate its flavors and textures in a nutritionally balanced fashion. By employing Conscious Cuisine techniques, I was able to recreate the flavor and appearance of the original—proving you can make and enjoy great-tasting foods that are good for you.

Ingredients
Makes 3 servings.

1/2 cup rock salt or coarse kosher salt
12 fresh oysters, top shells removed
1 teaspoon extra-virgin olive oil
1/2 cup chopped yellow onion (about 1 medium)
1 teaspoon minced garlic
6 cups packed fresh spinach, cleaned (about 1/2 pound)
2 tablespoons Pernod liqueur (licorice-flavored liqueur)
5 tablespoons reduced-fat cream cheese
1/4 cup bread crumbs
1/4 teaspoon ground nutmeg
1/4 teaspoon sea salt
Pinch of freshly ground black pepper
1 teaspoon finely grated Parmesan cheese

Garnish
Lemon wedges
Tabasco sauce
Coarse salt and tricolored peppercorns, optional

Preparation
Preheat the oven to 425°F (220°C).

Spread the rock salt on the bottom of a baking pan. Arrange the oysters on top of the salt.

Heat a medium sauté pan over medium-high heat and add the olive oil to lightly coat the bottom of the pan. Add the onion and garlic. Cook until the onion has softened, about 2 minutes. Add the spinach and cook for 2 minutes. Remove the pan from the heat and add the Pernod. Return the pan to the heat and ignite carefully—the flame may burn high. Cook until all the alcohol has burned off and the flames subside.

Place the spinach mixture, cream cheese, and bread crumbs in a food processor and puree until smooth. Season with nutmeg, salt, pepper, and Parmesan cheese.

Spoon 1 tablespoon of the spinach mixture on top of each oyster. Bake the oysters for 12 to 15 minutes or until lightly browned.

To serve: Fill four plates with coarse kosher salt and tricolored peppercorns if desired. Arrange 4 oysters on each plate. Garnish with lemon wedges and Tabasco sauce.

Ahi Tuna Sashimi

Per serving:
Calories 90; Protein 14g; Total Fat 2.5g;
Saturated Fat 0g; Carbohydrates 2g; Dietary
Fiber 0g; Cholesterol 25mg; Sodium 135mg

Per spoon:
Calories 10; Protein 1g; Total Fat 0g; Saturated
Fat 0g; Carbohydrates 0g; Dietary Fiber 0g;
Cholesterol 5mg; Sodium 25mg

If you are a lover of sushi and sashimi, you will surely enjoy this dish. One of the things that I find interesting about eating Japanese cuisine is the bold, fresh flavors and the creative and tempting presentations. The artful, simple, and clean presentation has persuaded many to try sashimi for the first time. This recipe has been a guest favorite at Miraval for years.

Ingredients
Makes 4 servings.

Tuna
*1 cup diced sushi-grade ahi tuna
  (saku maguro), about 8 ounces*
1/2 teaspoon toasted sesame oil
1 teaspoon Sriracha (chile) sauce
1 teaspoon tamari (soy) sauce
1/4 teaspoon grated fresh ginger
1 teaspoon chopped green onion
1 teaspoon seasoned rice wine vinegar

Vegetables
*1/4 cup peeled, finely chopped English
  cucumber*
1/4 cup finely chopped daikon radish
1/4 cup finely chopped avocado
2 teaspoons minced fresh cilantro
1/4 teaspoon toasted black sesame seeds
2 teaspoons seasoned rice wine vinegar

Garnish
*Pickled ginger, wasabi paste or tobiko
  (wasabi caviar), radish sprouts, and
  Sriracha sauce*

Preparation

For the Tuna: In a mixing bowl, combine the tuna and remaining ingredients. Adjust the seasonings to taste with additional Sriracha and soy sauce. Refrigerate the tuna until needed.

For the Vegetables: Combine the cucumber and daikon in a small bowl. Add the avocado to the cucumber mixture; stir in the cilantro, sesame seeds, and vinegar to season.

To assemble: To form the tower, use a 2-inch tall cylinder that is 2 inches in diameter or a small tomato paste can with both ends removed. If using the small can, use a spoon to place the ingredients into the can because the edges may still be sharp.

Place the cylinder on an appetizer plate. Spoon 1 heaping tablespoon of the tuna mixture into the cylinder, followed by 1 heaping tablespoon of the vegetable mixture. Then top with another 1 tablespoon of tuna. Repeat process. Press mixture firmly into the cylinder to mold. Lift the cylinder up, holding the tuna down with a spoon so the tuna tower remains on the plate. Repeat with remaining ingredients to form 3 more towers.

Garnish with a pinch of pickled ginger, wasabi paste or caviar, radish sprouts, and a drizzle of Sriracha sauce.

Second serving option: You can serve this appetizer in Asian soup spoons. Place 1 teaspoon of the tuna mixture in the back of each spoon. Place 1/2 teaspoon of the vegetable mixture in the front of each spoon. Garnish with a dollop of wasabi paste or caviar, a piece of radish sprout, and a dot of Sriracha sauce on the base of the spoon handle.

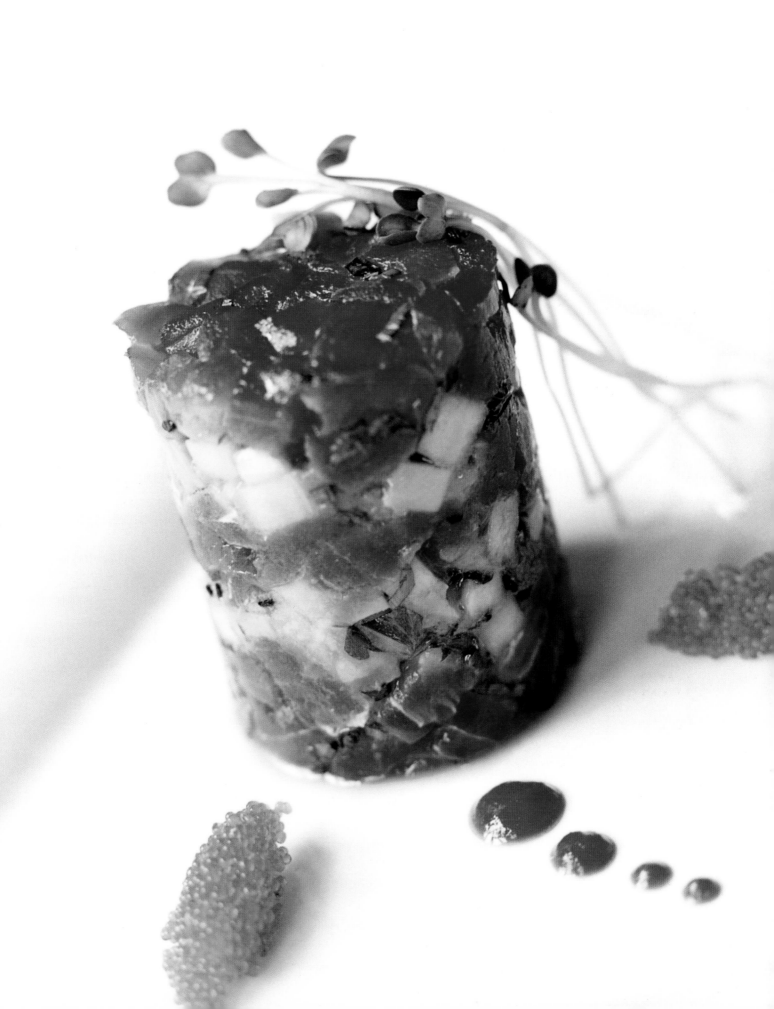

Fresh Vegetable Silo

Per serving:
Calories 90; Protein 2g; Total Fat 5g; Saturated
Fat 1g; Carbohydrates 9g; Dietary Fiber 2g;
Cholesterol 0mg; Sodium 640mg

This recipe is a tribute to the harvest of fresh and glorious tasting vegetables. I have penned the title, "vegetable silo," in reference to its tower presentation, as in the corn silos of the Midwest. The luscious contrasts in flavors and textures are as much fun to prepare as they are to eat.

Ingredients
Makes 4 servings.

Dressing
1 tablespoon Fresh Herb Mix (see page 39)
1 tablespoon extra-virgin olive oil
1/4 cup Fine Herb Vinegar (see page 118)
1 cup Thickened Vegetable Stock (see
  page 153)
1/8 teaspoon sea salt
1/8 teaspoon freshly ground black pepper

Vegetables
1/4 cup diced, peeled Roma (plum)
  tomatoes
1/4 cup diced, blanched asparagus
1/4 cup diced, peeled yellow tomato
1/4 cup diced avocado
1/4 cup fresh shiitake mushrooms, sautéed
  and cooled
1/4 cup diced, cooked artichoke hearts
1/4 cup diced, peeled jícama

Garnish
2 teaspoons Balsamic Reduction (see
  page 19)
1/4 cup radish or broccoli sprouts
1/4 cup shelled, blanched fava beans

Preparation

For the Dressing: Whisk together the herbs, olive oil, vinegar, and stock in a small bowl. Stir in salt and pepper.

For the Vegetables: To mold the salad, you will need 4 2-inch cylinder molds or small tomato paste cans with both ends removed so you can assemble 4 plates at a time. It is important to use a spoon to fill the cans because the edges may be sharp. Place molds in the centers of 4 large dinner plates.

In a mixing bowl, combine the Roma tomatoes with 4 teaspoons of the dressing. Carefully divide the tomatoes among the molds. Repeat, mixing the next vegetable with another 4 teaspoons of the dressing. Repeat with remaining ingredients. Add to the molds in the order the ingredients are listed, using the back of a spoon to pack down each layer. Carefully remove the molds to expose the layered vegetables.

Drizzle 1/2 teaspoon of the Balsamic Reduction onto each vegetable silo and plate.

Garnish with sprouts on top of the vegetable silos and sprinkle fava beans around.

Ragoût of Escargot

Per serving:
Calories 320; Protein 21g; Total Fat 2g;
Saturated Fat 0g; Carbohydrates 39g; Dietary
Fiber 5g; Cholesterol 40mg; Sodium 770mg

Garlic and herb butter is a wonderful and typical accompaniment to escargot. Its richness and complex flavor works wonders with the earthy flavor of the snails. In producing a French-style menu, I was inspired to create a healthy version of this culinary staple. Roasted Shallot Sauce instead of butter delivers flavor and substance and makes this treat a satisfying comfort food.

Ingredients
Makes 4 servings of 6 escargots each.

1/4 teaspoon extra-virgin olive oil
24 canned escargots, drained, rinsed
3/4 teaspoon minced garlic
12 broccoli florets
12 cauliflower florets
12 baby carrots, halved
4 artichoke hearts, cut into quarters
8 button mushrooms, stems removed and
   caps cut into quarters
1/4 cup brandy
1 1/3 cups Roasted Shallot Sauce (see
   page 30)
1/2 teaspoon sea salt
1/4 teaspoon freshly ground black pepper
1 teaspoon Fresh Herb Mix (see page 39)

Garnish
1 tomato, peeled, seeded, and cut into 16
   strips
8 triangles Chickpea Lavosh (see page 95)

Preparation
Heat a medium sauté pan over medium-high heat and add the olive oil to lightly coat the bottom of the pan. Add the escargots, garlic, broccoli, cauliflower, carrots, artichoke hearts, and mushrooms. Sauté for 1 minute. Carefully pour in the brandy, ignite, and cook until the alcohol has burned off, about 1 to 2 minutes. Add the shallot sauce. Season with salt, pepper, and herbs. Pour the ragoût into 4 serving bowls. Garnish with tomato strips and lavosh.

Chile Rellenos Filled with Two Cheeses and Spring Vegetables

Traditional chile rellenos are roasted and peeled green chiles filled with cheese then fried in a light egg batter. This version plays off the technique of roasting, peeling, and filling the chile with a mixture of rich cheese—and adds the season's best vegetables. Although the chile can be fried, I choose to serve it cold, eliminating the excess fat and achieving an awesome presentation of lovely southwestern-style vegetables.

Per 1 chile:
Calories 70; Protein 4g; Total Fat 4g; Saturated Fat 2g; Carbohydrates 9g; Dietary Fiber 2g; Cholesterol 10mg; Sodium 90mg

Per 2 slices:
Calories 30; Protein 1g; Total Fat 1.5g; Saturated Fat 0.5g; Carbohydrates 4g; Dietary Fiber 0g; Cholesterol 5mg; Sodium 35mg

Ingredients
Makes 6 servings.

Chiles
6 roasted Anaheim chiles (see page 38)

Filling
1/4 teaspoon extra-virgin olive oil
1 teaspoon minced garlic
1/4 cup finely chopped green onions
1/4 cup finely chopped tomatillos
1/4 cup finely chopped jícama
1/4 cup finely chopped zucchini
1/4 cup finely chopped fresh shiitake mushrooms
1/4 cup fresh or frozen corn kernels
2 teaspoons Fresh Herb Mix (see page 39)
1/8 teaspoon sea salt
1/8 teaspoon freshly ground black pepper
1/4 cup reduced-fat cream cheese
2 tablespoons goat cheese

Garnish
Sriracha sauce
Julienned red bell peppers
Cilantro

Preparation
For the Filling: Heat a medium saucepan over medium-high heat. Add the olive oil to coat the bottom of the pan. Add all the vegetables. Cook until they have just softened, about 3 minutes. Stir in the herbs, salt, and pepper.

Heat the cream cheese in a bowl in the microwave or over a small pot of boiling water. Whisk in the goat cheese and mix until softened. Add the vegetable mixture to the cheese mixture and stir to incorporate.

Peel the chiles and remove the seeds. Stuff each chile with 2 tablespoons of the cheese-vegetable mixture.

To serve: Arrange one chile on each serving plate. Garnish with Sriracha sauce, julienned red peppers, and cilantro.

Second serving option: You can slice each stuffed chile into 4–6 slices depending on the size of the chiles and serve on a platter.

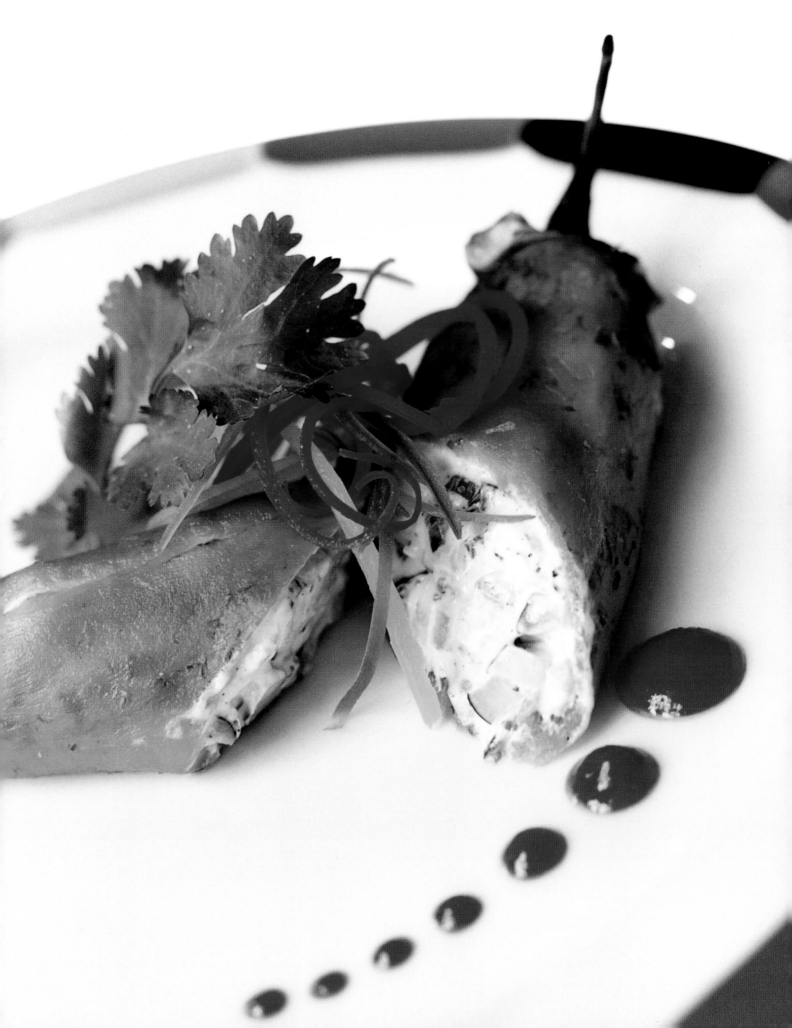

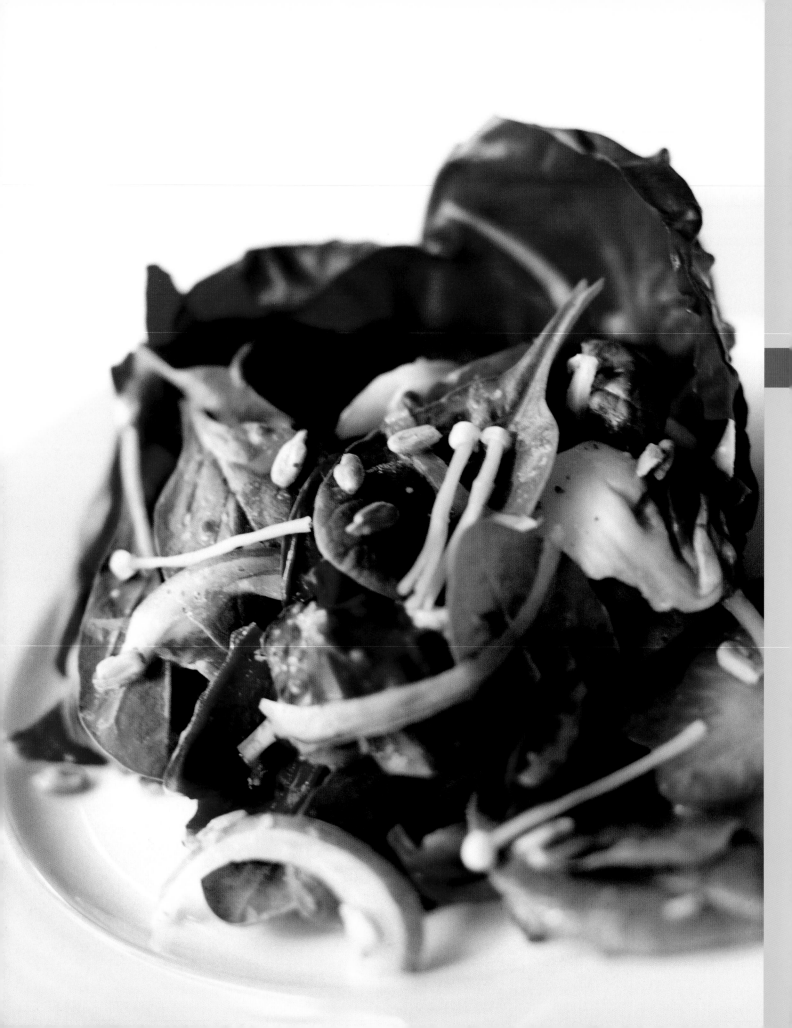

Scrumptious Salads, Flavored Oils, & Vinegars

chapter 6

Basil Oil

Carrot Oil

Bell Pepper Oil

Ginger-Lemongrass Vinegar

Mayonnaise Nouvelle

Caesar Dressing

Ranch Dressing

Fine Herb Vinaigrette

Balsamic Vinaigrette

Citrus-Anchovy Vinaigrette

Honey Mustard Dressing

Sesame Dressing

Summer Fruit Salad

Tabbouleh

Citrus and Jícama Salad

Spinach and Strawberry Salad with Honey Mustard Vinaigrette

Curried Potato Salad

Spicy Turkey and Cabbage Salad

Caesar Salad

Asparagus, Shrimp, and Mushroom Salad

Pico de Gallo Shrimp Salad

Vegetable Slaw

Apple-Barley Salad

Thai Roast Chicken and Vegetable Salad

Curried Cauliflower Salad

Southwestern Black Bean Salad

Bouquet of Organic Greens in a Garlic Herb Vase

Pictured at left: Spinach and Strawberry Salad with Honey Mustard Vinaigrette

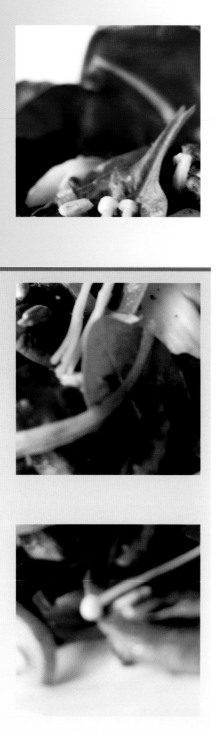

Too often, dinner salads are composed of almost nutrient-free lettuce with crudely cut vegetables and topped with salty vinaigrettes or heavy mayonnaise-based dressings. A Cobb or chef's salad lunch can be as fatty and caloric as a burger and fries. Typically, these salads are made with iceberg lettuce and topped with julienned (the chef salad) or chopped (the Cobb salad) ham, beef, salami, cheese, hard-cooked eggs, olives, and dressing. The chef's salad can have as many as 989 calories and 89 grams of fat, and extra dressing will raise the fat and calorie count even higher. (A McDonald's Quarter Pounder with Cheese contains 797 calories and 44 grams of fat.)

For a healthier lifestyle, ask questions when you're in a restaurant regarding the type and quantity of ingredients used. Alternatives such as a low-fat, low-calorie dressing are often available. Reducing or eliminating the meats, cheese, or egg is another option. Choosing a grilled breast of chicken or steak instead of the deli meats is a better choice. Requesting a half portion or saving half to eat at another time is another tool to make better conscious decisions when dining out.

While a salad is frequently the first course served in a restaurant, it is often overlooked when eating at home. A lovely salad not only offers a light, delicious sample of fresh seasonal produce, but it can also easily supply the same balance of nutrients found in a full meal.

This chapter will reveal the secrets of preparing herb- and vegetable-infused oils and vinegars, vinaigrettes, and dressings to consciously create sensational salads. You'll marvel at the stunning presentation and scrumptious taste of revised old favorites and new creations. This chapter will also highlight fresh seasonal produce and illustrate creative ways to prepare delightful, nutritious appetizer and main-course salads.

Basil Oil

Ingredients
Makes 2 cups.

2 cups packed fresh basil leaves
1 3/4 cups canola oil
1/4 cup extra-virgin olive oil
1/2 teaspoon sea salt

The intense flavor and vibrant color of herb-infused oils allow you to reduce the amount of oil used in vinaigrettes, providing a boost of essential flavor while reducing the amount of calories found in similar recipes. Infused oils such as basil, cilantro, chive, and tarragon can also be drizzled over a host of foods for a dramatic and colorful garnish that delivers on taste.

Preparation
Sterilize a glass container either by submerging in boiling water for 5 minutes or washing in a dishwasher.

Wash the basil and pat dry. Prepare a large bowl of water and ice; set aside. Bring a small amount of water to boil in a small saucepan over medium heat. Add the basil and boil for 1 minute. Drain the basil and submerge in the ice water to cool. Remove from the water and pat dry.

Heat the canola and olive oils in a small saucepan over medium heat until just warmed, about 3 minutes. Place the basil in a blender. With the blender on low, slowly pour in the oil through the hole in the lid. Puree until smooth. Season with the salt. Strain the mixture through a fine mesh strainer or a colander lined with cheesecloth.

Transfer the oil to the sterilized container and refrigerate until ready to use. The oil will keep in the refrigerator up to 1 week.

Variations
Cilantro Oil: Substitute 2 cups fresh cilantro leaves and stems for the basil.
Chive Oil: Substitute 2 cups fresh chives for the basil.
Tarragon Oil: Substitute 2 cups fresh tarragon for the basil.

Carrot Oil

Ingredients
Makes about 1 1/2 cups.

1/2 cup canola oil
1 cup carrot juice (about 3 carrots)
1/4 teaspoon sea salt

Infused vegetable oils are terrific as a base for vinaigrettes or drizzled over almost anything from salads to entrées. The cool pastel colors create a palette for making artful, stylish presentations. Try substituting other vegetables—such as beets, yellow tomatoes, and even horseradish—for the carrots in this recipe to make tantalizing variations with huge success. The neutral flavor of canola oil allows the flavor of the vegetable to dominate.

Preparation
Sterilize a glass container either by submerging in boiling water for 5 minutes or washing in a dishwasher.

Heat the canola oil in a small saucepan over medium heat until just warmed, about 3 minutes. Place the carrot juice in a blender. With the blender on low, slowly pour in the oil through the hole in the lid. Puree until smooth. Season with the salt. Strain the mixture through a fine mesh strainer or a colander lined with cheesecloth.

Transfer the oil to the sterilized container and refrigerate until ready to use. The oil will keep in the refrigerator for up to 1 week.

Bell Pepper Oil

Ingredients
Makes about 3 cups.

3 cups chopped red or yellow bell peppers
    (about 3 peppers)
1 3/4 cups canola oil
1/4 cup extra-virgin olive oil
1/4 teaspoon sea salt

The intense flavor and bright colors of red and yellow bell peppers provide a delicious alternative to salad dressings and sauces for seafoods and poultry.

Preparation

Sterilize a glass container either by submerging in boiling water for 5 minutes or washing in a dishwasher.

Prepare a large bowl of water and ice; set aside. Bring a small amount of water to boil in a small saucepan over medium heat. Add the bell peppers and boil for 3 minutes. Drain the bell peppers and submerge in the ice water to cool. Remove from the water and pat dry.

Heat the canola and olive oils in a small saucepan over medium heat until just warmed, about 3 minutes. Place the bell peppers in a blender. With the blender on low, slowly pour in the oil through the hole in the lid. Puree until smooth. Season with the salt. Strain the mixture through a fine mesh strainer or a colander lined with cheesecloth.

Transfer the oil to the sterilized container and refrigerate until ready to use. The oil will keep in the refrigerator for up to 1 week.

Ginger-Lemongrass Vinegar

Ingredients
Makes 1 cup.

1 cup seasoned rice wine vinegar
2 teaspoons sliced fresh ginger
1-inch piece lemongrass, cut in half
   lengthwise
1 garlic clove, thinly sliced
1 sprig fresh cilantro

Infused vinegars provide a delicious burst of flavor when lightly sprayed or drizzled over salads. Flavored vinegars also make an excellent base for creating "conscious" vinaigrettes and dressings. The intense flavors can enhance poultry, seafood, and meat dishes. I often save decorative food bottles to fill with attractively garnished infused vinegars. Seal the bottle with a cork and even cover with melted wax to create a lovely gift or decoration for the kitchen.

Preparation
Sterilize a glass container either by submerging in boiling water for 5 minutes or washing in a dishwasher.

In a small saucepan, heat the vinegar to a simmer.

Place the remaining ingredients into the sterilized container. Using a funnel, slowly pour the vinegar into the container and let cool.

Seal tightly and store at room temperature for at least 24 hours before serving. The vinegar will keep, stored in a cool dry place, for up to 2 months.

Variations

Fine Herb Vinegar
1 cup seasoned rice wine vinegar
1 garlic clove, thinly sliced
2 teaspoons fresh thyme (about 2 sprigs)
2 teaspoons fresh oregano (about 2 springs)
2 teaspoons fresh basil (about 4 leaves)
2 teaspoons fresh cilantro (about 2 sprigs)
1/4 teaspoon crushed black peppercorns

Raspberry Vinegar
1 cup red wine vinegar
1/4 cup fresh raspberries
3 mint leaves

Rosemary Vinegar
1 cup seasoned rice wine vinegar
2-inch piece fresh rosemary
1 garlic clove, thinly sliced

Strawberry Vinegar

1 cup seasoned rice wine vinegar
1/4 cup strawberries
3 mint leaves

Sun-Dried Tomato Vinegar

1 cup seasoned rice wine vinegar
1/4 cup dry-packed sun-dried tomatoes
2 garlic cloves, thinly sliced
1 basil leaf
1-inch piece fresh rosemary

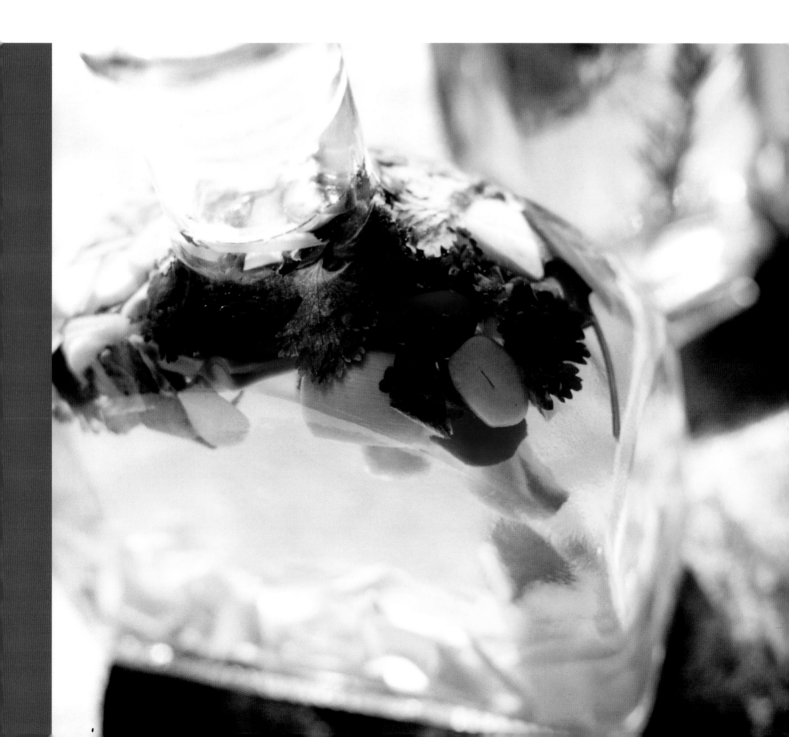

Mayonnaise Nouvelle

Per 2 tablespoons:
Calories 15; Protein 2g; Total Fat 0g; Saturated
Fat 0g; Carbohydrates 2mg; Dietary Fiber 0g;
Cholesterol 0mg; Sodium 115mg

I developed this mayonnaise substitute to prepare traditional dressings and salads without excess fat and calories. A traditional mayonnaise has 100 calories and 11 grams of fat per tablespoon. In contrast, the Mayonnaise Nouvelle is fat free and has only 15 calories per 2 tablespoons. The flavor is remarkably good, especially when used as a base with other ingredients. Use Mayonnaise Nouvelle when making tuna and chicken salad or any other recipe that calls for mayonnaise.

Ingredients
Makes 4 cups.

2 cups plain, fat-free yogurt
2 cups silken tofu (16 ounces)
1 tablespoon minced Roasted Garlic (see
   page 38)
2 tablespoons Fine Herb Vinegar (see
   page 118) or white wine vinegar
1 teaspoon Worcestershire sauce
1/2 teaspoon Tabasco sauce
1 teaspoon sea salt
1/2 teaspoon ground white pepper

Preparation

First, make yogurt cheese by draining the yogurt as follows. Line a colander with cheesecloth and place in a bowl. Spoon the yogurt into the colander. Refrigerate and let drain for at least 1 hour. Discard the liquid in the bowl.

In a food processor, combine the yogurt cheese, tofu, and garlic. Process until the mixture is pureed, about 3 minutes. Add the remaining ingredients. Process again to combine, about 3 minutes. Adjust the seasoning with additional salt or pepper to taste.

This dressing will keep for up to 2 weeks in an airtight container in the refrigerator.

Caesar Dressing

Per 2 tablespoons:
Calories 25; Protein 2g; Total Fat 1g; Saturated Fat 0g; Carbohydrates 2g; Dietary Fiber 0g; Cholesterol 0mg; Sodium 200mg

Ingredients

Makes 2 1/4 cups.

2 cups Mayonnaise Nouvelle (see page 120)
1 tablespoon minced Roasted Garlic (see page 38)
1 1/2 teaspoons minced fresh garlic
1 tablespoon anchovy paste or minced anchovy fillets
1 tablespoon Dijon mustard
1 tablespoon extra-virgin olive oil
1/2 teaspoon white miso (soybean paste)
1/8 teaspoon sea salt
1/2 teaspoon freshly ground black pepper
1 teaspoon minced fresh parsley

Caesar salad has long been a favorite of American diners. It has evolved from the tableside preparation of fine dining restaurants to a garlicky dressing that's topped with chicken, steak, or even shrimp.

This recipe was created to rival the zesty flavors of the classic Caesar salad dressing. A traditional Caesar salad can have as many as 426 calories and 42 grams of fat. You will be delighted with this version of Caesar salad dressing; it's so comparable in flavor, texture, and satisfaction that the traditional dressing will no longer be an option. Hail Caesar!

Preparation

In a food processor, combine the Mayonnaise Nouvelle, roasted garlic, fresh garlic, anchovies, Dijon mustard, olive oil, and miso. Process until the garlic is incorporated into the dressing. Pulse in the salt, pepper, and parsley. The dressing will be thick and creamy. The miso offers a lovely Parmesan flavor.

This dressing will keep for 2 to 3 days in an airtight container in the refrigerator.

Ranch Dressing

This is one of my favorite recipes—it shows how Conscious Cuisine can surpass the flavors of traditional recipes. This dressing also serves well as a vegetable dip. By adding chopped tomatoes, spinach, or cooked mushrooms, you can create new and exciting dressings and condiments.

Ingredients

Makes 2 1/4 cups.

2 cups Mayonnaise Nouvelle (see
    page 120)
1 tablespoon minced Roasted Garlic
    (see page 38)
1 teaspoon minced fresh garlic
1 tablespoon chopped green onion
1 teaspoon chopped fresh parsley
1 teaspoon chopped fresh oregano
1 teaspoon chopped fresh basil
1 teaspoon chopped fresh chives
1/2 cup low-fat buttermilk
1/4 teaspoon sea salt
1/8 teaspoon freshly ground black pepper

Preparation

In a food processor, combine the Mayonnaise Nouvelle, roasted garlic, fresh garlic, green onion, parsley, oregano, basil, and chives. Process until the garlic and herbs are pureed.

With the processor on, slowly pour in the buttermilk and season with the salt and pepper. The dressing will be thick and creamy.

This dressing will keep for 2 to 3 days in an airtight container in the refrigerator.

Fine Herb Vinaigrette

Per 2 tablespoons:
Calories 25; Protein 0g; Total Fat 1g; Saturated
Fat 0g; Carbohydrates 4g; Dietary Fiber 0g;
Cholesterol 0mg; Sodium 75mg

This dressing's bright green color and light taste are derived from focusing on the freshness and distinct flavor profile of each herb. Thickened Vegetable Stock is used in place of oil to provide volume and body. High-quality extra-virgin olive oil is used as an optional ingredient, and only to provide seasoning as you would salt or pepper.

Keep this vinaigrette on hand to use as a marinade for meats, poultry, and fish. Rub it on vegetables prior to grilling or roasting in place of oil to prevent the veggies from sticking to the grill and to provide a zesty flavor.

Ingredients
Makes 3 cups.

2 tablespoons honey
3 tablespoons Dijon mustard
2 tablespoons chopped Roasted Garlic
    (see page 38)
1 tablespoon chopped Roasted Shallots
    (see page 38)
1/2 teaspoon minced fresh garlic
1/4 cup chopped fresh basil
1/4 cup chopped fresh cilantro
1/4 cup chopped fresh parsley
1/4 cup chopped fresh oregano
1 tablespoon chopped fresh rosemary
2 cups Thickened Vegetable Stock (see
    page 153)
1/4 cup unsweetened apple juice
1 tablespoon extra-virgin olive oil
1/4 teaspoon sea salt
1/4 teaspoon freshly ground black pepper

Preparation

In a blender, combine the honey, mustard, roasted garlic, roasted shallots, fresh garlic, and herbs with the vegetable stock. Process on low speed until smooth.

With the blender on low, slowly pour in the apple juice and olive oil through the hole in the lid. Season with the salt and pepper.

This dressing will keep for 2 to 3 days in an airtight container in the refrigerator.

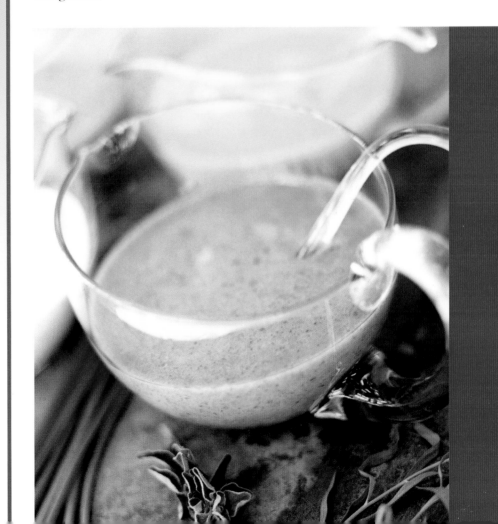

Balsamic Vinaigrette

The use of Dijon mustard, shallots, and garlic provides the base to build this luscious vinaigrette. Balsamic vinegar, made from unfermented grapes, is prized for its complex flavor. It is aged in wooden casks for one to seventy-five years, developing a sweet and intensively flavored vinegar that has a host of applications. Inexpensive, less-aged balsamic vinegar can be used in vinaigrettes or reduced for sauces. The well-aged vinegar is thick and syrupy and should be used sparingly, simply drizzled over greens, meats, cheeses, and fruits.

Ingredients

Makes 3 cups.

3 tablespoons Dijon mustard
1 teaspoon chopped fresh oregano
1 teaspoon finely shredded fresh basil
1 tablespoon minced Roasted Garlic (see page 38)
1 1/2 teaspoons minced shallots
2 tablespoons honey
2 cups Thickened Vegetable Stock (see page 153)
1/4 cup balsamic vinegar
2 tablespoons extra-virgin olive oil
1/2 teaspoon sea salt
1/4 teaspoon ground black pepper

Preparation

In a blender, combine the mustard, herbs, garlic, shallots, honey, and stock. Process on low speed until the garlic is incorporated. With the blender on, slowly pour in the balsamic vinegar and olive oil through the hole in the lid. Season with the salt and pepper.

This dressing will keep for 2 to 3 days in an airtight container in the refrigerator.

Citrus-Anchovy Vinaigrette

Per 2 tablespoons:
Calories 20; Protein 1g; Total Fat 0.5g;
Saturated Fat 0g; Carbohydrates 4g; Dietary
Fiber 0g; Cholesterol 0mg; Sodium 270mg

The varied and complex flavors of the ingredients in this recipe blend well to produce a delicious, tart dressing. This vinaigrette makes a light complement to bitter greens or an interesting sauce for grilled seafood and poultry.

Ingredients
Makes 4 1/2 cups.

2 teaspoons minced fresh garlic
3 tablespoons minced Roasted Garlic (see page 38)
2 tablespoons minced anchovy paste
1/2 cup Dijon mustard
1/4 cup frozen orange juice concentrate, thawed
2 cups Thickened Vegetable Stock (see page 153)
1/2 cup Fine Herb Vinegar (see page 118) or seasoned rice wine vinegar
1 tablespoon extra-virgin olive oil
1 teaspoon freshly grated orange zest
1 teaspoon freshly grated lemon zest
1/2 teaspoon sea salt
1/4 teaspoon freshly ground black pepper
1 tablespoon minced fresh parsley
1 tablespoon minced fresh oregano

Preparation

In a blender, combine the fresh garlic, Roasted Garlic, anchovy paste, mustard, orange juice concentrate, Thickened Vegetable Stock, and Fine Herb Vinegar. With the blender on low speed, slowly pour in the olive oil through the hole in the lid. Add the zests, salt, pepper, parsley, and oregano. Blend for 10 seconds.

This dressing will keep for 2 to 3 days in an airtight container in the refrigerator.

Honey Mustard Dressing

Per 2 tablespoons:
Calories 45; Protein 0g; Total Fat 1g; Saturated Fat 0g; Carbohydrates 8g: Dietary Fiber 0g; Cholesterol 0mg; Sodium 220mg

I will proudly put this dressing up against any commercially made honey-mustard dressing on the market. It is not overly sweet and is delicious on a chilled or warmed spinach salad. It also makes a wonderful glaze on grilled chicken and vegetables.

Ingredients

Makes 2 1/2 cups.

1/4 cup Dijon mustard
1/2 cup whole-grain mustard
2 tablespoons minced Roasted Shallots
   (see page 38)
1 tablespoon minced Roasted Garlic (see
   page 38)
1 1/2 teaspoons fresh garlic
1/2 cup honey
1/3 cup apple cider vinegar
1/2 cup Thickened Vegetable Stock (see
   page 153)
1 tablespoon extra-virgin olive oil
1/4 teaspoon sea salt
1/8 teaspoon white pepper
1 teaspoon chopped fresh chives

Preparation

In a medium bowl, whisk together the mustards, Roasted Shallots, Roasted Garlic, fresh garlic, honey, and vinegar. Add the Thickened Vegetable Stock, oil, salt, pepper, and chives. Whisk until the Thickened Vegetable Stock and oil are incorporated. The dressing will be thick and creamy.

This dressing will keep for 2 to 3 days in an airtight container in the refrigerator.

Sesame Dressing

If you are a fan of Asian-style salads, this dressing is a must. The classic flavors of the three *G*s—garlic, ginger, and green onions—provide the background that enables the flavors of sesame and tamari to shine. Pure, natural tamari is used instead of standard soy sauce. Notice that Thickened Vegetable Stock is used to reduce the amount of toasted sesame oil needed. Sriracha sauce is an Asian chile sauce with a balance of heat from chiles and tartness from vinegar that is just right. Play around with this dressing by using peanut butter instead of sesame seed paste or add citrus juice and zest to create a new twist for dressings or dipping sauces.

Ingredients
Makes 3 1/2 cups.

1 teaspoon minced fresh garlic
2 teaspoons minced fresh ginger
1/4 cup seasoned rice wine vinegar
1 tablespoon tahini (sesame seed paste)
2 tablespoons tamari (soy) sauce
2 cups Thickened Vegetable Stock (see page 153)
1 tablespoon toasted sesame oil
1/2 teaspoon Sriracha (chile) sauce
1/2 teaspoon sea salt
1/4 teaspoon freshly ground black pepper
1 tablespoon chopped green onion
2 teaspoons finely chopped fresh cilantro

Preparation

In a blender, combine the garlic, ginger, vinegar, tahini, tamari, and vegetable stock. Process until the garlic is incorporated. With the blender on low, add in the toasted sesame oil, Sriracha sauce, salt, and pepper through the hole in the lid. Add the green onion and cilantro. Blend just until the cilantro is chopped, about 1 minute.

This dressing will keep for 2 to 3 days in an airtight container in the refrigerator.

Summer Fruit Salad

This salad should be in everyone's repertoire to take advantage of the summer's best fruits and berries. Serve as a salad, an appetizer, over cereal, or as a magnificent dessert by itself or over ice cream.

Ingredients
Makes 6 servings.

Dressing
1/4 cup honey
1/2 vanilla bean, split lengthwise
1 tablespoon finely shredded fresh mint

Salad
3 cups diced melon, such as cantaloupe, honeydew, or mixed (about 1 small)
1 cup diced papaya (about 1/2 medium)
1 1/2 cups diced pineapple (about 1/2 small)
1/2 cup halved fresh strawberries (about 5 medium)
1/2 cup fresh blueberries

Preparation

For the Dressing: Scrape the seeds from the vanilla bean pod and combine with the honey in a small saucepan over medium heat. (The remaining pod can be put to another use such as flavoring vanilla sugar, see page xix.) Simmer for 5 minutes. Allow the honey to cool, about 10 minutes. Stir in the mint.

For the Salad: Combine all the fruits in a medium bowl and mix gently. Carefully fold the honey into the fruit mixture.

Chill for at least 30 minutes before serving.

Tabbouleh

Tabbouleh is a traditional Middle Eastern bulgur wheat salad. In this recipe, the mint and parsley add a refreshing twist. It is delicious as a salad or as a side dish with an entrée of roasted lamb, chicken, or beef.

Per 1 cup:
Calories 230; Protein 8g; Total Fat 3g; Saturated Fat 0g; Carbohydrates 48g; Dietary Fiber 12g; Cholesterol 0mg; Sodium 170mg

Ingredients
Makes 8 servings.

Salad
3 3/4 cups Vegetable Stock (see page 152)
    or water
3 cups bulgur wheat
1 small red onion, diced
3 medium tomatoes, diced
1/4 cup chopped green onion

Dressing
1/2 cup fresh lemon juice
1 tablespoon extra-virgin olive oil
1/2 teaspoon sea salt
1/4 teaspoon freshly ground black pepper
1 cup chopped fresh parsley
1/2 cup chopped fresh mint

Preparation

For the Salad: In a medium saucepan, bring the stock to a boil. Add the bulgur wheat and cover. Reduce heat to low and simmer for 10 minutes. Remove from heat and let stand, covered, for 5 minutes. Gently stir the bulgur with a fork to fluff. Transfer the mixture to a large bowl.

Add the red onion, tomatoes, and green onion to the bulgur. Mix well.

For the Dressing: Whisk together all the dressing ingredients in a small bowl.

Pour the dressing over the bulgur mixture and stir to combine. Cover and chill for at least 30 minutes before serving.

Citrus and Jícama Salad

Per serving:
Calories 150; Protein 3g; Total Fat 5g;
Saturated Fat 1g; Carbohydrates 25g; Dietary
Fiber 5g; Cholesterol 0mg; Sodium 5mg

Jícama, a white-fleshed tuber, has a crisp texture and slightly sweet flavor. It closely resembles a turnip in color and a pear in taste. Its smooth brown skin peels away rather easily. In Mexico, jícama is cut into sticks, drizzled with lime juice and chile powder, and sold as street food. I adapted the recipe from my good friend and comrade, Rene Robles, who makes jícama salsa to serve with his luscious sandwiches.

Ingredients
Makes 4 servings.

Salad
4 teaspoons toasted, shelled pumpkin
    seeds
1/2 teaspoon chile powder
2 oranges, peeled, segmented
2 blood oranges, peeled, segmented
1 grapefruit, peeled, segmented
1/2 cup julienned jícama (about half
    of a jícama)
1/2 head romaine lettuce, cut into thin,
    diagonal slices

Dressing
1 cup unsweetened orange juice
1 tablespoon fresh lime juice
2 teaspoons fresh lemon juice
1/4 teaspoon chile powder

1/2 avocado, cut into 8 slices

Preparation

For the Salad: Sprinkle the pumpkin seeds with the 1/2 teaspoon chile powder. In a large bowl, toss together the oranges, grapefruit, jícama, lettuce, and pumpkin seeds.

For the Dressing: Whisk together the citrus juices and the 1/4 teaspoon chile powder in a medium bowl.

Toss the salad with the dressing. To serve, divide the salad among 4 plates. Lay 2 slices of avocado on top of each serving.

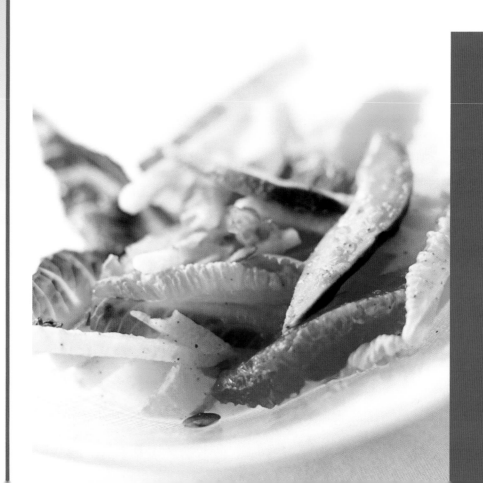

Spinach and Strawberry Salad with Honey Mustard Vinaigrette

Per serving:
Calories 45; Protein 1g; Total Fat 1g; Saturated Fat 0g; Carbohydrates 10g; Dietary Fiber 1g; Cholesterol 0mg; Sodium 110mg

To notice the contrast in flavors—from the astringency of shaved onions and the slight bitterness of spinach and radicchio to the sweetness of honey and strawberries—is an act of "conscious" eating. This salad uses fresh, seasonal ingredients to create a refreshing, light, and satisfying meal that's attractive and can be prepared on a moment's notice. Photo on page 112.

Ingredients
Makes 8 servings.

Salad
6 cups spinach, washed, and thoroughly
   dried
1 1/2 cups sliced strawberries
1 tablespoon sunflower seeds
1 small red onion, thinly sliced

Dressing
1 tablespoon seasoned rice wine vinegar
2 tablespoons honey
2 teaspoons Dijon mustard
Sea salt and freshly ground pepper, to taste

1 head radicchio lettuce, washed and
   leaves separated
1/3 cup enoki mushrooms (about
   2 ounces)

Preparation
For the Salad: Tear the spinach into bite-sized pieces and place in a large bowl. Add the strawberries, sunflower seeds, and onion.

For the Dressing: In a small bowl, whisk together the vinegar, honey, mustard, salt, and pepper.

To serve: Pour the dressing over the salad and toss to combine. Place 1 radicchio leaf on each plate. Place 1 cup of spinach salad in each radicchio cup and garnish with enoki mushrooms.

Curried Potato Salad

I love this salad for its simplicity of preparation and its complex flavor, textures, and aroma. I sometimes serve this with a rosette of smoked salmon for a spectacular entrée salad. The photo at the right shows Curried Potato Salad served with a smoked salmon rosette.

Ingredients

Makes 6 servings.

Salad

4 cups chopped, cooled, cooked Yukon gold potatoes (about 1 1/2 pounds)
1/2 cup golden raisins
2 tablespoons chopped green onion (about 4)
1 Granny Smith apple, chopped
2 tablespoons chopped pistachio nuts

Dressing

1 tablespoon curry powder
1/4 cup apple cider or unfiltered apple juice
1 cup plain, fat-free yogurt
1/2 teaspoon sea salt
1/4 teaspoon freshly ground black pepper

6 leaves Bibb lettuce

Preparation

For the Salad: Place the potatoes in a bowl with the raisins, green onion, apple, and pistachios.

For the Dressing: In a small bowl, mix the curry powder with the apple juice. Stir in the yogurt, salt, and pepper. Gently stir the dressing into the potato mixture.

Refrigerate for 30 minutes before serving.

To serve: Place 1 lettuce leaf on each plate. Place 1 cup of potato salad in each lettuce leaf.

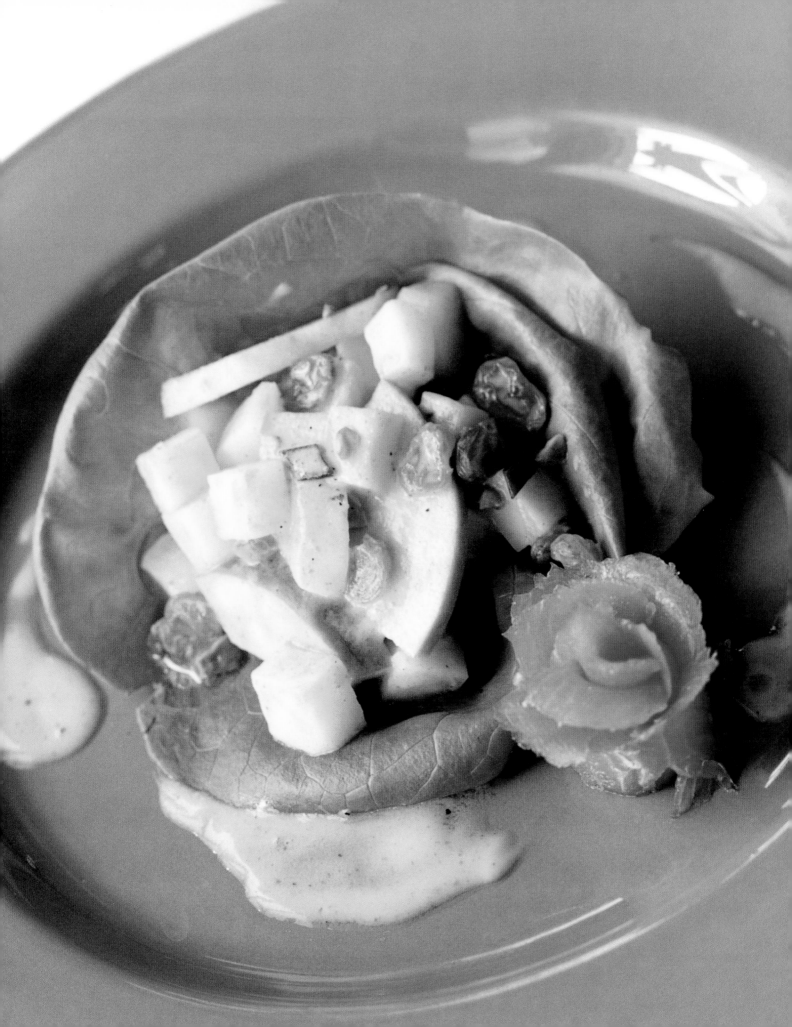

Spicy Turkey and Cabbage Salad

Per serving:
Calories 60; Protein 7g; Total Fat 0.5g;
Saturated Fat 0g; Carbohydrates 8g; Dietary
Fiber 2g; Cholesterol 15mg; Sodium 510mg

Looking for ideas to use up roast turkey? Try this colorful combination of turkey, cabbages, and carrots seasoned with an oriental touch and sparked with chile sauce. Another great combination is to substitute baked tofu for the turkey. This salad tastes great wrapped in a soft tortilla for a fast lunch.

Ingredients
Makes 4 or 5 servings.

Salad
3/4 cup julienned, cooked turkey breast
   (about 3 ounces)
2 1/2 cups shredded green cabbage
1 cup shredded red cabbage
1/2 cup julienned carrots (about 1 small)

Dressing
1/4 teaspoon toasted sesame oil
1/4 teaspoon Sriracha (chile) sauce
1/4 cup seasoned rice wine vinegar
2 tablespoons tamari (soy) sauce

Preparation
For the Salad: In a large bowl, combine the turkey, cabbages, and carrots.

For the Dressing: In a small bowl, whisk together all the dressing ingredients. Pour the dressing over the salad and toss well to combine.

Refrigerate for 30 minutes before serving.

Caesar Salad

Per Serving:
Calories 80; Protein 5g; Total Fat 2.5g;
Saturated Fat 0.5g; Carbohydrates 10mg;
Dietary Fiber 2g; Cholesterol 5mg; Sodium
290mg

This salad, whose dressing is based on a mayonnaise substitute made of tofu and yogurt, rivals the classic Caesar salad without the saturated fat and cholesterol of egg yolks. Artfully arrange the romaine hearts in the center of the plate to create an appealing presentation for this new wave Caesar. The photo shows each Parmesan Crisp cut into four pieces and displayed between the tomato slices.

Ingredients
Makes 4 servings.

6 cups torn romaine lettuce
1/2 cup Caesar Dressing (see page 121)
1/4 cup bagel chips
4 slices yellow tomato
4 slices red tomato
4 Parmesan Crisps

Parmesan Crisps
Makes 4 Crisps.
4 teaspoons finely grated Parmesan cheese

Preparation

Toss the romaine with the dressing and divide among 4 plates. Garnish each salad with the bagel chips, tomatoes, and a Parmesan Crisp.

For the crisps: Preheat the oven to 350°F (175°C). Line a baking sheet with a nonstick baking liner or parchment paper. Carefully spoon 1 teaspoon of the cheese into a long thin strip about 4 inches long by 1/2 inch wide. Repeat to make 3 more strips. Bake for 8 minutes or until golden brown and crispy. Cool completely before removing from the pan.

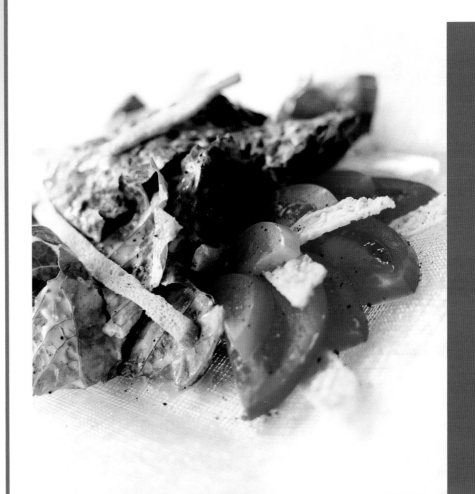

Asparagus, Shrimp, and Mushroom Salad

Per serving:
Calories 90; Protein 9g; Total Fat 3g; Saturated Fat 0g; Carbohydrates 9g; Dietary Fiber 2g; Cholesterol 50mg; Sodium 220mg

This is a lovely use of fresh asparagus when it is in season. For an appetizer, serve wrapped in a leaf of butter lettuce.

Ingredients
Makes 7 servings.

Salad
1/2 pound peeled, cooked medium shrimp
3 cups chopped asparagus spears, blanched and cooled (about 1 bunch)
1 pint teardrop or cherry tomatoes, cut in half
1 1/2 cups chopped mushrooms, such as chanterelle, oyster, or button (about 2 ounces)

Dressing
1 cup fresh lemon juice
1/2 cup Thickened Vegetable Stock (see page 153)
1 tablespoon extra-virgin olive oil
1 tablespoon minced fresh parsley
1 tablespoon minced fresh thyme
1/2 teaspoon sea salt
1/2 teaspoon freshly ground black pepper

Preparation
For the Salad: Cut the shrimp in half lengthwise. In a large bowl, combine the shrimp, asparagus, tomatoes, and mushrooms. Toss together gently.

For the Dressing: In a small bowl, whisk together all the dressing ingredients until well blended. Adjust the seasoning with additional salt, pepper, and olive oil, to taste. Pour the dressing over asparagus mixture and toss to combine.

Refrigerate for at least 30 minutes before serving.

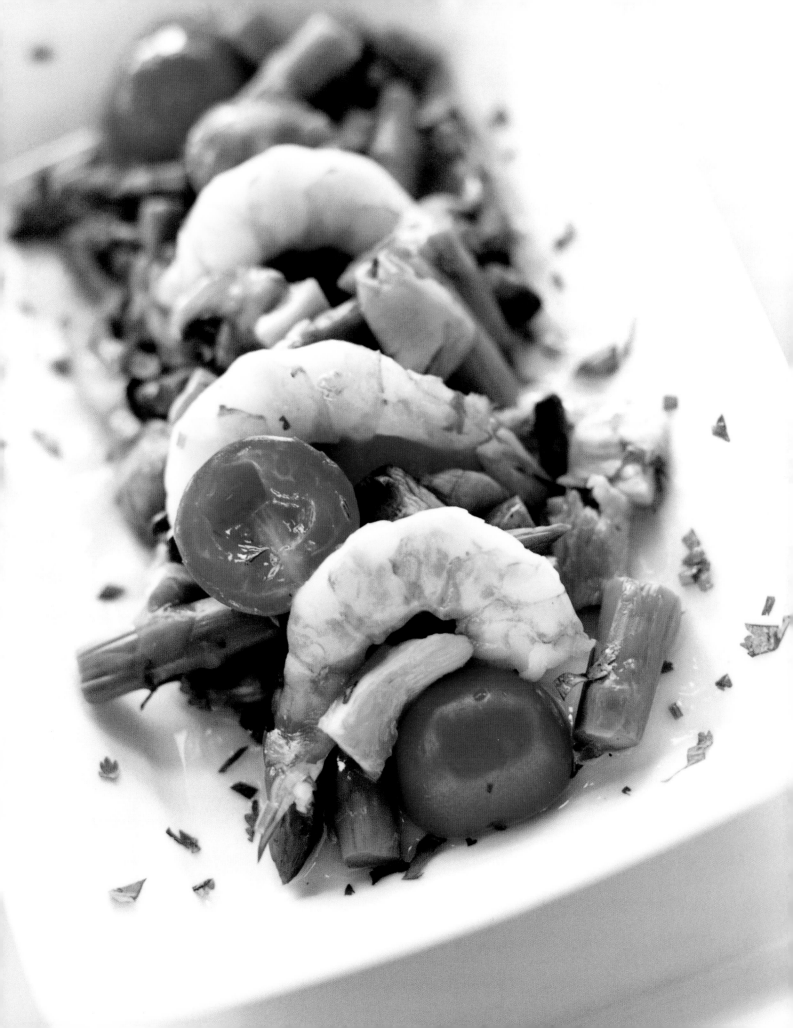

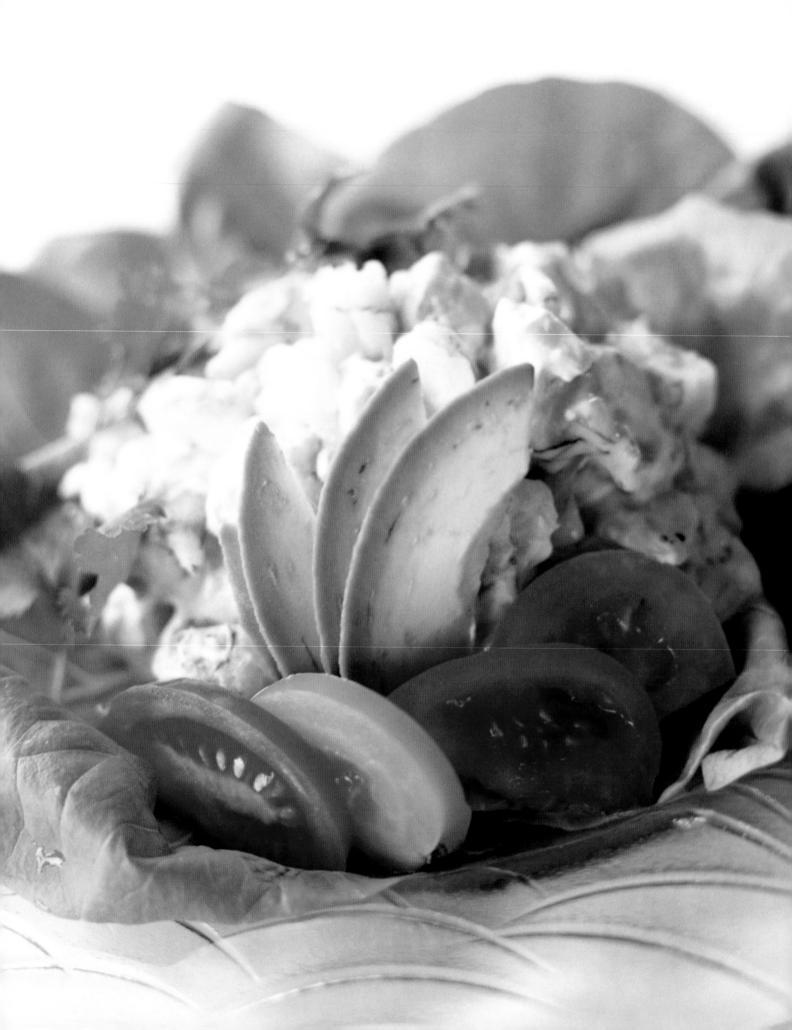

Pico de Gallo Shrimp Salad

Per serving:
Calories 110; Protein 15g; Total Fat 1.5g;
Saturated Fat 0g; Carbohydrates 8g; Dietary
Fiber 0g; Cholesterol 90mg; Sodium 400mg

The name *pico de gallo* refers to a condiment of chopped tomatoes, chiles, and cilantro. Adding cooked shrimp or sea scallops and a simple dressing creates a taste sensation that's a sure crowd-pleaser. Try this refreshing shrimp salad as an entrée with sliced avocado or presented in a large bowl for a festive brunch or poolside treat.

Ingredients
Makes 4 servings.

Salad
1/2 pound peeled, cooked medium shrimp
1 cup chopped tomato (about 1 medium)
1/4 cup chopped red onion
2 teaspoons minced jalapeño chile
2 tablespoons minced fresh cilantro

Dressing
6 tablespoons fat-free sour cream
1/3 cup reduced-fat cream cheese,
   softened
1 1/2 tablespoons fresh lime juice (about
   2 small)
1/2 teaspoon sea salt
1/4 teaspoon ground white pepper

Preparation
For the Salad: Combine all of the salad ingredients in a large bowl and refrigerate while the dressing is prepared.

   For the Dressing: Combine all of the dressing ingredients in a small bowl and stir vigorously until smooth. Gently stir the dressing into the shrimp mixture.

   Refrigerate for 30 minutes before serving.

Variation for Serving
Place lettuce cups on each plate. Scoop salad into cups. Garnish with sliced red and yellow tomatoes and avacado.

Vegetable Slaw

Per serving:
Calories 90; Protein 3g; Total Fat 3g; Saturated Fat 0g; Carbohydrates 15g; Dietary Fiber 4g; Cholesterol 0mg; Sodium 105mg

This light, refreshing slaw replaces the traditional mayonnaise-based coleslaw. The natural sugars of the jícama and carrot give it a slightly sweet and intriguing flavor. The wonderful colors of each vegetable make this salad an attractive complement to any luncheon sandwich or entrée.

Ingredients

Makes 6 or 7 servings.

Salad

2 1/2 cups finely shredded green cabbage
1 1/4 cups shredded zucchini (1 medium)
1 1/2 cups finely shredded jícama
1 small carrot, finely shredded
1 cup fresh corn kernels, cooked
2 tablespoons chopped green onion
2 tablespoons toasted, shelled sunflower
   seeds

Dressing

1/4 cup fresh lime juice
1/2 tablespoon extra-virgin olive oil
1/4 cup Thickened Vegetable Stock (see
   page 153)
1/2 tablespoon honey
1 tablespoon minced fresh oregano
1 tablespoon minced fresh parsley
1/4 teaspoon sea salt
1/8 teaspoon freshly ground black pepper

Preparation

For the Salad: In a medium bowl, toss together the vegetables and sunflower seeds.

For the Dressing: In a small bowl, whisk together the dressing ingredients. Pour the dressing over the salad and toss to coat.

Refrigerate for at least 30 minutes before serving.

Apple-Barley Salad

Per serving:
Calories 210; Protein 6g; Total Fat 2g;
Saturated Fat 0g; Carbohydrates 45g; Dietary
Fiber 10g; Cholesterol 0mg; Sodium 260mg

Barley gives body to this salad while adding a boost of energy through its complex carbohydrates and B vitamins. When laced with sweet and tart apples or pears, it creates a taste sensation that kids will love—just don't tell them that it's good for them.

Ingredients
Makes 4 to 5 servings.

Salad
1 cup barley
2 cups Vegetable Stock (see page 152)
1/4 cup minced fresh parsley
1/4 cup finely shredded fresh mint
*1 medium apple (Red Delicious or Granny
    Smith or half of each), cored and diced*

Dressing
2 tablespoons fresh lemon juice
2 teaspoons extra-virgin olive oil
1/4 cup unsweetened apple juice
1/3 cup seasoned rice wine vinegar
1/2 tablespoon honey
1/8 teaspoon sea salt
Pinch freshly ground black pepper

Preparation

For the Salad: Toast the barley in a dry medium saucepan over medium heat. Stir constantly until lightly browned, about 3 minutes. Add the stock and bring to a boil. Cover, reduce heat, and simmer for 25 minutes or until the barley is soft. Remove from heat and drain.

In a mixing bowl, combine the cooked barley with the parsley, mint, and apple.

For the Dressing: In a small bowl, whisk together the dressing ingredients. Pour the dressing over the barley mixture and toss to coat.

Refrigerate for at least 30 minutes before serving.

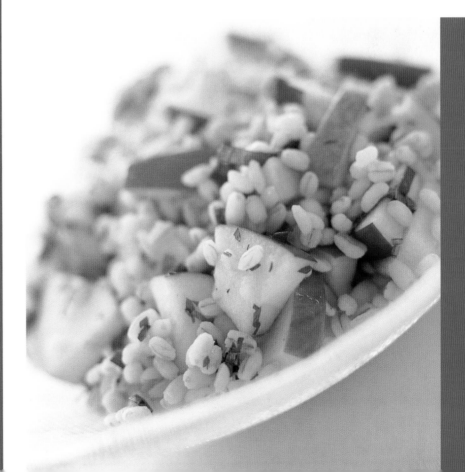

Thai Roast Chicken and Vegetable Salad

Per serving:
Calories 130; Protein 13g; Total Fat 2g;
Saturated Fat 0g; Carbohydrates 14g; Dietary
Fiber 2g; Cholesterol 30mg; Sodium 610mg

An Asian-inspired dressing provides delicious flavor for this salad of cooked chicken and fresh vegetables. The recipe can easily be adapted into an entrée with the addition of stir-fried vegetables, steamed rice, or pasta.

Ingredients
Makes 6 servings.

Salad
*2 cups julienned, cooked chicken breasts
(2 chicken breasts grilled, baked, or
poached)
1 cup julienned red bell pepper
(1 medium)
1 cup julienned yellow bell pepper
(1 medium)
1 cup julienned zucchini (1 medium)
1 cup julienned yellow summer squash
(1 medium)
1 cup julienned carrots (2 medium)
1 cup sliced fresh shiitake mushrooms
(3 1/2 ounces)*

Dressing
*1/2 cup unsweetened orange juice
1 teaspoon tahini (sesame seed paste)
1 tablespoon tamari (soy) sauce
1 tablespoon seasoned rice wine vinegar
1 teaspoon minced fresh ginger
1/2 teaspoon minced fresh garlic
1/4 teaspoon Sriracha (chile) sauce
1/8 teaspoon ground star anise*

Preparation
For the Salad: In a large bowl, combine the chicken and vegetables. Set aside.

For the Dressing: In a small bowl, whisk together all the dressing ingredients. Toss the chicken mixture with the dressing.

Divide the salad among 6 serving plates.

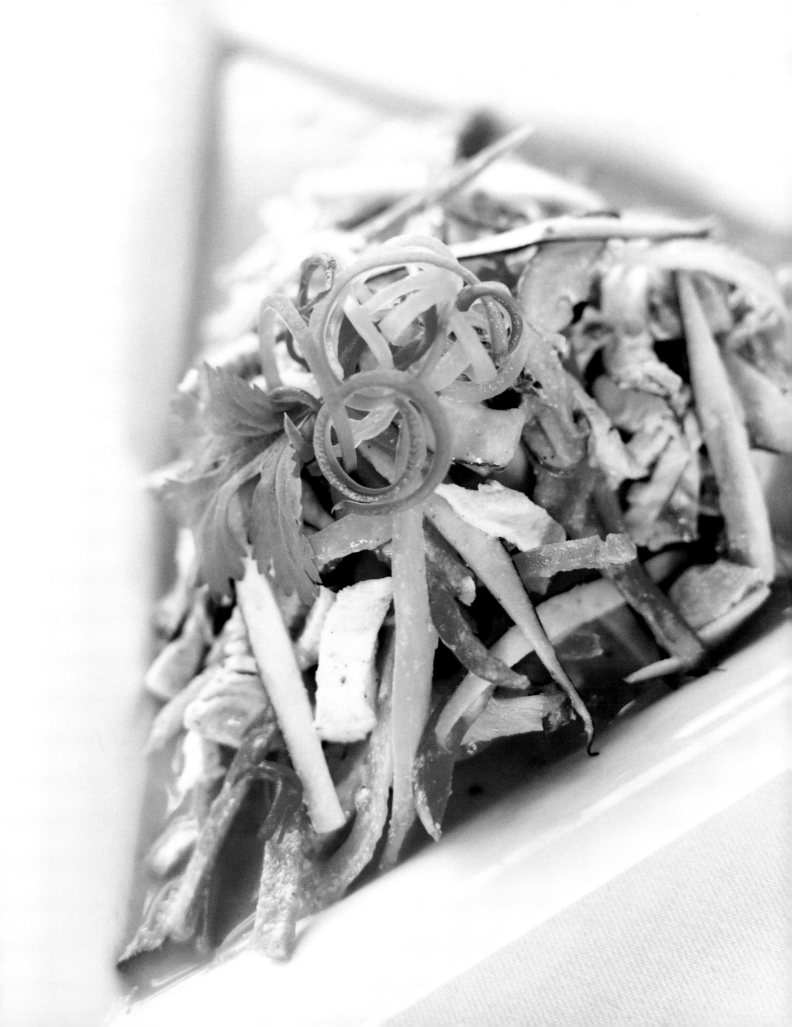

Curried Cauliflower Salad

Per serving:
Calories 70; Protein 6g; Total Fat 3g; Saturated
Fat 0g; Carbohydrates 6g; Dietary Fiber 2g;
Cholesterol 0mg; Sodium 90mg

This zippy salad has it all—vitamins and fiber from the cauliflower and protein from the baked tofu. The curry powder and red bell pepper make the flavors come alive, glorifying the underutilized cauliflower.

Ingredients
Makes 4 to 5 servings.

1/2 head cauliflower, broken into florets
1/2 tablespoon curry powder
1/2 teaspoon extra-virgin olive oil
1 1/2 tablespoons seasoned rice wine
    vinegar (divided)
1/2 cup julienned red bell pepper
1/2 cup thin strips baked tofu
1/8 teaspoon sea salt
1/8 teaspoon freshly ground black pepper

Preparation
Preheat oven to 350°F (175°C). Spray a baking sheet with cooking spray.

In a large bowl, combine the cauliflower, curry powder, olive oil, and 1/2 tablespoon of the vinegar. Place on the prepared baking sheet and bake for 10 minutes or until the cauliflower is just starting to soften. Cool on a rack for about 10 minutes and return to the bowl.

Add the bell pepper and tofu to the cauliflower mixture. Toss with the remaining 1 tablespoon rice wine vinegar, salt, and pepper.

Refrigerate for at least 30 minutes before serving.

Southwestern Black Bean Salad

Per serving:
Calories 90; Protein 4g; Total Fat 0.5g;
Saturated Fat 0g; Carbohydrates 17g; Dietary
Fiber 1g; Cholesterol 0mg; Sodium 290mg

Beans are a terrific way to achieve necessary protein in your diet without meats, poultry, or fish. The sweetness of the corn and fresh flavor of the cilantro make this a terrific salad and an enjoyable relish to serve as an accompaniment to a host of grilled foods.

Ingredients
Makes 4 or 5 servings.

Salad
3/4 to 1 cup canned or cooked black
   beans, drained
1/4 cup diced red onion
1/4 cup diced tomatoes
1/4 cup diced green bell pepper
1/4 cup chopped green onion
3/4 cup cooked corn kernels
1/2 tablespoon chopped fresh cilantro

Dressing
2 tablespoons Fine Herb Vinegar (see page
   118) or seasoned rice wine vinegar
1/2 teaspoon chile powder
1/8 teaspoon sea salt
1/8 teaspoon freshly ground pepper

Preparation

For the Salad: In a mixing bowl, combine the beans, vegetables, and cilantro. Toss gently to combine.

For the Dressing: In a small bowl, stir together the dressing ingredients. Pour the dressing over the salad and mix well.

Refrigerate for at least 30 minutes before serving.

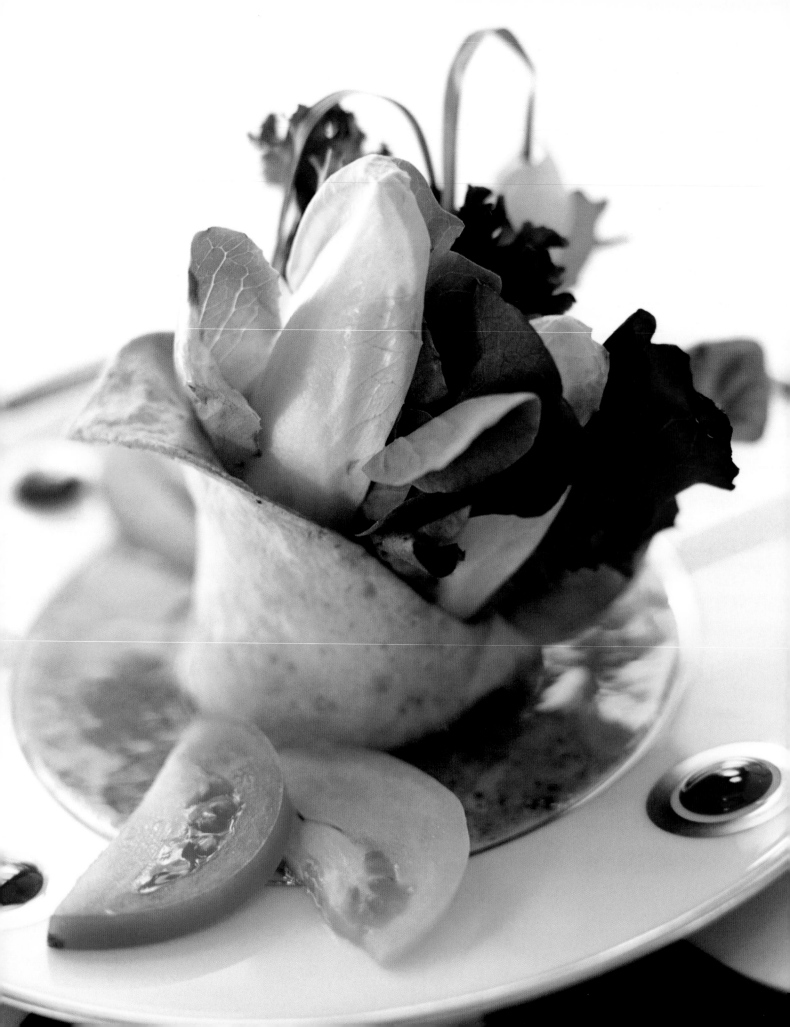

Bouquet of Organic Greens in a Garlic Herb Vase

Per serving:
Calories 160; Protein 6g; Total Fat 1g;
Saturated Fat 0g; Carbohydrates 34g; Dietary
Fiber 3g; Cholesterol 0mg; Sodium 340mg

This is one of my favorite salads. I have always marveled at the glorious colors and shapes of fresh baby lettuces, which remind me of beautiful flowers. Gathering an arrangement of fresh greens and tying them together with a chive or green onion makes a stunning bouquet of the garden's best. For special occasions, try making this garlic herb vase to hold the lettuces upright.

Ingredients
Makes 8 servings.

Garlic Herb Vase
2 tablespoons Roasted Garlic (see page 38)
1/2 cup diced yellow onion (about 1 medium)
1 to 1 1/2 cups unbleached all-purpose flour
3/4 cup semolina flour
1 tablespoon white wine vinegar
1 tablespoon Fresh Herb Mix (see page 39)
1 tablespoon cracked black pepper
1 teaspoon sea salt

Greens
4 cups mixed, organic field greens
1/2 cup Fine Herb Vinaigrette (see page 123)

Garnish
1 tablespoon Fresh Herb Mix
1 red tomato, thinly sliced and slices cut in half (16 slices)
1 yellow tomato, thinly sliced and slices cut in half (16 slices)

Preparation

For the Garlic Herb Vase: In a food processor, combine the Roasted Garlic and onion. Process until the onion is liquefied—this is a key step because this is the liquid that binds the dough together. Add the remaining ingredients to the food processor and pulse until a ball of dough is formed. Remove from the processor bowl and place on a floured board.

Knead the dough until it is smooth and elastic, about 5 minutes. Cover with a towel and let rest for 45 minutes.

Preheat the oven to 300°F (150°C).

On a floured board, roll the dough out to an 1/8-inch thick rectangle of about 8 1/2 x 15 inches. Cut 8 triangles with 6-inch bases and 5-inch sides. To prevent the dough from bubbling, prick it with a fork. Cut parchment paper or waxed paper into eight 2 x 6 inch strips.

Shape the vases in a muffin pan as follows. Bend the base of a dough triangle to form a little "crown," pressing the points together and placing it inside a muffin cup. Bend a paper strip into a ring and place it inside the vase at the bottom of the muffin cup. Fill with pie weights or dry beans to hold the paper out against the inside of the vase and to help stabilize it. Repeat with remaining triangles to make 8 vases.

Bake for 10 minutes or until crisp. Cool completely before removing from the muffin pan.

For the Greens: Artfully gather baby greens together as you would to assemble a bouquet of flowers.

To assemble: Ladle 2 tablespoons of Fine Herb Vinaigrette onto each plate. Place a vase on each of eight salad plates. Fill the vases with the dressed greens. Garnish each plate with the herbs and tomato slices.

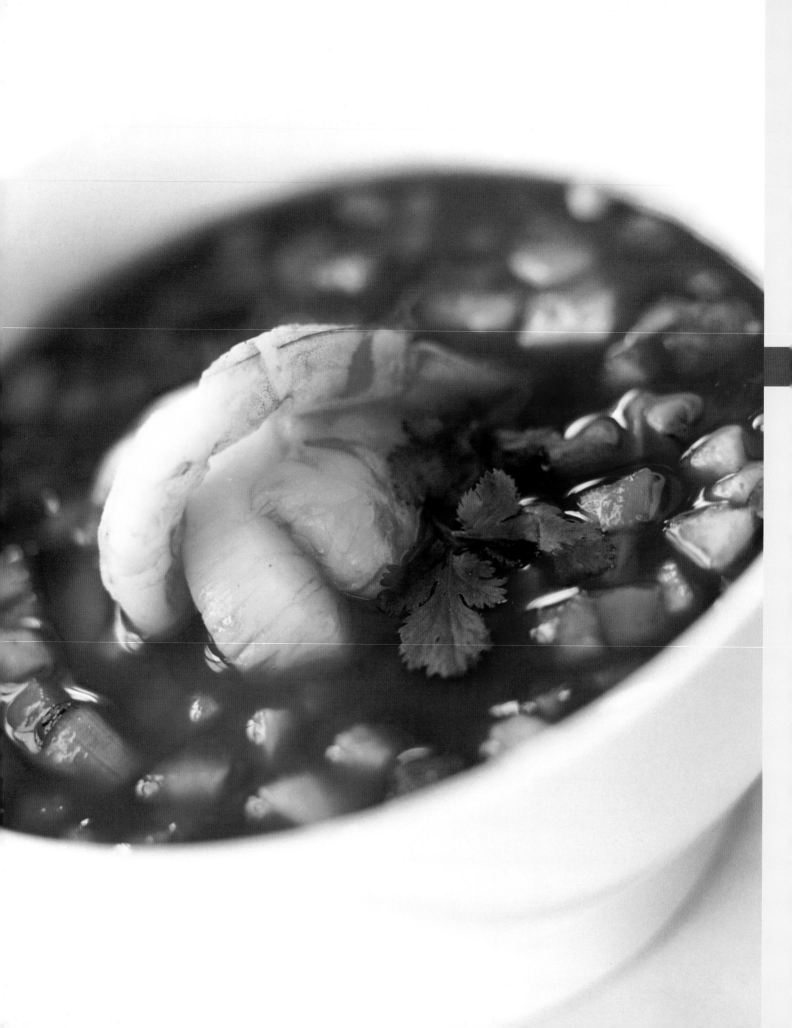

Smart Stocks & Soups

Pictured at left: Shrimp and Scallop Gazpacho

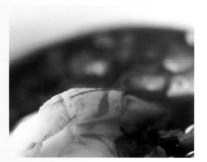

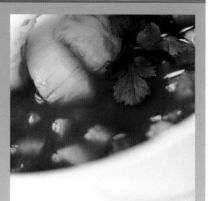

When I held the position of saucier at La Tour Restaurant in the Park Hyatt Hotel Chicago, I was responsible for preparing food from the hot, busy sauté station. But my main responsibility was sauce-making. It was my duty to prepare every stock and glacé used by the entire hotel. I was also responsible for preparing over twenty sauces and two soups for each night's dinner service. I was ecstatic to be entrusted with the task of preparing mouth-watering sauces to complement the daily specials created by my talented chef de cuisine. The best thing about sauce-making is the limitless opportunity to create something new or revive something old each day. I've studied and experimented with hundreds of different soups and sauces, which may be hot, cold, savory, or sweet, and the foundation of 98 percent of these soups and sauces is a flavorful stock or glacé.

Stocks

Stocks and glacés are the simplest to prepare, least understood, and most critical elements used in preparing fine foods. A stock is a highly flavored broth produced from a key main ingredient. This is an essential flavor source used to produce a wide range of delightful recipes, from basic soups and stews to slowly braised meats and vegetables and complex sauces. Stocks provide the base upon which recipes are built. Stocks are also nutritious and can be extremely low in calories and fat.

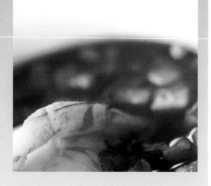

When you reduce a veal stock by half its volume, you create a demi-glace—a ready-to-use, naturally thickened sauce. When you reduce the demi-glace in half once again, you produce a meat glaze called a glacé de viande. This meat glaze can be added to sauces to enhance flavor or combined with water to make stock in an instant.

This chapter will help you gain a greater understanding of the preparation and use of stocks and glacés in all of your cooking, which will be the key to producing delicious and healthful foods. I have included recipes for some of the most common stocks.

Although stocks are one of the simplest and most basic items in cookery, they are time-consuming to make. If time prohibits you from venturing into stock-making, you will be able to find a wide range of stocks, broths, and bases at your local grocer with ease. Please read the labels carefully and select only those with a minimum amount of sodium. Try to select products that are made with natural ingredients rather than imitation flavorings. I have found a wonderful natural product made by More Than Gourmet (see page 326) that I recommend to home and professional cooks who are in need of a quality base product.

Soups

Soup-making has always been one of my favorite areas of cooking. A soup course is representative of the creative abilities of a chef and sets the stage for what is yet to come from his or her kitchen. For years I relished the opportunity to showcase my passion in soup-making. I carefully selected the finest and richest ingredients without any regard for excess fats and calories. I trademarked my style by finishing soups and chowders with crème frâiche, reduced cream, butter, and liqueurs, producing incredibly rich and delicious soups that were a feast for the eyes as well as the taste buds.

I now take my passion for creating fanciful soups to new heights, but without the excess fat. It delights me to prepare and teach others how to prepare soups that are made smartly—soups that deliver on satisfaction, consistency, and delicious flavors while providing a significant amount of nutrients and fewer fats and calories than my previous recipes. Smartly made soups are rewarding to the cook who makes them and to the diner who enjoys the refreshing and comforting pleasures that they provide. Soup is satisfying and makes you feel full quickly—it is great to eat when you've come to the table ravenous. Soups are a wonderful and healthful way to start a meal, or they can be enjoyed as the main entrée.

Through *Conscious Cuisine* you will learn how to successfully prepare soups, chowders, stews, and consommés from quality ingredients. Preparing fresh soups is a gratifying way to enjoy seasonal whole foods that are vibrant with flavor and nutritional value. It is also a convenient way to use up scraps and leftover fruits, vegetables, grains, and proteins. Try the hearty Vegetarian Chili, the revised classics of Onion Soup Nouveau and Clam Chowder, and the beautiful Eclipse Soup—a duet of spicy Black Bean Soup and seasonal Butternut Squash Soup. Use these as models for endless possibilities of soups made consciously.

If you enjoy cream-style soups, you'll see that they can be prepared in a healthful manner by utilizing potatoes and grains that, when pureed, produce a smooth, creamy consistency and light color, eliminating the need for a roux.

Soups, served hot or cold, are tremendously versatile. They provide the opportunity to enjoy a variety of colorful ingredients, subtle aromas, and complex flavors and textures all in one glorious spoonful. The soothing character of soups entices us to slow down and savor the unique seasoning of spices and herbs, the silky smoothness of pureed soups, the chewiness of chowders, or the satisfaction of an intensely flavored consommé.

Vegetable Stock

I find this stock indispensable for many recipes. It is naturally fat-free and full of flavor. Vegetable stock is an excellent source of flavor for soups, for braising meats and vegetables, or for preparing sauces and even salad dressings. Vegetable stocks can be made with a dominant single flavor such as mushroom, fennel, or carrot, or can be light and balanced in flavor from multiple ingredients, such as in this recipe.

Ingredients
Makes 8 cups.

1 1/2 teaspoons dried parsley
1 1/2 teaspoons dried thyme
1 1/2 teaspoons dried oregano
1 tablespoon black peppercorns
3 medium onions, chopped
2 celery ribs, chopped (no leaves)
3 medium carrots, chopped
1 medium leek, chopped
10 medium mushrooms, quartered
2 tomatoes, quartered
4 garlic cloves, halved
1 small fennel bulb, chopped, optional
About 2 quarts filtered water

Preparation

Place the herbs and peppercorns in a 10-inch piece of cheesecloth and tie with a 3-inch piece of butcher's twine to make a sachet; this makes removing them much easier.

Heat a large stockpot over medium heat and add the vegetables. Cook, stirring occasionally to prevent scorching, until the vegetables are softened, 3 to 5 minutes. Add the herb sachet to the stockpot and enough water to cover the vegetables. Bring to a boil, reduce heat, and simmer uncovered for 2 hours, skimming off impurities as needed.

Strain the stock through a colander lined with cheesecloth or a fine mesh strainer.

Use the stock immediately or cool down in an ice bath. The stock will keep for up to 1 week in an airtight container in the refrigerator or up to 1 month in the freezer.

Thickened Vegetable Stock

To eliminate or drastically reduce the amount of oil used to make salad dressings, I thicken vegetable stock to the consistency of oil and replace the oil with the cool stock. Thickened vegetable stock can provide the volume for a dressing or vinaigrette without adding excess fat, and the neutral flavors marry well with high-quality vinegars, herbs, fruits, and vegetables. A splash of high-quality oil can be added at the end to season the dressing and to add a boost of flavor.

Ingredients
Makes 2 cups.

2 cups Vegetable Stock (see page 152)
4 tablespoons cornstarch mixed with
   4 tablespoons Vegetable Stock or water

Preparation

In a medium saucepan, bring the stock to a rolling boil. Whisk in the cornstarch mixture and boil, whisking constantly, until the mixture is smooth and the consistency of thick oil.

Cool the thickened stock in an ice bath. Cover and refrigerate for at least 1 hour before using. Stir well before each use.

The thickened stock will keep for up to 1 week in an airtight container in the refrigerator.

Chicken Stock

This is the mother of all stocks. In some cultures, the use of chicken soup as "penicillin" dates back to the twelfth century. There is medical evidence to support the fact that consuming chicken soup can relieve the symptoms of a variety of illnesses, including the common cold. The nutrients found in chicken bones, paired with vegetables, have an anti-inflammatory effect that can relieve the symptoms of upper respiratory tract infections. The photo at the right is of assorted stocks.

Ingredients
Makes 2 quarts.

2 garlic cloves, halved
1 bay leaf
1 tablespoon dried thyme
1 teaspoon dried tarragon
2 tablespoons whole black peppercorns
4 large onions, chopped
2 celery ribs, chopped (no leaves)
1 medium leek (white part only), chopped
3 pounds chicken bones or 3 carcasses, thoroughly washed, excess fat removed
About 3 quarts filtered water

Preparation
Place the garlic, herbs, and peppercorns in a 10-inch piece of cheesecloth and tie with a 3-inch piece of butcher's twine to make a sachet; this makes removing them much easier.

Heat a large stockpot over medium heat and add the vegetables. Cook, stirring occasionally to prevent scorching, until the vegetables are softened, 3 to 5 minutes. Stir in the chicken bones and herb sachet. Add enough water to cover the bones and the vegetables. Bring contents to a boil, reduce heat, and simmer uncovered for 4 hours. Use a slotted spoon to skim off any impurities, such as foam and fat, throughout the cooking process.

Strain stock through a colander lined with cheesecloth or through a fine mesh strainer, discarding the bones and vegetables.

Use the stock immediately or cool down in an ice bath. The stock will keep for up to 1 week in an airtight container in the refrigerator or up to 1 month in the freezer.

Variation
Turkey Stock: Substitute turkey bones or carcasses for the chicken.

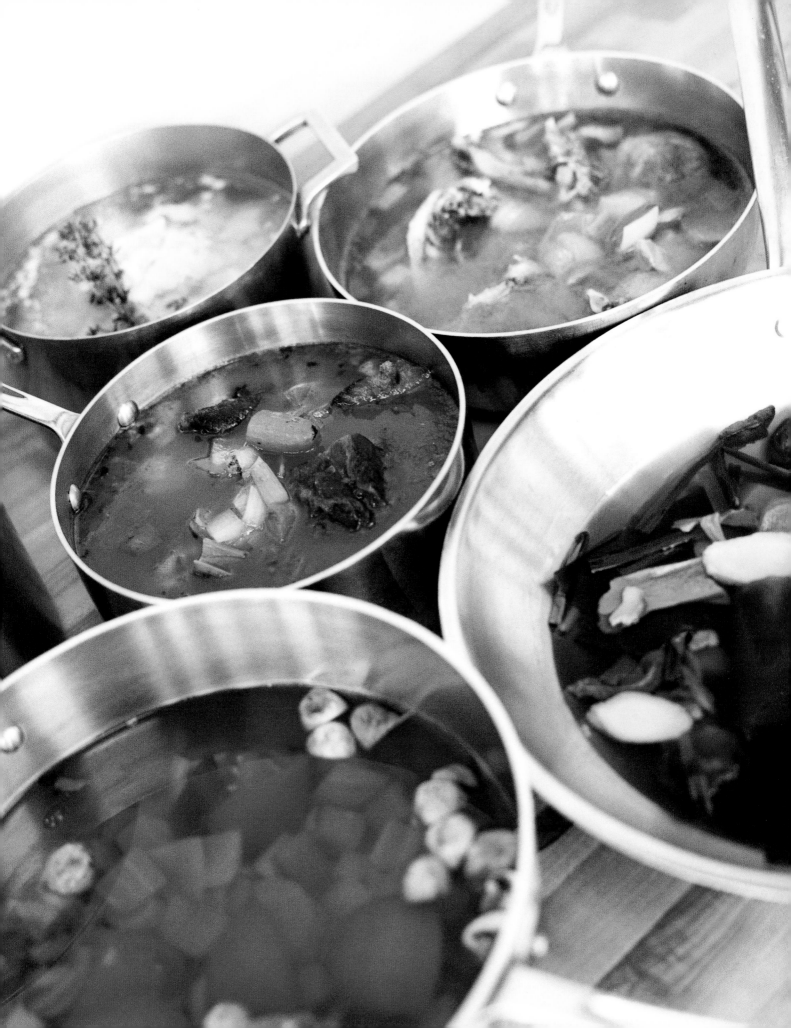

Asian Stock

You will love this stock; it provides a fragrant and complex flavor profile for building Asian-style soups, sauces, and hot pots. Kombu seaweed is not essential to the recipe, but it adds a wonderful flavor and minerals to the stock. Kombu can be purchased at Asian grocery stores; it also is used to cook dried beans.

Ingredients
Makes 3 cups.

8 dried shiitake or black mushrooms,
    rinsed
6 green onions, cut into 3 pieces
2 medium carrots, peeled and cut into
    3 pieces
3 cups filtered water
3/4 teaspoon sea salt (divided)
1/4-inch piece kombu seaweed
2 teaspoons tamari (soy) sauce
1/4 teaspoon raw cane sugar
1 teaspoon sake or white wine
1/2 teaspoon toasted sesame oil

Preparation

In a medium saucepan, combine the mushrooms, onions, carrots, and water. Add 1/2 teaspoon of the salt. Cover and simmer over low heat for 30 minutes. Add the kombu and simmer until stock has a medium brown color, about 5 minutes.

Strain the stock through a colander lined with cheesecloth or a fine mesh strainer. Stir in the remaining 1/4 teaspoon salt, tamari, sugar, sake, and toasted sesame oil.

Use the stock immediately or cool down in an ice bath. The stock will keep for up to 1 week in an airtight container in the refrigerator or up to 1 month in the freezer.

Fish Stock

Per 1 cup:
Calories 80; Protein 3g; Total Fat 0g; Saturated Fat 0g; Carbohydrates 8g; Dietary Fiber 0g; Cholesterol 5mg; Sodium 40mg

Do not throw out the bones from bass, sole, snapper, or other white fish—use them to prepare this simple, flavor-packed broth. You can also ask your local fish market for bones—just be sure they are from white fish, not from stronger fish such as salmon. This stock is invaluable for preparing seafood soups, stocks, and sauces.

Ingredients
Makes 2 quarts.

4 garlic cloves, halved
1 bay leaf
1/4 bunch fresh thyme (about 6 stems)
1/4 bunch parsley (about 6 stems)
1/4 bunch fresh tarragon (about 6 stems)
1 tablespoon fresh black peppercorns
2 medium onions, chopped
1 medium leek (white part only), chopped
2 ribs celery, chopped (no leaves)
1 medium fennel bulb, chopped
5 pounds white fish bones, chopped and
    washed well
About 3 quarts filtered water
2 cups white wine

Preparation
Place the garlic, herbs, and peppercorns in a 10-inch piece of cheesecloth and tie with a 3-inch piece of butcher's twine to make a sachet; this makes removing them much easier.

Heat a large stockpot over medium heat and add the vegetables. Cook, stirring occasionally to prevent scorching, until the vegetables are softened, 3 to 5 minutes. Stir in the fish bones, water, wine, and herb sachet. Bring to a boil, reduce heat, and simmer uncovered for 45 minutes. Use a slotted spoon to skim off any impurities, such as foam and fat, throughout the cooking process.

Strain the stock through a colander lined with cheesecloth or a fine mesh strainer, discarding the bones and vegetables.

Use the stock immediately or cool down in an ice bath. The stock will keep for up to 1 week in an airtight container in the refrigerator or up to 1 month in the freezer.

Variation
To produce a strong glacé (glacé de poisson), simmer slowly until the strained fish stock is reduced to one-fourth of its original volume. This is easy to store and freeze and is a great flavor enhancer.

Veal Stock

Rich, aromatic, versatile, and indispensable is a good description of veal stock to a chef. This dark brown meat broth is used to create countless sauces, stews, and braised entrées. I have always simmered the stock for twenty-four hours. This produces a deeply flavorful *fond de veau* or "stock of veal."

Ingredients
Makes 2 gallons.

10 pounds veal neck and knuckle bones
3 cups burgundy wine
1 tablespoon dried thyme
1 bay leaf
1 tablespoon dried tarragon
1 tablespoon dried rosemary
1 tablespoon black peppercorns, crushed
4 medium onions, peeled and chopped
6 medium carrots, peeled and chopped
3 celery ribs, chopped (no leaves)
2 medium leeks, chopped
12 garlic cloves, halved
25 mushrooms, quartered
1 cup tomato paste
3 gallons cold water

Preparation
Preheat the oven to 375°F (190°C).

Rinse the bones and place in a roasting pan. Roast the bones in the oven for about 1 hour or until a deep brown color. Using tongs, remove the bones from the pan and place in a large bowl.

Add the wine to the roasting pan (deglaze) and scrape up the browned bits and sediments from the bottom of the pan. Reserve this wine mixture.

Place the herbs and peppercorns in a 10-inch piece of cheesecloth and tie with a 3-inch piece of butcher's twine to make a sachet; this makes removing them much easier.

Heat a large stockpot over medium heat and add the vegetables. Cook, stirring occasionally to prevent scorching, until the vegetables are softened, 3 to 5 minutes. Add the browned veal bones, wine mixture, and herb sachet. Stir in the tomato paste and water.

Bring the stock to a boil, reduce heat, and simmer for 24 hours. Use a slotted spoon to skim off any impurities, such as foam and fat, throughout the cooking process. As the stock cooks, check the water level periodically. You will need to add additional cold water to maintain the volume of liquid in the stockpot.

You may cook the stock in intervals if leaving the pot on the heat for 24 hours is not an option. Remove the stock from the heat and cool down completely in a ice bath between each cooking period. Then bring the stock to a boil again, reduce heat, and simmer; continue until cooking time is complete.

Strain the stock through a colander lined with cheesecloth or a fine mesh strainer, discarding the bones and vegetables.

Use the stock immediately or cool down in an ice bath. The stock will keep for up to 1 week in an airtight container in the refrigerator or up to 1 month in the freezer.

Veal Glacé

A glacé is a stock that has been reduced until highly concentrated. The reduced volume makes it convenient to store these flavor enhancers for future use. Pour the reduced stock into plastic freezer bags and lay flat to freeze into thin, stackable packs. Another great way to store glacés is in plastic ice cube trays. This provides convenient individual cubes of concentrated stock that can be used as is to add a burst of flavor to a dish or diluted with water to create an instant stock.

Ingredients
Makes 1 1/2 quarts.

3 quarts Veal Stock (see page 158)

Preparation
In a large stockpot, bring the stock to a boil. Reduce heat and simmer until the stock is reduced by half. Use to make sauces or stews.

Variations
Vegetable Glacé: Reduce 3 quarts Vegetable Stock (see page 152) to 1 1/2 quarts.

Per 2 tablespoons:
Calories 10; Protein 0g; Total Fat 0g; Saturated Fat 0g; Carbohydrates 3g; Dietary Fiber 0g; Cholesterol 0mg; Sodium 5mg

Chicken Glacé: Reduce 3 quarts Chicken Stock (see page 154) to 1 1/2 quarts.

Per 2 tablespoons:
Calories 10; Protein 1g; Total Fat 0g; Saturated Fat 0g; Carbohydrates 2g; Dietary Fiber 0g; Cholesterol 105mg; Sodium 0mg

Fish Glacé: Reduce 2 quarts Fish Stock (see page 157) to 1 quart.

Per 1 cup:
Calories 15; Protein 1g; Total Fat 0g; Saturated Fat 0g; Carbohydrates 1g; Dietary Fiber 0g; Cholesterol 75mg; Sodium 5mg

Cream of Asparagus Soup

Springtime brings us the fresh flavor and color of bright green (and white) spears of asparagus. Using vegetable stock instead of chicken stock makes this a vegetarian recipe. Potatoes are used for thickening; they give this lovely soup a silky smooth consistency and a creamy pastel color.

Ingredients

Makes 6 1-cup servings.

1/4 teaspoon extra-virgin olive oil
1 cup diced yellow onion (about 1 large)
1/2 cup chopped celery (1 medium rib)
4 cups chopped, peeled asparagus (about 2 pounds)
1/2 teaspoon minced garlic
1 bay leaf
1 teaspoon fresh thyme
3 cups diced, peeled potatoes
4 cups Vegetable Stock (see page 152)
1/2 teaspoon grated nutmeg
1 teaspoon sea salt
1/4 teaspoon freshly ground black pepper

Preparation

Heat a medium stockpot over medium-high heat. Add the olive oil to lightly coat the bottom of the pan. Add the onion, celery, and asparagus. Cook until the asparagus is bright green, about 2 minutes. Add the garlic and cook 1 minute. Stir in the bay leaf, thyme, and potatoes. Add enough of the stock to cover the vegetables. Bring to a boil. Reduce heat and simmer until the potatoes are soft, 20 to 25 minutes. Add the nutmeg, salt, and pepper. Remove the bay leaf.

Carefully ladle the soup into a blender and process until pureed and smooth. Strain through a fine mesh strainer or colander lined with cheesecloth to remove any asparagus strings. Return the strained soup to a pan over low heat. Taste and adjust the seasoning with additional salt, pepper, and nutmeg, if desired. Add a little more stock or water to give the soup a creamy consistency if it seems too thick.

Variation

Add sautéed, fresh morel mushrooms to the finished soup for a magnificent garnish and upscale presentation.

Artichoke Soup

Per serving:
Calories 120; Protein 5g; Total Fat 0g;
Saturated Fat 0g; Carbohydrates 27g; Dietary
Fiber 7g; Cholesterol 0mg; Sodium 180mg

Fresh artichokes are a summertime favorite. If time doesn't permit the preparation of fresh artichokes (see Chef's Tip below), this recipe also works well with canned or frozen artichokes.

Ingredients
Makes 8 1-cup servings.

1/4 teaspoon extra-virgin olive oil
4 cups fresh, frozen, or canned,
    water-packed artichoke hearts,
    quartered
1 cup diced yellow onion (about 1 large)
1 cup chopped celery (3 medium ribs)
2 teaspoons minced garlic
3 cups chopped, peeled potatoes
1 bay leaf
1/2 teaspoon dried thyme
1 teaspoon dried oregano
4 cups Vegetable Stock (see page 152)
1/4 teaspoon sea salt
1/4 teaspoon freshly ground black pepper

Preparation

Heat a medium stockpot over medium-high heat. Add the olive oil to lightly coat the bottom of the pan. Add the artichokes, onion, and celery. Cook until the onion has softened, about 2 minutes. Add the garlic and cook 1 minute. Stir in the potatoes, bay leaf, thyme, and oregano. Add enough stock to cover the vegetables and bring to a boil. Reduce heat and simmer until the potatoes are soft, 20 to 25 minutes. Season with the salt and pepper. Remove the bay leaf.

Carefully ladle the soup into a blender and process until pureed and smooth. Strain the soup through a fine mesh strainer or a colander lined with cheesecloth to remove any pulp. Return the strained soup to a pan over low heat. Taste and adjust the seasoning. Add a little more stock or water to give the soup a creamy consistency if it seems too thick.

Variation

I love to stir fresh, sliced truffles into this soup right before serving for a dramatic flavor combination.

Chef's Tip: *To cook fresh artichokes, first remove the stems and all the tough outer leaves. Simmer the artichokes in water seasoned with lemon, thyme, bay leaves, and peppercorns until the bottoms are fork-tender, about 30 minutes. Cool the artichokes in the cooking liquid and spoon out the hairy chokes. Cut the hearts into quarters.*

Black Bean Soup

Per serving:
Calories 200; Protein 11g; Total Fat 1.5g;
Saturated Fat 0g; Carbohydrates 37g; Dietary
Fiber 11g; Cholesterol 0mg; Sodium 160mg

Hearty, satisfying, and complex, aromatics and chiles make this soup a classic in Latin and southwestern-style food. I prefer to strain the soup and use the resulting bean and vegetable pulp as a delicious dip or spread. Photo on page 164.

Ingredients

Makes 5 1-cup servings.

1/4 teaspoon extra-virgin olive oil
1/2 cup diced yellow onion (about
   1 medium)
1/2 cup diced celery (1 medium rib)
1/2 cup diced carrot
1 teaspoon minced garlic
3 cups canned black beans
   (2 15-ounce cans, drained and rinsed)
1 tablespoon chopped jalapeño chile
   (with seeds)
1 bay leaf
1/2 teaspoon dried thyme
1/2 teaspoon ground cumin
1/2 teaspoon ground coriander
4 cups Vegetable Stock (see page 152)
1/4 cup chile sauce
1/4 cup chopped fresh cilantro
1/4 teaspoon sea salt
1/4 teaspoon freshly ground black pepper

Preparation

Heat a medium stockpot over medium-high heat. Add the olive oil to lightly coat the bottom of the pan. Add the onion, celery, carrot, garlic, and beans. Cook until the onion has softened, about 2 minutes. Add the jalapeño, bay leaf, thyme, cumin, and coriander. Cook 1 minute. Add the stock and chile sauce. Bring to a boil. Reduce heat and simmer for 30 minutes. Stir in the cilantro, salt, and pepper. Remove the bay leaf.

Carefully ladle the soup into a blender and process until pureed and smooth. Strain the soup through a fine mesh strainer or a colander lined with cheesecloth to remove any bean pulp. Return the strained soup to a pan over low heat. Taste and adjust the seasoning. Add a little more stock or water to give the soup a creamy consistency if it seems too thick.

Butternut Squash Soup

Per serving:
Calories 120; Protein 3g; Total Fat 1g;
Saturated Fat 0g; Carbohydrates 30g; Dietary
Fiber 8g; Cholesterol 0mg; Sodium 290mg

Although it has a high sugar content, butternut squash is a healthful carbohydrate. This wonderfully sweet fall vegetable should be a staple in every kitchen. If you have whole nutmeg, grate some on top of this soup for an aromatic and delicious touch that will warm up the winter. Photo on page 164.

Ingredients

Makes 5 1-cup servings.

1/4 teaspoon extra-virgin olive oil
4 to 5 cups diced, peeled butternut squash
1 cup chopped yellow onion (about
    1 large)
1 cup chopped celery (3 medium ribs)
1 bay leaf
4 cups Vegetable Stock (see page 152)
2 tablespoons minced fresh oregano
1/4 teaspoon ground nutmeg
1/2 teaspoon sea salt
1/4 teaspoon freshly ground black pepper

Preparation

Heat a medium stockpot over medium-high heat. Add the olive oil to lightly coat the bottom of the pan. Add the squash, onion, and celery. Cook until the onion has softened, about 2 minutes. Add the bay leaf and cook for 2 minutes. Add enough of the stock to cover the vegetables and bring to a boil. Reduce heat and simmer until the squash is very soft, 20 to 25 minutes. Stir in the oregano, nutmeg, salt, and pepper. Remove the bay leaf.

Carefully ladle the soup into a blender and process until pureed and smooth. Strain through a fine mesh strainer or a colander lined with cheesecloth to remove any squash pulp. Return the strained soup to a pan over low heat. Taste and adjust the seasoning with additional salt, pepper, and nutmeg, if desired. Add a little more stock or water to give the soup a creamy consistency if it seems too thick.

Eclipse Soup

Per serving:
Calories 160; Protein 7g; Total Fat 1g;
Saturated Fat 0g; Carbohydrates 34g; Dietary
Fiber 10g; Cholesterol 0g; Sodium 250mg

Create a culinary masterpiece by serving Black Bean Soup and Butternut Squash Soup side by side in the same bowl. The appealing color contrast of bright gold with shiny black is surpassed only by the contrast of the black beans' spiciness with the natural sweetness of the butternut squash. I serve this soup with a dollop of Red Pepper Puree to represent an eclipse of the sun. It's as much fun for you to see your guests sit in awe of the beautiful presentation as it is for them to decide how to eat this magnificent combination.

Ingredients
Makes 1 serving.

1/2 cup Black Bean Soup (see page 162)
1/2 cup Butternut Squash Soup (see page 163)
1 tablespoon Red Pepper Puree (see page 36)

Preparation
Simultaneously ladle the two soups into opposite sides of a soup plate or bowl. Spoon the red pepper puree into the center. Using a wooden skewer or toothpick, pull the red pepper puree into the soups to resemble the sun's rays.

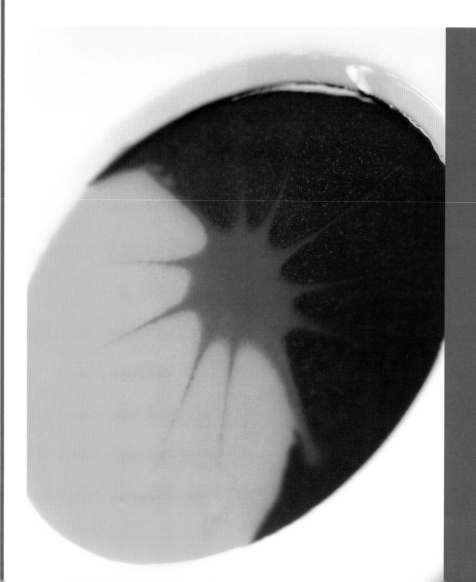

Vegetarian Chili

Per serving:
Calories 150; Protein 6g; Total Fat 1g;
Saturated Fat 0g; Carbohydrates 32g; Dietary
Fiber 8g; Cholesterol 0mg; Sodium 410mg

Three types of beans, diced vegetables, and oven-toasted barley make this chili a hearty meal and a sensational treat for lunch or dinner. Vegetarian Chili has had the honor of being Miraval's most requested recipe from the first day that we opened our doors. When making it at home, I use canned beans to shorten the preparation time.

Ingredients

Makes 16 1-cup servings.

1/4 teaspoon extra-virgin olive oil
*1 cup chopped yellow onion (about
    1 large)*
1 cup chopped celery (3 medium ribs)
*1 cup chopped, peeled carrot (about
    2 medium)*
1 teaspoon minced garlic
1 cup chopped green bell pepper
1 cup fresh or frozen corn kernels
*1 28-ounce can diced, stewed tomatoes,
    undrained*
*1 1/2 cups cooked pinto beans, drained,
    rinsed (1 15-ounce can)*
*1 1/2 cups cooked red kidney beans,
    drained, rinsed (1 15-ounce can)*
*1 1/2 cups cooked black beans, drained,
    rinsed (1 15-ounce can)*
1/2 cup toasted barley (see page 194)
1/2 teaspoon cayenne powder
1 tablespoon chile powder
1/2 teaspoon ground cumin
1 teaspoon ground coriander
1 bay leaf
1 teaspoon dried basil
2 teaspoons dried oregano
1 teaspoon sea salt
1/2 teaspoon freshly ground black pepper
3 5.5-ounce cans tomato juice or V8
6 cups Vegetable Stock (see page 152)
1 cup chopped zucchini
1 cup chopped yellow squash

Preparation

Heat a medium stockpot over medium-high heat. Add the olive oil to lightly coat the bottom of the pan. Add the onion, celery, carrot, garlic, and bell pepper. Cook until the onion has softened, about 2 minutes.

Stir in the corn, tomatoes, beans, barley, spices, herbs, salt, pepper, tomato juice, and stock. Bring to a boil. Reduce heat and simmer for 20 to 25 minutes. Stir in the zucchini and yellow squash. Taste and adjust the seasoning with additional salt, pepper, and chile powder, if desired.

The chili will keep for up to 3 days in an airtight container in the refrigerator or up to 1 month in the freezer. If stored in the refrigerator, you may need to add additional water or stock to reheat the chili because the beans and barley will soak up some of the liquid as it sits.

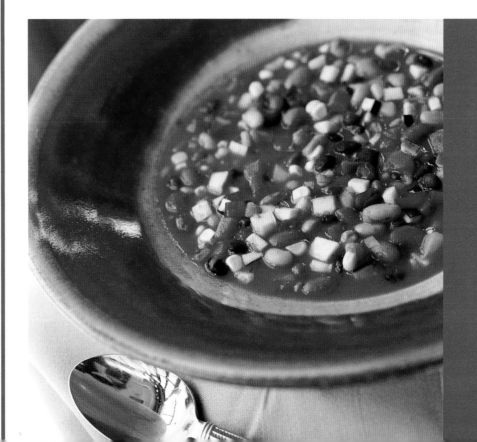

Sweet Corn, Barley, and Bean Soup

This comforting soup is not only complex in flavor and texture, but also loaded with nutrients. Sorrel is a dark, triangular leafy green that is tart when enjoyed raw and slightly sour when cooked. Stir into cooked soup to add a delicate flavor; if sorrel is not available, use spinach, kale, napa cabbage, or Swiss chard.

Ingredients

Makes 8 1-cup servings.

1/4 teaspoon extra-virgin olive oil
1 cup chopped yellow onion (about
  1 large)
1/2 cup chopped celery (1 medium rib)
1/2 cup chopped carrot
1 teaspoon minced garlic
2 cups fresh or frozen corn kernels
1/2 cup toasted barley (see page 194)
1/2 teaspoon dried basil
1/2 teaspoon dried marjoram
1 bay leaf
8 cups Vegetable Stock (see page 152)
1 1/2 cups cooked navy beans, drained,
  rinsed (1 15-ounce can)
1 cup julienned sorrel, spinach, kale, napa
  cabbage, or Swiss chard
1/2 teaspoon sea salt
1/2 teaspoon freshly ground black pepper

Preparation

Heat a medium stockpot over medium-high heat. Add the olive oil to lightly coat the bottom of the pan. Add the onion, celery, carrot, and garlic. Cook until the onion has softened, about 2 minutes. Stir in the corn, barley, herbs, bay leaf, and stock. Bring to a boil. Reduce heat and simmer until the barley is softened, 20 to 25 minutes.

Remove the bay leaf. Mix in the beans and sorrel and season with the salt and pepper. Heat through and serve.

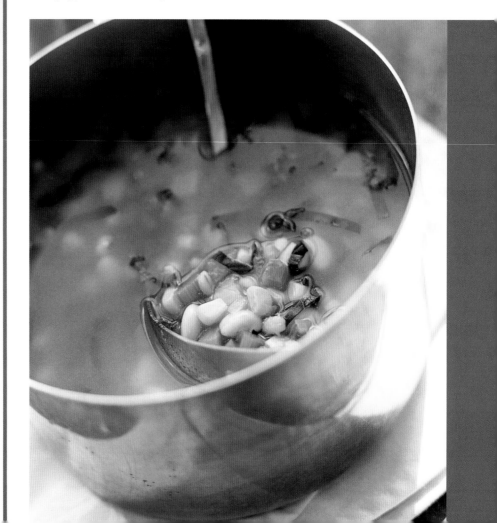

Miso Soup

Light, quick, easy to make, and packed with nutrients and complex flavors, there is no wonder why the delicacy of miso soup has been enjoyed by the sophisticated palettes of Asian communities for centuries.

Ingredients
Makes 8 1-cup servings.

1/4 cup dried arame seaweed
6 1/2 cups water (divided)
1 cup diced firm tofu (12 ounces, drained)
1/2 teaspoon minced garlic
1/2 teaspoon minced fresh ginger
1/2 cup sliced, peeled carrot (1 medium)
2 green onions, chopped
1 cup chopped greens, tightly packed
*   (Swiss chard, kale, mustard, or Chinese*
*   cabbage)*
3 tablespoons red miso paste
3 tablespoons tamari (soy) sauce

Preparation
In a small bowl, soak the arame in 1/2 cup of the water for about 5 minutes. Drain the arame and chop into 1/2-inch pieces. Divide the arame and diced tofu among 8 serving bowls.

In a medium saucepan, bring the remaining 6 cups of water to a low boil. Add the garlic, ginger, and carrot. Reduce heat and simmer just until the carrot starts to soften, about 5 minutes. Add the green onions and greens and cook 1 minute. Remove from heat and add the miso and tamari, stirring gently to dissolve the miso. Let rest for 2 minutes, then pour the soup into the prepared bowls and serve.

Variations
Try adding diced potato and shiitake mushrooms to the above recipe. Experiment with other vegetable combinations, such as substituting wakame for the arame seaweed, turnips for the carrots, or leeks for the green onions.

Tomato-Roasted Garlic Soup

Per 1 cup:
Calories 130; Protein 5g; Total Fat 1g;
Saturated Fat 0g; Carbohydrates 32g; Dietary
Fiber 5g; Cholesterol 0mg; Sodium 1060mg

Ingredients
Makes 4 1-cup servings.

1/4 teaspoon extra-virgin olive oil
1 bulb Roasted Garlic, about 10 medium
   cloves (see page 38)
1 cup chopped yellow onion (about
   1 large)
1 cup chopped celery (3 medium ribs)
2 28-ounce cans diced, stewed tomatoes,
   undrained
1 bay leaf
2 teaspoons dried basil
1 teaspoon dried oregano
1 teaspoon dried thyme
1/2 teaspoon sea salt
1/2 teaspoon freshly ground black pepper

As a child growing up on the south side of Chicago, a piping hot bowl of Campbell's tomato soup and a sandwich was my favorite lunch during the cold Chicago winters. For my first soup-skills test at Washburne Trade School, I developed a tomato soup that I felt was a notch above Campbell's. My classmates and I were sure that I beat out Campbell's for the title of tomato soup champion. However, my instructor, Wally Lebin, thought it was good but fell short of an *A+*. Ever since, I've sought that elusive tomato soup title. I'm sure you will agree that this soup, with its earthy flavors of roasted garlic and zesty fresh herbs, has finally earned me the crown of new champion soup-maker.

Preparation
Heat a medium stockpot over medium-high heat. Add the olive oil to lightly coat the bottom of the pan. Add the garlic, onion, and celery. Cook until the onion has softened, about 3 minutes. Stir in the tomatoes and herbs. Bring to a boil. Reduce heat and simmer for 12 to 15 minutes, skimming off any foam that comes to the surface. Remove the bay leaf. Season with the salt and pepper, and heat through.

Carefully ladle the soup into a blender and process until smooth.

Exotic Mushroom and Millet Soup

Per serving:
Calories 210; Protein 8g; Total Fat 2g;
Saturated Fat 0g; Carbohydrates 38g; Dietary
Fiber 7g; Cholesterol 0 mg; Sodium 390mg

Mushrooms are one of my favorite foods—they add a rustic flavor and texture to appetizers, salads, entrées, and soups. I relish choosing among the bountiful variety of flavors, shapes, and colors that mushrooms offer, whether domestic, exotic, or wild. This soup calls for three of the most commonly used exotic mushrooms.

Toasted millet is used to thicken the soup instead of a roux; its earthy and nutty flavor adds complexity to the soup, plus a boost of vitamin B, copper, and iron.

Ingredients

Makes 7 1-cup servings.

1 cup millet
1/4 teaspoon extra-virgin olive oil
1 cup chopped yellow onion (about
    1 large)
1 cup chopped celery (3 medium ribs)
1 teaspoon minced garlic
2 cups packed, sliced shiitake mushrooms
    (7 ounces)
2 cups packed, sliced oyster mushrooms
    (7 ounces)
3 cups packed, sliced portobello mush-
    rooms, gills removed (about 3 large
    mushrooms)
2 teaspoons dried thyme
1 bay leaf
7 cups Vegetable Stock (see page 152)
1 teaspoon sea salt
1/2 teaspoon freshly ground black pepper

Garnish
Enoki mushrooms and chives, optional

Preparation

In a large sauté pan, toast the millet over medium heat until it is one shade darker and there is a popcorn smell, 3 to 5 minutes. Remove from the heat and set aside.

Heat a medium stockpot over medium-high heat. Add the olive oil to lightly coat the bottom of the pan. Add the onion, celery, garlic, and half of each type of mushroom. Cook until the onion has softened and the mushrooms have started to release their juices. Add the remaining mushrooms and cook 2 minutes.

Add the millet, thyme, and bay leaf. Stir in the stock and simmer until the millet has softened, about 20 minutes. Remove the bay leaf.

Carefully ladle the soup into a blender and process until smooth. Strain the soup through a fine mesh strainer or a colander lined with cheesecloth to remove any pulp. Return the strained soup to a pan, season with salt and pepper, and heat through.

Garnish with enoki mushrooms and chives, if desired.

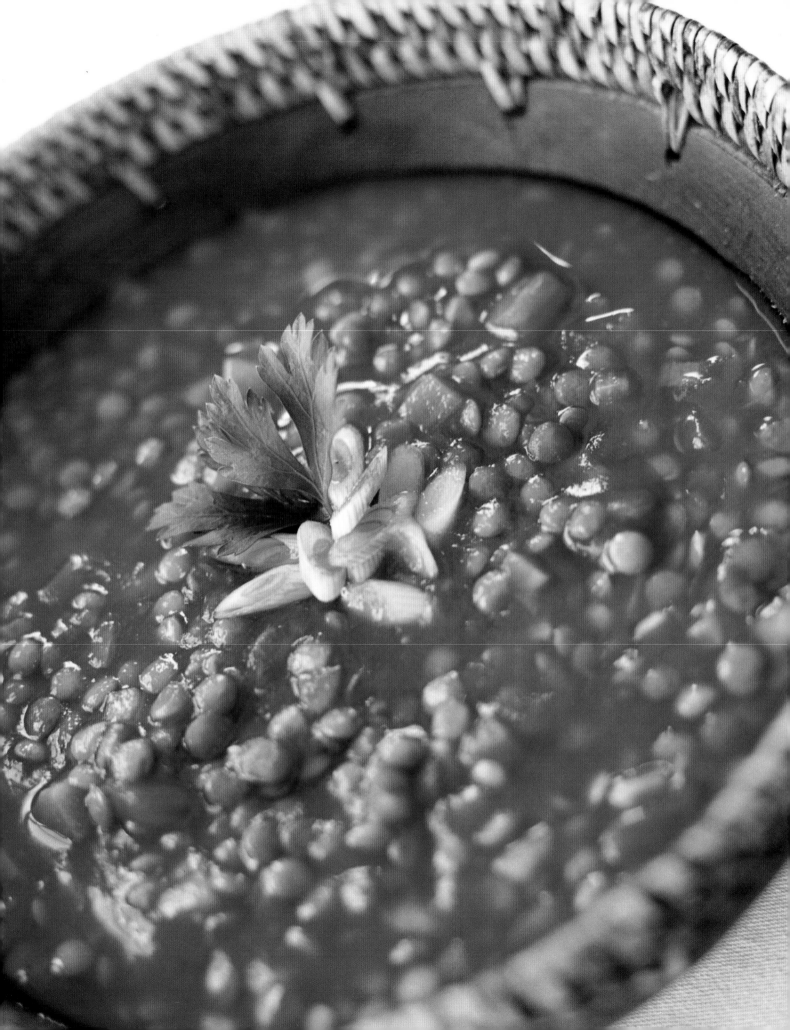

Spicy Lentil Soup

Per serving:
Calories 170; Protein 11g; Total Fat 1g;
Saturated Fat 0g; Carbohydrates 33g; Dietary
Fiber 7g; Cholesterol 0mg; Sodium 400mg

Lentils—of red, brown, or green hue—cook quickly and never require soaking. Lentils are packed with protein, vitamins, and other nutrients. This rich, spicy soup cooks in minutes and works well as an appetizer or as an entrée.

Ingredients

Makes 12 1-cup servings.

1/4 teaspoon extra-virgin olive oil
1 cup chopped yellow onion (about
   1 large)
1 cup chopped, peeled carrot (about
   2 medium)
1 cup chopped celery (3 medium ribs)
1 teaspoon minced garlic
2 cups lentils (about 1 pound), washed
1 28-ounce can diced, stewed tomatoes
   in their juice
8 cups Vegetable Stock (see page 152)
1 bay leaf
1/2 teaspoon cayenne
1 teaspoon chile powder
1/2 teaspoon ground cumin
1 teaspoon paprika
1 teaspoon dried basil
1 teaspoon sea salt
1/2 teaspoon freshly ground black pepper

Preparation

Heat a medium stockpot over medium-high heat. Add the olive oil to lightly coat the bottom of the pan. Add the onion, carrot, celery, and garlic. Cook until the onion has softened, about 2 minutes.

Stir in the lentils, tomatoes, stock, bay leaf, cayenne, chile powder, cumin, paprika, basil, salt, and pepper. Bring to a boil, reduce heat, and simmer until the lentils have softened, about 20 minutes. Remove the bay leaf before serving.

Pear-Parsnip Soup

Per serving:
Calories 260; Protein 5g; Total Fat 1.5g;
Saturated Fat 0g; Carbohydrates 62g; Dietary
Fiber 13g; Cholesterol 0mg; Sodium 340mg

Parsnips are ivory-colored root vegetables that resemble carrots. Their flavor is closer to that of celery, and their nutritional benefits include vitamin C. When parsnips are harvested late in the season, their starch turns to sugar, which produces a luscious, sweet vegetable. I've found that organic parsnips are dependably sweet and flavorful. Even if organic parsnips are not available, the addition of pears in this recipe provides sweetness and a touch of tartness.

Ingredients

Makes 8 1-cup servings.

1/4 teaspoon extra-virgin olive oil

2 cups chopped yellow onion (about 2 large)

9 cups chopped, peeled parsnips (about 4 1/2 pounds)

4 cups chopped, peeled pears (about 6 medium)

3 cups diced, peeled potatoes (about 3/4 pound)

8 to 9 cups Vegetable Stock (see page 152)

1 teaspoon freshly grated nutmeg

2 teaspoons chopped fresh thyme

1 teaspoon sea salt

1/2 teaspoon white pepper

Preparation

Heat a medium stockpot over medium-high heat. Add the olive oil to lightly coat the bottom of the pan. Add the onion, parsnips, pears, and potatoes. Cook until the onion has softened, about 2 minutes. Add the stock and bring to a boil. Reduce heat and simmer until the parsnips and potatoes are soft, 15 to 20 minutes. Stir the nutmeg and thyme into the simmering soup.

Carefully ladle the soup into a blender and process until smooth. Strain the soup through a fine mesh strainer or a colander lined with cheesecloth to remove any pulp. Return the strained soup to a pan and heat through. Season with the salt and white pepper.

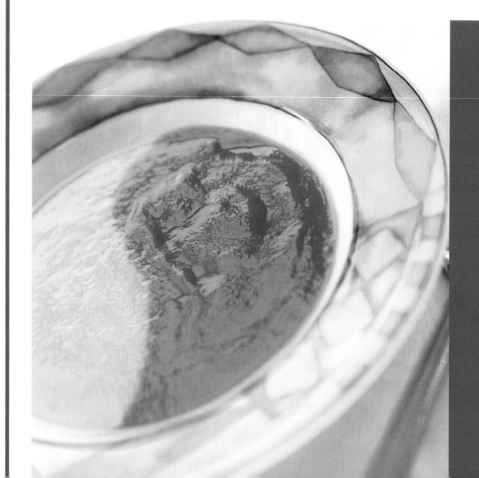

Carrot-Ginger-Apple Soup

I love the sweet, peppery, and refreshing flavors found in carrot-ginger-apple juice and was certain that it would make a fabulous soup. Chef Al Chase, an organic vegetarian chef and founder of the Center of Culinary Awakening in Santa Fe, showed me the clever use of oatmeal in soup. The oatmeal not only provides a wealth of vital nutrients to the soup, it also thickens it and gives it a creamy color and mouth feel. Thanks to Chef Al, I'm culinarily awakened.

Ingredients
Makes 5 1-cup servings.

1/4 teaspoon extra-virgin olive oil
4 cups chopped carrots
1 cup chopped yellow onion (about
    1 large)
1/2 teaspoon minced garlic
1 teaspoon minced fresh ginger
1 1/2 cups chopped, peeled Granny Smith
    apples
5 cups Vegetable Stock (see page 152)
1/2 cup oatmeal
1 teaspoon ground nutmeg
1 teaspoon dried thyme
1/2 teaspoon sea salt
1/4 teaspoon freshly ground pepper

Preparation

Heat a medium stockpot over medium-high heat. Add the olive oil to lightly coat the bottom of the pan. Add the carrots, onion, garlic, ginger, and apples. Cook until the onion has softened, about 2 minutes. Add the remaining ingredients and bring to a boil. Reduce heat and simmer until the carrots are soft, about 20 minutes.

Carefully ladle the soup into a blender and process until smooth. Strain the soup through a fine mesh strainer or a colander lined with cheesecloth to remove pulp. Return the strained soup to a pan and heat through. Taste and adjust the seasoning with additional salt and pepper, if desired. Add a little more stock or water to give the soup a creamy consistency if it seems too thick.

Chef's Tip: *The Pear-Parsnip and Carrot-Ginger-Apple soups are great separate, but make a wonderful fall dish when served together. Simultaneously ladle the two soups into opposite sides of the soup plate or bowl. Photo on page 172.*

Onion Soup Nouveau

The key to good onion soup is to caramelize the onions until they are a dark brown color, releasing as much of the natural sugars as possible. Chefs use various stocks to flavor this soup. A classic preparation is to top the soup with a thick buttered crouton and mounds of melted Gruyère and Parmesan cheeses. Reduced cream may be used to make a rich, creamy version of the classic, creating a wonderful soup that's ridiculously high in fat and calories.

Try this nouveau presentation that pairs the classic look and taste of rich, sweet onions in a dark broth with a delicious, creamy version.

Ingredients

Makes 10 servings of 5 cups Dark Onion Soup and 7 cups Creamy Onion Soup.

Onion Base
1/4 teaspoon extra-virgin olive oil
16 cups julienned yellow onions (about 4 pounds)
1 teaspoon dried thyme
1 tablespoon minced garlic

Creamy Onion Soup
1/2 recipe Onion Base
2 cups chopped, peeled potatoes (1 pound)
1 teaspoon dried thyme
1 bay leaf
1/4 teaspoon freshly ground black pepper
1 cup sherry
1 teaspoon sea salt
4 cups Vegetable Stock (see page 152)

Dark Onion Soup
1/2 recipe Onion Base
1 teaspoon dried thyme
1 bay leaf
1/4 teaspoon freshly ground black pepper
1 cup sherry
1 teaspoon sea salt
4 cups Vegetable Stock (see page 152)

10 Parmesan Crisps (see page 135), to serve

Preparation

For the Onion Base: Heat a medium stockpot over medium heat. Add the olive oil to lightly coat the bottom of the pan. Add the onions and cook until they have caramelized, stirring occasionally, about 15 minutes. Stir in the thyme and garlic. Cook 1 minute. Remove from heat. Divide the onions between two medium saucepans.

For the Creamy Onion Soup: Heat the onion base in a medium saucepan over medium-high heat. Add the potatoes, thyme, bay leaf, and pepper. Stir in the sherry. Boil until the pan is almost dry, about 2 minutes. Add the salt and stock and simmer until the potatoes have softened, about 15 minutes. Remove the bay leaf.

Carefully ladle the soup into a blender and process until smooth. Strain the soup through a fine mesh strainer or a colander lined with cheesecloth to remove pulp. Return the strained soup to a pan and heat through to serve.

For the Dark Onion Soup: Heat the onion base in a medium saucepan over medium-high heat. Add the thyme, bay leaf, and pepper. Stir in the sherry. Boil until the pan is almost dry, about 2 minutes. Add the salt and stock and simmer for 15 minutes. Remove the bay leaf.

To serve: Ladle 1/2 cup of the creamy soup into each bowl. Carefully ladle 1/2 cup of the dark soup into the center of the creamy soup. Serve with a Parmesan Crisp as a garnish.

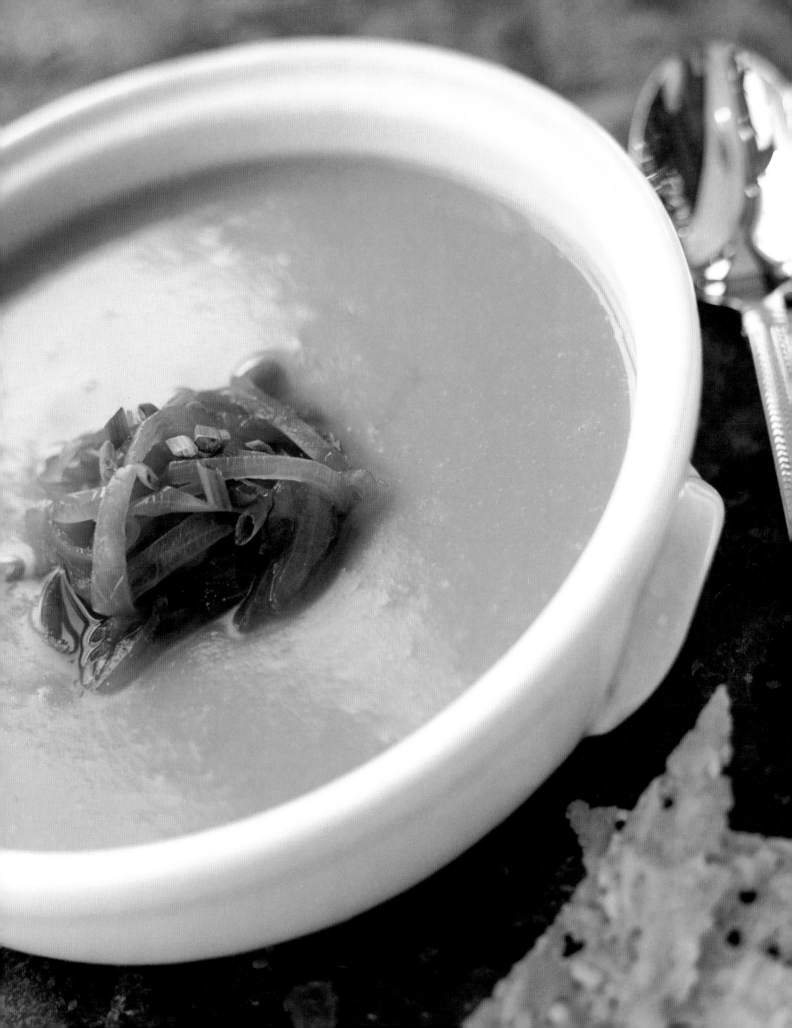

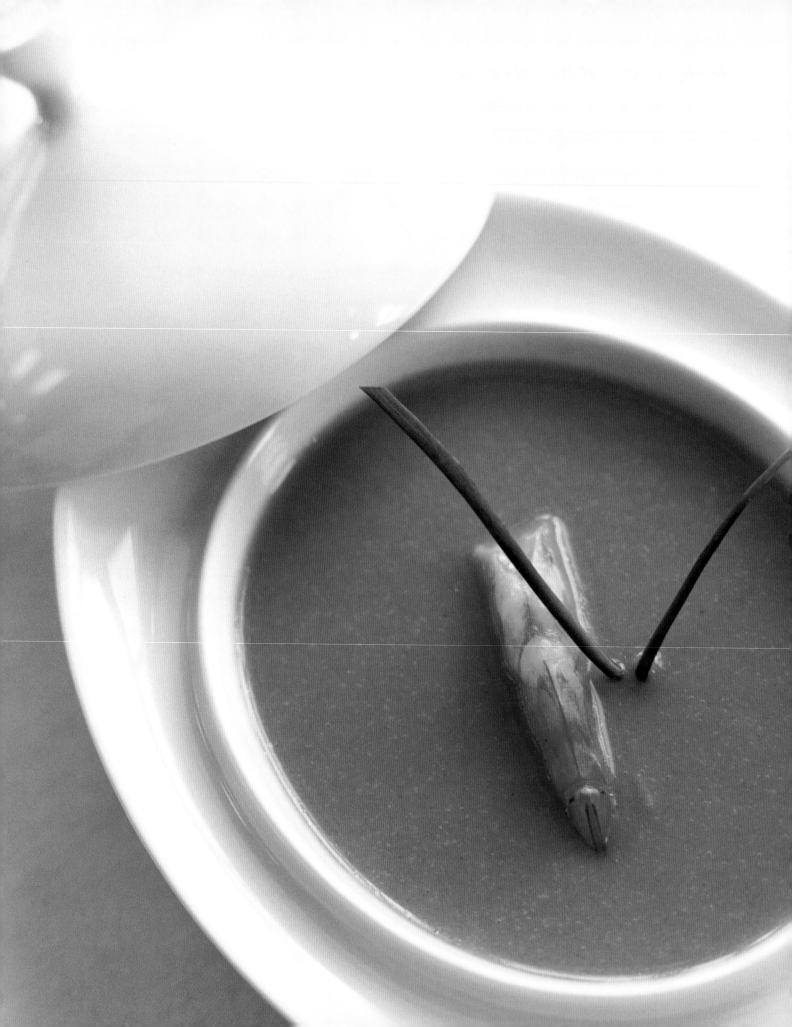

Thai Coconut and Shrimp Bisque

This soup offers a successful marriage of unique ingredients that delivers boldly on flavor, complexity, and satisfaction. Coconut milk is delicious, but high in fat. Using a light version reduces the fat. Arborio rice is prized for its starchy consistency; it is put to work here to thicken the soup. If making a stock is not convenient, I have listed the phone number of More Than Gourmet (see page 326), a company that produces stocks of excellent quality and will ship anywhere across the United States.

Ingredients
Makes 6 1-cup servings.

8 cups Fish Stock (see page 157)
1/4 teaspoon extra-virgin olive oil
2 cups small shrimp with shells
1 cup chopped yellow onion (about
   1 large)
1 cup chopped celery (3 medium ribs)
1/4 cup finely chopped lemongrass
1 teaspoon minced garlic
1 teaspoon minced fresh ginger
1 tablespoon chopped jalapeño chile
1 cup arborio rice
1/4 cup brandy
1/3 cup white wine
1/3 cup tomato paste
1 tablespoon red curry paste
1/4 cup chopped fresh cilantro
1/2 cup reduced-fat coconut milk
1/2 teaspoon sea salt

Garnish
Cooked shrimp and chives, optional

Preparation

In a medium saucepan, bring the stock to a low boil. Reduce heat and let simmer until needed.

Heat a medium stockpot over medium-high heat. Add the olive oil to lightly coat the bottom of the pan. Add shrimp and saute until bright pink. Add the onion, celery, lemongrass, garlic, ginger, and chile. Cook until the onion has softened, about 2 minutes. Add the rice and cook 1 minute.

Carefully pour in the brandy, ignite, and cook until the alcohol has burned off, about 1 or 2 minutes. (Be very careful, the flame may burn high.) Add the wine and boil until the wine is reduced by half, about 3 minutes. Stir in the hot stock, tomato paste, and curry paste. Cook until the rice has softened and absorbed about 1/3 of the liquid, about 20 minutes.

Carefully ladle the soup into a blender and process until smooth. Strain the soup through a fine mesh strainer or a colander lined with cheesecloth to remove any pulp. Return the strained soup to a pan. Stir in the cilantro, coconut milk, and salt. Heat through.

Ladle into bowls and garnish with shrimp and chives, if desired.

Clam Bisque

Per serving:
Calories 190; Protein 18g; Total Fat 2g;
Saturated Fat 0g; Carbohydrates 23g; Dietary
Fiber 3g; Cholesterol 30mg; Sodium 190mg

This smartly prepared soup delivers all the flavor and richness of a classic bisque while eliminating the excess fat and calories. This bisque can also serve as the base for a creamy Clam Chowder (see page 179).

Ingredients

Makes 5 1-cup servings.

6 thyme sprigs
1 bay leaf
1/2 teaspoon whole peppercorns
1/4 teaspoon extra-virgin olive oil
1 cup chopped yellow onion (about
   1 large)
1 teaspoon minced garlic
2 cups chopped, peeled red-skinned or
   Yukon gold potatoes (about 4 medium)
3 8-ounce jars clam juice or 3 cups Fish
   Stock (see page 157)
1 6 1/2-ounce can chopped clams,
   undrained
1/4 teaspoon sea salt
1/8 teaspoon cayenne

Preparation

Place the thyme, bay leaf, and peppercorns in a 10-inch piece of cheesecloth and tie with a 3-inch piece of butcher's twine to make a sachet; this makes removing them much easier.

Heat a medium saucepan over medium-high heat. Add the olive oil to lightly coat the bottom of the pan. Add the onion, garlic, and potatoes. Cook, stirring constantly, until the onion has softened, about 2 minutes. Add the clam juice and the clams with their liquid. Stir in the salt, cayenne, and herb sachet. Bring to a boil, reduce heat, and simmer until the potatoes are tender, about 20 minutes.

Remove the herb sachet. Carefully ladle the potato mixture into a blender and process until smooth and creamy. Return the soup to a saucepan and heat through to serve.

Clam Chowder

Clam chowder has always been one of my favorite soups to make. A true clam chowder has a thin base thickened slightly by the starch from the potatoes that it's cooked with, but I have always enjoyed a thick, rich chowder that's hearty and plentiful with small chunks of vegetables and baby clams.

Per serving:
Calories 260; Protein 25g; Total Fat 3g; Saturated Fat 1g; Carbohydrates 32g; Dietary Fiber 5g; Cholesterol 60mg; Sodium 510mg

Ingredients
Makes 5 servings.

1/4 teaspoon extra-virgin olive oil

3/4 cup chopped yellow onion (about 1 medium)

3/4 cup chopped celery (2 medium ribs)

3/4 cup diced, blanched red-skinned potatoes (about 1/2 pound)

3/4 cup chopped red or yellow bell pepper (1 medium)

1/4 teaspoon minced garlic

1 6 1/2-ounce can whole clams, undrained

1 recipe Clam Bisque (see page 178)

1 bay leaf

1/4 teaspoon sea salt

1/4 teaspoon freshly ground black pepper

1/2 teaspoon chopped fresh thyme

Preparation

Heat a medium stockpot over medium-high heat. Add the olive oil to lightly coat the bottom of the pan. Stir in the onion, celery, potatoes, bell pepper, and garlic. Cook until the onion has softened, about 2 minutes. Add the clams with their liquid, Clam Bisque, and bay leaf. Simmer, stirring occasionally, until the potatoes have softened, about 20 minutes. Remove the bay leaf. Season with the salt, pepper and fresh thyme.

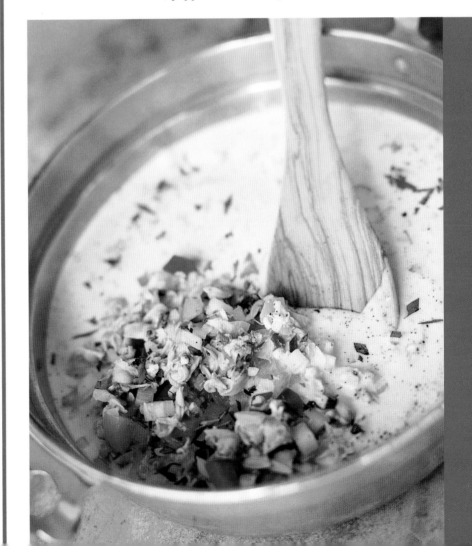

Corn and Oyster Chowder

Per serving:
Calories 210; Protein 9g; Total Fat 3g;
Saturated Fat 0.5g; Carbohydrates 40g; Dietary
Fiber 6g; Cholesterol 35mg; Sodium 320mg

I love the delicate flavor of fresh oysters. Although there is a risk in eating them raw, flash-freezing fresh oysters or thoroughly cooking them will kill any harmful bacteria. Shucked oysters packed in plastic tubs or jars are readily available—I suggest using them and their liquid to add flavor to your stock.

Ingredients

Makes 8 1-cup servings.

Chowder Base

1/4 teaspoon extra-virgin olive oil
2 cups fresh or frozen corn kernels
2 cup chopped, peeled potatoes
1 cup chopped yellow onion (about 1 large)
1/2 cup chopped celery (1 medium rib)
1/2 teaspoon minced garlic
1 teaspoon dried thyme
4 cups Vegetable Stock (see page 152)
1 cup shucked fresh oysters

Chowder

1/4 teaspoon extra-virgin olive oil
1/2 teaspoon minced garlic
1 cup chopped yellow onion (about 1 large)
1 cup chopped celery (3 medium ribs)
1 cup chopped, peeled potatoes (about 1/2 pound)
1/4 cup diced red bell pepper
1/4 cup diced green bell pepper
2 cups fresh or frozen corn kernels
1 cup shucked fresh oysters
1 bay leaf
1 teaspoon dried thyme
1/2 teaspoon sea salt
1/4 teaspoon freshly ground black pepper

Preparation

For the Chowder Base: Heat a medium stockpot over medium-high heat. Add the olive oil to lightly coat the bottom of the pan. Add the corn, potatoes, onion, celery, garlic, and thyme. Cook until the onion has softened, about 2 minutes. Stir in the stock and 1 cup of the oysters and bring to a boil. Reduce heat and simmer until the potatoes are soft, about 20 minutes.

Carefully ladle the soup into a blender and process until smooth. Strain through a fine mesh strainer to remove any pulp. Return the strained soup to a pan and keep warm while the remaining chowder ingredients are prepared.

For the Chowder: Heat a medium stockpot over medium-high heat. Add the olive oil to lightly coat the bottom of the pan. Add the vegetables and cook until the onion has softened, about 3 minutes. Add the oysters, bay leaf, thyme, salt, pepper, and prepared chowder base. Bring to a boil. Reduce heat and simmer until the potatoes are soft, about 20 minutes. Remove bay leaf before serving.

Cilantro and Chicken Consommé

Per serving:
Calories 100; Protein 8g; Total Fat 2.5g;
Saturated Fat 0.5g; Carbohydrates 11g; Dietary
Fiber 1g; Cholesterol 15mg; Sodium 540mg

Ingredients

Makes 7 1-cup servings.

10 cups Chicken Stock (see page 154)
    —or—10 cups water plus 5 tablespoons
    of chicken stock base (see page 326)
3 ounces boneless, skinless chicken breast
1 cup chopped yellow onion (about
    1 large)
1/2 cup chopped celery (1 medium rib)
1/2 cup chopped carrot
1 medium tomato, chopped
2 garlic cloves
4 large egg whites
1 tablespoon fresh thyme
1 bay leaf
1/4 teaspoon black peppercorns, cracked
1/2 cup chopped fresh cilantro
1/2 teaspoon ground coriander
1/2 teaspoon sea salt
1/4 teaspoon white pepper

A consommé is a crystal clear, intensely flavored broth. Consommé has long been viewed as a difficult soup to make; however, it is not complicated. The secret to a successful consommé is to use a good, tasty stock for flavor and egg whites to clarify the soup. Egg whites are combined with finely chopped vegetables and added to the warm stock. They form a solid layer, which chefs call a "raft," to hold the vegetables afloat and to absorb the sediments from the stock. This procedure both flavors and clarifies the consommé. A consommé makes an attractive light starter to any meal.

Preparation

Bring the Chicken Stock (or water and chicken stock base) to a boil in a medium saucepan. Turn the heat down to low to keep the stock just warm. You want to make sure the stock is not too hot because it will cook the eggs too soon; cold stock will cause the eggs to fall to the bottom of the pot and scorch.

Pulse the chicken in a food processor until chopped. Add the onion, celery, carrot, tomato, and garlic. Pulse until finely chopped. Add the egg whites, thyme, bay leaf, peppercorns, cilantro, and coriander, and pulse to combine.

Whisk the egg white mixture into the warm stock. Bring the stock to a boil; reduce heat to a low simmer. The egg white and chicken mixture will form a solid layer.

Once the egg white mixture is set, gently stir it to ensure that all of the egg whites cook. Simmer gently until the egg white mixture is solid again. Spoon a hole in the center of the egg white mixture to vent out the steam and so you can see when the stock is clear. Simmer for 8 to 10 minutes. Keep a watchful eye on the consommé so it doesn't boil too fast or scorch.

Line a strainer with cheesecloth or a coffee filter. Carefully ladle the stock out through the hole in the egg white mixture and into the strainer. When you get close to the bottom, gently pour out the remaining stock. The consommé should be crystal clear and very flavorful. Place in a clean saucepot to reheat and season with the salt and white pepper.

Melon Duet

Per serving:
Calories 60; Protein 1g; Total Fat 0g; Saturated Fat 0g; Carbohydrates 15g; Dietary Fiber 1g; Cholesterol 0mg; Sodium 35mg

This is an elegant and outrageously delicious soup to serve at the height of summer when melons are at their peak of freshness and flavor. The presentation is impressive, but the preparation is quick and requires no cooking. You'll find that the addition of freshly grated ginger provides a mysteriously refreshing flavor-enhancer.

Ingredients
Makes 4 1-cup servings.

1/2 medium cantaloupe, peeled, seeded, coarsely chopped (about 12 ounces)
1 tablespoon fresh lime juice, divided
1/4 teaspoon fresh, grated ginger, divided
1/4 medium honeydew, peeled, seeded, coarsely chopped (about 12 ounces)

Garnish
Mint sprigs, optional

Preparation
In a blender, puree the cantaloupe with half of the lime juice and half of the ginger. Transfer to a bowl. Rinse out the blender. Puree the honeydew with the remaining lime juice and ginger.

Simultaneously pour 1/2 cup of each melon mixture into opposite sides of a soup bowl. Garnish each serving with a mint sprig, if desired.

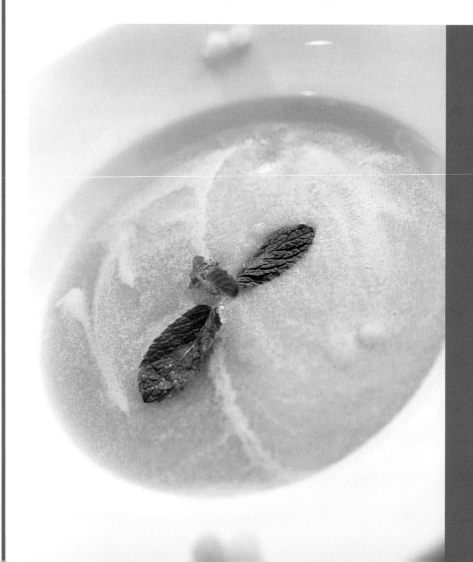

Chilled English Pea and Mint Soup

Per serving:
Calories 120; Protein 7g; Total Fat 0.5g;
Saturated Fat 0g; Carbohydrates 22g; Dietary
Fiber 6g; Cholesterol 0mg; Sodium 290mg

Fresh English peas inspired the creation of this cool, delicious soup, but frozen green peas work magnificently as well. The addition of fresh mint and creamy yogurt makes this soup a refreshing warm-weather treat.

Ingredients
Makes 8 1-cup servings.

1/4 teaspoon extra-virgin olive oil
1/2 cup chopped yellow onion (about
*   1 medium)*
1 teaspoon minced garlic
1 1/2 teaspoons minced fresh ginger
6 cups shelled fresh or frozen green peas
*   (2 1-pound bags)*
4 cups Vegetable Stock (see page 152)
2 tablespoons julienned fresh mint leaves
1/4 cup plain, fat-free yogurt
1/2 teaspoon sea salt
1/4 teaspoon white pepper

Garnish
Plain, fat-free yogurt, optional
Mint sprigs, optional

Preparation

Heat a medium saucepan over medium-high heat. Add the olive oil to lightly coat the bottom of the pan. Add the onion, garlic, and ginger. Cook until the onion has softened, about 2 minutes. Add the peas and cook 1 minute, then add the stock and bring to a boil. Reduce heat and simmer until the peas have just softened and are still bright green, 8 to 10 minutes.

Carefully ladle the soup, mint leaves, and yogurt into a blender and process until smooth. Strain the soup through a fine mesh strainer or a colander lined with cheesecloth to remove any pulp. Season with the salt and white pepper. Chill for 1 hour. Serve the soup cold, garnished with a dollop of yogurt, if using, and a mint sprig.

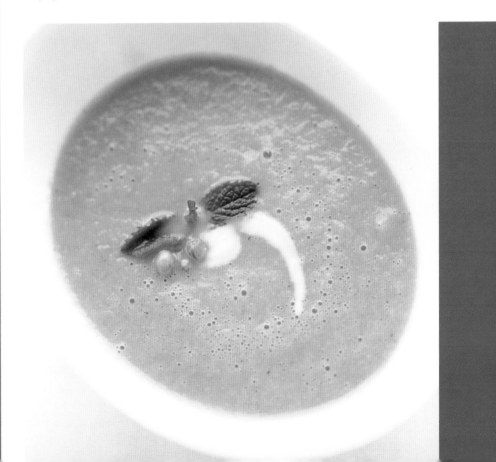

Chilled Vegetable Chowder

Per serving:
Calories 100; Protein 6g; Total Fat 2g;
Saturated Fat trace; Carbohydrates 17g; Dietary
Fiber 3g; Cholesterol 0mg; Sodium 300mg

This soup is a favorite among my chefs. The refreshing cucumbers and yogurt serve as a base to highlight the best vegetables of the garden. Finish the soup with fine shreds of fresh basil and a hint of fine extra-virgin olive oil to make this subtle, chilled chowder sing with robust flavors and textures.

Ingredients

Makes 6 1-cup servings.

3 medium English cucumbers, peeled and
   chopped
2 cups plain, fat-free yogurt
1/2 teaspoon sea salt
1/2 teaspoon ground white pepper
1/2 cup chopped, seeded, peeled, vine-
   ripened, red tomatoes (1 small)
1/2 cup chopped, seeded, peeled, vine-
   ripened, yellow tomatoes (1 small)
1/4 cup chopped yellow squash
1/4 cup chopped zucchini
1/4 cup chopped fresh or frozen corn
   kernels (cooked and drained if fresh)
1/4 cup chopped jícama
1/4 cup chopped, cooked, peeled potatoes
2 tablespoons chopped green onion
1 tablespoon seasoned rice wine vinegar

Garnish

2 teaspoons extra-virgin olive oil
2 tablespoons finely shredded basil

Preparation

Place the cucumbers, yogurt, salt, and white pepper into a blender and process to puree the cucumbers. Chill while you prepare the remaining ingredients.

In a large bowl, combine the remaining vegetables and rice wine vinegar. Stir in the yogurt mixture. Cover and chill for 2 hours before serving.

To serve, ladle the soup into bowls, drizzle with the olive oil, and sprinkle with the basil.

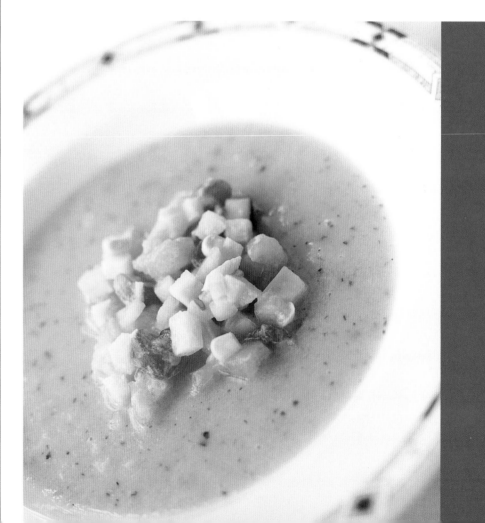

Shrimp and Scallop Gazpacho

Per serving:
Calories 130; Protein 10g; Total Fat 4g;
Saturated Fat 0.5g; Carbohydrates 12g; Dietary
Fiber 2g; Cholesterol 35mg; Sodium 1220mg

The vegetables can be cut easily, quickly, and safely with a mandoline vegetable cutter. Run the cucumbers, jícama, tomatillos, green peppers, and celery through the fine julienne blade, stack, and cut into 1/4-inch cubes. This produces beautiful, small chunks of vegetable that will be laced with the spicy flavors of tomatoes, chiles, and aromatic fresh cilantro. Stir in cooked shrimp and scallops or use them as a garnish to make a gloriously designed soup. Whip this up for your next barbecue to make a delicious splash on the scene. Photo on page 148.

Ingredients
Makes 4 1-cup servings.

1 teaspoon pureed Roasted Garlic (see
   page 38)
4 cups tomato juice
1 teaspoon fresh lemon juice
1/4 cup finely diced red onion
1/4 cup finely diced cucumber
1/4 cup finely diced jícama
1/4 cup finely diced tomatillos
1/4 cup finely diced green pepper
1/4 cup finely diced celery
1/2 cup diced, steamed sea scallops
1/2 cup diced, steamed medium shrimp
1/2 teaspoon minced jalapeño chile
1/4 teaspoon minced garlic
1 tablespoon red wine vinegar
1 tablespoon extra-virgin olive oil
2 tablespoons minced fresh cilantro
3/4 teaspoon sea salt
1/4 teaspoon freshly ground black pepper

Preparation
Combine all the ingredients in a medium bowl. Cover and chill before serving. Taste and adjust seasoning with additional jalapeño, salt, and pepper, if desired.

Yellow Gazpacho

The summer months bring us brightly colored yellow tomatoes—extra sweet and less acidic than their red counterparts. For this gazpacho, the tomatoes are pureed with yellow bell peppers to make a smooth backdrop for the diced vegetables.

By adding additional vinegar and oil, you can turn this soup into a beautiful dressing for butter lettuce or grilled seafood.

Ingredients

Makes 5 1-cup servings.

3 cups chopped, peeled yellow tomatoes
    (see Chef's Tip below)
1 teaspoon extra-virgin olive oil
1 tablespoon seasoned rice wine vinegar
    or Fine Herb Vinegar (see page 118)
1 tablespoon chopped fresh cilantro
1 teaspoon minced jalapeño chile
1 teaspoon minced garlic
1/3 cup chopped yellow bell pepper
1 cup Vegetable Stock (see page 152)
1/3 cup diced cucumber
1/3 cup diced red onion
1/3 cup diced tomatillos
1/3 cup diced jícama
1/3 cup diced celery
1/2 teaspoon sea salt
1/4 teaspoon white pepper

Preparation

Place the tomatoes, olive oil, vinegar, cilantro, chile, garlic, and yellow bell pepper into a large blender (or blend in batches). Add enough stock to cover the vegetables and process until smooth; reserve remaining stock.

Transfer the pureed tomato mixture to a medium mixing bowl. Stir in the cucumber, red onion, tomatillos, jícama, celery, salt, and white pepper. If soup seems too thick, adjust the consistency with the remaining Vegetable Stock. Cover and chill before serving. Taste and adjust the seasoning with additional salt and white pepper, if desired.

Chef's Tip: *To peel tomatoes easily, bring a large pot of water to a boil and prepare a bowl of ice water. Cut a small X on the bottom of each tomato. Carefully place tomatoes, a few at a time, into the boiling water and heat for 30 seconds. Using a slotted spoon or strainer, transfer the tomatoes to the ice water to cool. The skins should slip off easily.*

Red Gazpacho

Per serving:
Calories 70; Protein 2g; Total Fat 1.5g;
Saturated Fat 0g; Carbohydrates 13g; Dietary
Fiber 3g; Cholesterol 0mg; Sodium 360mg

When your prized tomatoes begin to soften and become overly ripe, do not discard them—make this refreshing soup to tantalize your taste buds. For a dramatic presentation, serve side by side in the same bowl with the Yellow Gazpacho (see page 186) and garnish with baked tortilla straws and a sprig of fresh cilantro.

Ingredients

Makes 6 1-cup servings.

3 cups chopped, peeled tomatoes (see
    Chef's Tip, page 186)
1 teaspoon extra-virgin olive oil
1 tablespoon red wine vinegar
2 cups vegetable juice cocktail or tomato
    juice
1/4 cup chopped fresh cilantro
1/3 cup chopped red bell pepper
1 teaspoon minced garlic
1 teaspoon finely chopped jalapeño chile
1/3 cup diced red onion
1/3 cup diced cucumber
1/3 cup diced tomatillos
1/3 cup diced jícama
1/3 cup diced celery
1/2 teaspoon sea salt
1/4 teaspoon white pepper

Preparation

Combine the tomatoes, olive oil, vinegar, vegetable juice, cilantro, bell pepper, garlic, and chile in a large blender (or blend in batches). Puree until smooth, then transfer to a mixing bowl.

Stir in the onion, cucumber, tomatillos, jícama, celery, salt, and white pepper. Cover and chill for 30 minutes before serving. Taste and adjust the seasoning with additional salt and white pepper, if desired.

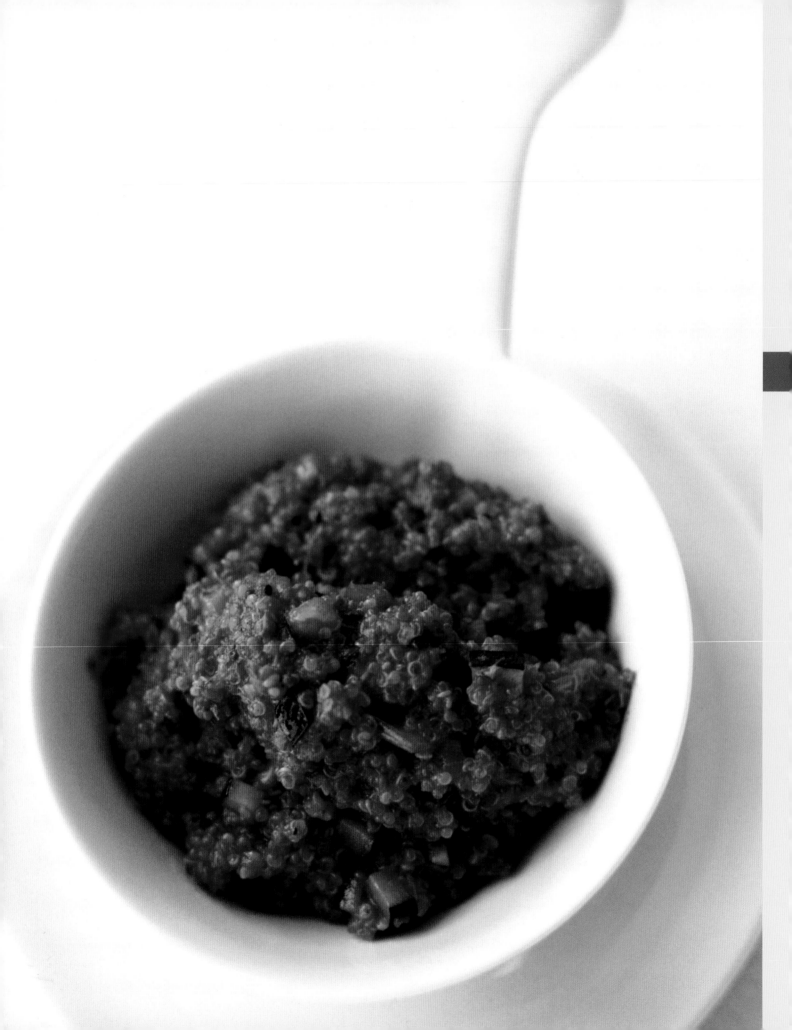

Great Grains & Legumes

chapter 8

Beet Couscous

Carrot Quinoa

Fried Brown Rice

Barley Risotto with Wild Mushrooms

Bulgur Pilaf with Asparagus and Sun-Dried Tomatoes

Millet-Polenta Quenelles

Buckwheat and Wild Rice Stuffing

Spelt-Stuffed Roasted Peppers

Orzo Griddle Cakes

Vegetable Sushi Rolls

Red Rice with Apples and Almonds

Black Bean Griddle Patties

Roasted Vegetable and Lentil Purses

Baked Falafel

Spinach Risotto with Roquefort Cheese

Fava Bean, Roasted Garlic, and Truffle Potato Patties

Edamame Ragoût

Homemade Tofu

Pictured at left: Carrot Quinoa

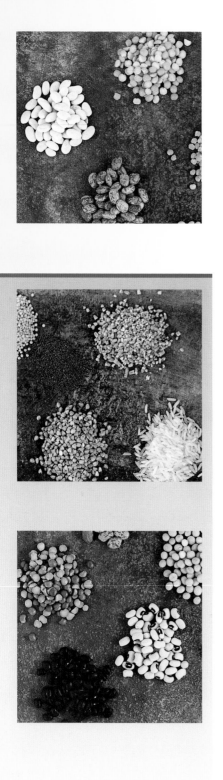

Conscious Cuisine emphasizes the use of grains and legumes as a vital component in achieving a balanced diet. Whole-grain products and beans contain complex carbohydrates, which are extremely effective in providing the body with fuel.

The USDA suggests that Americans should get at least 55 percent of their daily calories from carbohydrates to maintain a healthy lifestyle. The only questions are what type of carbohydrates you choose to eat and how you want to prepare them.

I encourage you to limit your consumption of highly processed grains which might provide a boost of energy, but in most cases are laden with sugars or fats—empty calories with little nutritional value. When paired with vegetables and proteins, whole grains create a balanced and satisfying meal.

When I talk with guests about whole grains and legumes, one issue that always comes up is the length of time that these ingredients require to cook. As you can see from the charts page on 191 illustrating the cooking times of many whole grains and legumes, cooking these foods does require time, but the actual preparation time is short, most can be cooked ahead, and beans and grains can simmer while you do other things. It will be worth it to invest the time to eat properly. It may save you fifteen minutes to cook a pot of instant rice versus cooking regular rice, but the instant rice has been precooked and stripped of most of its nutrients. Instant rice is far less nutritious and flavorful than a pot of brown rice that takes, in the end, only about twenty minutes to cook.

Legumes are not only high in complex carbohydrates, they are also high in protein and, in most cases, iron as well. Legumes are digested slowly, providing a controlled rise in blood sugar. Although beans are the best plant source for protein, most lack one or two amino acids needed to make a complete protein. Soybeans are the only beans that are, by themselves, a complete protein. All others can become complete quite easily by pairing them with grains, thus the reliable beans and rice. At one time, combinations of whole grains and legumes were common staples in almost every type of cuisine regardless of its ethnic origin. Many of these grains and legumes have been eliminated from our diet and replaced with highly processed foods.

This chapter highlights creative methods of introducing whole grains and legumes into your diet, from the sweet and nutty Carrot Quinoa or the comforting Barley Risotto with Wild Mushrooms to the dramatic presentation and delicious flavor of Roast Vegetables and Lentil Purses. Old favorites are also revisited, providing a healthy approach to Fried Brown Rice and Chickpea Falafel.

Legumes are sometimes considered to be hearty wintertime fare, but they can be incorporated into dishes throughout the year. Fava beans are plentiful in the summer months and make wonderful Fava Bean, Roasted Garlic, and Truffle Potato Patties. Black-Bean Griddle Patties, good at any time, provide a southwestern and Latin touch, and my favorite Edamame Ragoût provides a fanciful, quick, and delicious way to enjoy Asian-style foods all year long.

Grains

- With the exception of pearled barley, bulgur wheat, couscous, cracked or rolled oats, and kasha, wash all grains before cooking. Cover the grains with cold water, and swirl your fingers in the water to loosen any debris. Replace cloudy water with clear water. Repeat the process until the water remains clear.
- Add a pinch of salt for every 1 cup of grain to be cooked. Generally, grains are cooked in a two-part water to one-part grain ratio.

Cooking Grains

GRAIN	LIQUID	SIMMER
1 cup long grain brown rice	2 cups	45 minutes
1 cup short grain brown rice	2 cups	50 minutes
1 cup white rice long or short	2 cups	30 minutes
1 cup pearl barley	3 cups	35 to 45 minutes
1 cup millet	3 cups	35 minutes
1 cup raw buckwheat	3 cups	15 to 20 minutes
1 cup steel-cut oats	3 cups	30 minutes
1 cup quinoa	2 cups	20 minutes
1 cup bulgur wheat	2 cups	10 minutes
1 cup couscous	1 to 1 1/2 cups	10 minutes

Legumes

- All legumes should be sorted to remove any stones and debris and then washed to remove dirt and dust.
- With the exception of lentils, split peas, and adzuki beans, all legumes should be soaked in cold water in the refrigerator for six to eight hours prior to cooking. Drain and cook in fresh water.
- Simmer legumes completely covered in liquid. Rapid boiling causes the skin to fall off and the beans to break apart.
- Legumes double in size during cooking.
- Proportions for soup: add 1 cup dry legumes to 5 cups of water.
- Proportions for entrées or side dishes: add 1 cup dry legumes to 4 cups of water.

Cooking Legumes

GRAIN	LIQUID	SIMMER
1 cup adzuki beans	3 cups	60 minutes
1 cup black beans	3 cups	50 to 60 minutes
1 cup black-eyed peas	4 cups	1 to 1 1/2 hours
1 cup chickpeas	3 cups	1 1/2 to 3 hours
1 cup kidney beans	4 cups	50 to 60 minutes
1 cup lima beans	4 cups	50 to 60 minutes
1 cup navy beans	4 cups	1 to 1 1/2 hours
1 cup pinto beans	4 cups	50 to 60 minutes
1 cup red or green lentils	2 cups	20 to 30 minutes
1 cup split peas	2 cups	45 minutes

Beet Couscous

Frequent use of the vegetable juicer (as illustrated in chapter 4: Breakfast: Breaking the Fast) inspired me to create many wonderful vegetable-infused grain recipes. This is my favorite—its vibrant color and sweet flavor make you forget that beets are good for you and provide vitamin C, potassium, and iron. I recommend using Israeli couscous because of its large, round grains. Couscous is not a true grain, but a pasta made from ground hard durum wheat or "semolina." Photo on page 244.

Per 1/2 cup:
Calories 180; Protein 6g; Total Fat 0g; Saturated Fat 0g; Carbohydrates 38g; Dietary Fiber 2g; Cholesterol 0mg; Sodium 260mg

Ingredients
Makes 10 1/2-cup servings.

1/4 teaspoon extra-virgin olive oil
1/4 cup diced red onion
1 cup Israeli couscous
1/2 cup unsweetened apple juice
1 1/2 cups fresh beet juice (about 15
   medium beets) or other vegetable juice
1/2 teaspoon cinnamon
1/4 teaspoon sea salt
1/8 teaspoon white pepper

Preparation
Heat a medium saucepan over medium-high heat and add the olive oil to lightly coat the bottom of the pan. Stir in the onion and cook until it begins to soften, about 2 minutes. Add the couscous, apple juice, beet juice, and seasonings. Mix well and bring to a boil. Reduce the heat to a low simmer and cover the pot.

Steam until the liquid is absorbed and the couscous is bright red, 30 to 35 minutes.

Carrot Quinoa

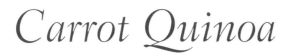

Although unknown to many Americans, quinoa has been cultivated continuously for over five thousand years. It is often referred to as a super-grain for its high iron, protein, and potassium content, to list just a few of its nutritional benefits. To help introduce this awesome whole grain to my patrons, I created a highly flavorful dish that tastes great and just happens to be good for you. In this recipe, we suggest that first you lightly toast the grain to give it a nutty flavor. The addition of carrot juice adds natural sweetness and a beautiful hue to the finished product. Photo on page 188.

Per 1/2 cup:
Calories 160; Protein 6g; Total Fat 2.5g; Saturated Fat 0g; Carbohydrates 30g; Dietary Fiber 3g; Cholesterol 0mg; Sodium 180mg

Ingredients
Makes 5 1/2-cup servings.

1 cup quinoa
1/4 teaspoon extra-virgin olive oil
1/2 cup chopped yellow onion (about
   1 medium)
1/2 cup chopped zucchini (1 small)
1/2 cup chopped celery (1 medium rib)
2 cups carrot juice (about 10 medium)
1/2 teaspoon nutmeg
1/4 teaspoon sea salt
1/4 teaspoon freshly ground black pepper

Preparation
Heat a saucepan over medium heat. Add the quinoa and toast it, stirring constantly, until the grain turns light brown and smells nutty, about 3 minutes. Remove the quinoa from the pan and return the pan to the stovetop.

Add the olive oil to lightly coat the bottom of the pan. Add the onion, zucchini, and celery. Cook until the onion has just softened, about 2 minutes. Add the carrot juice and bring to a low boil. Stir in the toasted quinoa, nutmeg, salt, and pepper. Bring to a boil, reduce heat to low, cover, and simmer until the quinoa has absorbed the carrot juice and is fluffy, 25 to 30 minutes.

Fried Brown Rice

Per 1/2 cup:
Calories 140; Protein 8g; Total Fat 3.5g;
Saturated Fat 0g; Carbohydrates 20g; Dietary
Fiber 5g; Cholesterol 0mg; Sodium 180mg

This is a great way to use up leftover brown rice. The clever addition of edamame makes this a balanced meal in itself. It also makes a perfect accompaniment to any Asian-style entrée—the classic flavors marry well with grilled scallops, marinated duck, or pan-seared tofu. Photo on page 243.

Ingredients
Makes 6 servings.

1/4 teaspoon extra-virgin olive oil
1 large egg white
1 tablespoon chopped yellow onion
1 tablespoon chopped celery
1 tablespoon chopped red bell pepper
1/2 teaspoon minced garlic
1/2 teaspoon minced fresh ginger
1 tablespoon chopped yellow squash
1 tablespoon chopped broccoli
2 tablespoons chopped snow peas
1/2 cup edamame (shelled green soybeans)
2 cups cooked brown rice
1 tablespoon chopped green onion
1 tablespoon tamari (soy) sauce

Preparation

Heat a medium sauté pan over medium-high heat and add the olive oil to lightly coat the bottom of the pan. Add the egg white and scramble. Remove the egg from the pan and set aside.

To the sauté pan over medium heat, add the yellow onion, celery, bell pepper, garlic, ginger, squash, broccoli, snow peas, and edamame. Sauté until the onion has softened, about 2 minutes.

Add the rice and stir until heated through, about 3 minutes. Stir in the green onion, tamari, and scrambled egg white.

Barley Risotto with Wild Mushrooms

Per serving:
Calories 130; Protein 5g; Total Fat 1g;
Saturated Fat 0g; Carbohydrates 26g; Dietary
Fiber 6g; Cholesterol 0mg; Sodium 90mg

Although arborio rice is used most often to make risotto, "risotto" refers to the method of cooking grains, not the rice itself. Barley has twice the protein and fiber of rice and is touted to lower blood cholesterol because it contains soluble fiber. Toasting barley in a dry sauté pan or in the oven gives it a wonderful nutty flavor, delightful in combination with fresh wild mushrooms such as shiitake and oyster. This recipe uses part toasted and part untoasted barley to create a lovely contrast of flavors, colors, and textures. Photo on page 235.

Ingredients

Makes about 5 servings.

3/4 cup organic barley
1/4 teaspoon extra-virgin olive oil
1/4 cup chopped yellow onion
1/2 teaspoon minced garlic
1 1/2 cups (about 2 ounces) assorted
    seasonal fresh mushrooms (shiitake,
    oyster, portobello, chanterelle)
1 bay leaf
3 to 3 1/2 cups Vegetable Stock (see
    page 152), heated
1/2 teaspoon chopped fresh thyme
1 teaspoon chopped fresh oregano
1/8 teaspoon sea salt
Pinch freshly ground black pepper
1 tablespoon shredded Parmigiano-
    Reggiano cheese, optional

Preparation

Place 1/2 cup of the barley in a dry medium sauté pan. Toast the barley, stirring constantly, over medium heat until it is golden brown and has a roasted nutty smell, 3 to 5 minutes. Remove the barley from the pan to stop the cooking process and set aside.

Heat a medium saucepan over medium-high heat and add the olive oil to lightly coat the bottom of the pan. Add the onion and garlic. Cook until the onion has just softened, about 2 minutes. Add the mushrooms and cook for 1 minute. Stir in the toasted barley, the remaining 1/4 cup of barley, and the bay leaf.

Stir 1/2 cup of the hot stock into the barley and reduce the heat to a simmer. (Keep the remaining stock hot.) Cook, stirring constantly, until the barley has absorbed all the liquid. Continue adding 1/2 cup of the hot stock at a time to the barley mixture, stirring until absorbed. Cook until the barley is tender, 20 to 30 minutes. Stir in the thyme, oregano, salt, pepper, and cheese (if using). Remove the bay leaf and serve.

Bulgur Pilaf with Asparagus and Sun-Dried Tomatoes

Bulgur wheat is a beloved staple in Middle Eastern cuisine. It is available in fine, medium, and coarse grind. It has a nutty flavor, extremely light texture, and marries well with a variety of foods, from robust spices, curries, fruits, and grilled meats to luscious salads. Accompany this delicious and colorful pilaf with your favorite foods. Or add olive oil and lemon juice to create a light and delicious salad.

Ingredients
Makes 5 servings.

1 1/2 cups Vegetable Stock (see page 152)
1 cup bulgur wheat, fine or medium grind
1/2 cup julienned asparagus
1/2 teaspoon minced garlic
2 minced kalamata olives
1/4 cup julienned, dry-pack sun-dried
　　tomatoes
1/2 tablespoon minced fresh parsley
1/2 teaspoon minced fresh oregano
1/4 teaspoon sea salt
1/4 teaspoon freshly ground black pepper

Preparation
Bring the stock to a low boil in a small saucepan.

In a medium heat-proof bowl, combine the bulgur wheat, asparagus, garlic, olives, and tomatoes. Stir the hot stock into the bulgur mixture and cover the bowl with plastic wrap. Allow to stand until the liquid is completely absorbed by the grain, 10 to 15 minutes. Remove the plastic wrap and season the bulgur with the parsley, oregano, salt, and pepper. The asparagus will become *al dente* and the tomatoes will soften nicely as the bulgur "steams" in the stock.

Millet-Polenta Quenelles

The tiny grains of millet date back to the Middle Ages. It's still widely consumed and valued in North Africa, India, and Asia as a nutritious source of B vitamins, copper, and iron. Its neutral flavor combines well with almost any seasoning. Toasting the millet brings out a nutty, corn-like flavor. Millet can be used for hot cereals, polenta, pilafs, or in an Ethiopian flatbread called *injera*.

This recipe uses the cooking technique employed in making polenta. Presented as French quenelles, the millet mixture is shaped into attractive oval nuggets of complex flavor to enhance stews or protein entrées. Photo on page 239.

Ingredients
Makes 8 servings.

1 cup millet
3 cups Vegetable Stock (see page 152)
1/4 teaspoon extra-virgin olive oil
1/4 cup chopped yellow onion
1 teaspoon minced garlic
1/4 cup chopped carrot
1/4 cup chopped celery
1/4 teaspoon sea salt
1/4 teaspoon freshly ground black pepper
1 tablespoon crumbled Roquefort cheese

Preparation

Toast the millet in a 350°F (175°C) oven or in a dry sauté pan on the stove until lightly browned or toasted, about 4 minutes.

Bring the stock to a low boil in a small saucepan.

Heat a medium saucepan over medium heat. Add the olive oil to lightly coat the bottom of the pan. Add the onion, garlic, carrot, and celery. Cook until the onion has just softened, about 2 minutes. Stir in the toasted millet, salt, and pepper.

Add the hot stock to the millet mixture, cover, and simmer until the millet is soft and sticky, the texture of polenta, 15 to 20 minutes. Stir in the cheese.

To form the quenelles (oval shaped dumplings): Preheat the oven to 350°F (175°C). Coat 2 large spoons with cooking spray. Scoop out some of the millet polenta on one spoon, and use the second spoon to shape the top of the oval. Shift the quenelle to the second spoon. Repeat this process until you have a neat, oval-shaped dumpling. Repeat with remaining polenta. Place the dumplings on a baking sheet coated with cooking spray. Bake for 10 minutes or until the quenelles are light brown and crispy.

Buckwheat and Wild Rice Stuffing

Per 1/2 cup:
Calories 180; Protein 7g; Total Fat 1g;
Saturated Fat 0g; Carbohydrates 38g; Dietary
Fiber 5g; Cholesterol 0mg; Sodium 170mg

Ingredients
Makes 8 servings.

1 cup raw buckwheat
1 cup wild rice
1/4 teaspoon extra-virgin olive oil
1/2 cup diced yellow onion (1 medium)
1/2 cup diced celery (1 medium rib)
1/2 teaspoon minced garlic
2 tablespoons chopped fresh parsley
1 tablespoon chopped fresh thyme
5 cups Vegetable Stock (see page 152),
    heated
1/2 teaspoon sea salt
1/2 teaspoon freshly ground black pepper

This recipe calls for whole, raw buckwheat groats. Its name is misleading because buckwheat is not related to wheat and is not a true grain. It's a fruit from the sorrel and rhubarb family. The groats have a triangular shape, an assertive flavor, and are high in essential amino acids and magnesium. When toasted, buckwheat's nutty flavor marries well with roasted meats and root vegetables. The earthy flavor of wild rice and the tart and sweet dried cherries make this a wonderful stuffing for poultry dishes. Photo on page 251.

Preparation
Heat a medium saucepan over medium-high heat. Add the buckwheat and toast until it has a toasty, nutty smell, about 2 minutes. Transfer the buckwheat to a mixing bowl and combine with the wild rice.

Return the saucepan to the heat. Add the olive oil to lightly coat the bottom of the pan. Add the onion, celery, and garlic, and cook until the onion has just softened, about 2 minutes. Add the parsley, thyme, and buckwheat-rice mixture. Stir in the hot stock, salt, and pepper. Bring to a boil. Reduce the heat to low, cover, and simmer until the stock is absorbed and the rice is *al dente*, 30 to 35 minutes. Season with additional salt and pepper, to taste.

Spelt-Stuffed Roasted Peppers

Spelt is a variety of wheat that is claimed to cure almost every human ailment. I cannot verify these claims, but I can say that this highly nutritious grain packs a lot of flavor. It has a light, chewy texture that's similar to rice, and provides a nice foil for the flavors of portobello mushrooms, butternut squash, and arugula. Stuffing the mixture inside roasted bell peppers creates an attractive presentation as an entrée or vegetable accompaniment.

Ingredients

Makes 4 servings.

3 cups Vegetable Stock (see page 152)
1 cup spelt or wheat berries
1/4 teaspoon extra-virgin olive oil
1/2 cup finely chopped red onion (about
   1 medium)
1 cup finely chopped portobello mushrooms, gills removed
1 cup finely chopped butternut squash
1 cup chopped teardrop or cherry
   tomatoes
1 cup chopped arugula
2 teaspoons Fresh Herb Mix (see page 39)
2 whole Roasted Yellow Bell Peppers (see
   page 38), tops and seeds removed
2 whole Roasted Red Bell Peppers (see
   page 38), tops and seeds removed

Preparation

Combine the stock with the spelt in a medium saucepan and bring to a boil over medium-high heat. Reduce the heat to low, cover, and simmer until most of the stock has been absorbed and the spelt is *al dente*, 35 to 40 minutes. Transfer the cooked spelt to a medium mixing bowl.

Heat a medium sauté pan over medium-high heat. Add the olive oil to lightly coat the bottom of the pan. Add the onion, mushrooms, and butternut squash and cook until the onion has just softened, about 2 minutes. Remove from the heat and add to the spelt. Mix in the tomatoes, arugula, and herbs.

Preheat the oven to 350°F (175°C). Arrange the Roasted Peppers on a baking sheet. Carefully fill each pepper with 3/4 cup of the filling. Bake until heated through, about 10 minutes.

Orzo Griddle Cakes

Per cake:
Calories 160; Protein 5g; Total Fat 1g;
Saturated Fat 0g; Carbohydrates 32g; Dietary
Fiber 2g; Cholesterol 0g; Sodium 115mg

I have included some of my favorite pastas—such as couscous and orzo—in the grains chapter to dispel the myth that pasta is a calorie-laden filler. A pasta dish becomes high in fat and calories when it's topped with an excessive amount of cheese and high-fat sauces. The attractive shape of orzo pasta mixed with fresh herbs and colorful vegetables makes this dish as beautiful as it is tasty. The cakes have a crisp crust, a soft, chewy interior, and can be topped with steamed vegetable bundles or your choice of protein.

Ingredients

Makes 6 servings.

1 1/2 cups Vegetable Stock (see page 152)
1/4 teaspoon extra-virgin olive oil
1/2 pound orzo pasta
1/4 cup finely chopped celery
1/4 cup finely chopped carrots
1/4 cup finely chopped red onion
1/2 tablespoon Fresh Herb Mix (see page 39)
1/4 teaspoon sea salt
1/8 teaspoon freshly ground black pepper

Preparation

Bring the stock to a boil in a small saucepan.

Heat a large sauté pan over medium-high heat. Add the olive oil to lightly coat the bottom of the pan. Stir in the orzo and vegetables and sauté, stirring constantly, until the orzo is just toasted, about 1 minute. Slowly add the stock to the pan and bring to a boil. Reduce the heat and simmer until the stock has been absorbed and the pasta is *al dente*, about 7 minutes. Stir in the Fresh Herb Mix and season with the salt and pepper.

Line an 11 x 7-inch baking pan with parchment or waxed paper, and coat with cooking spray. Spread the cooked pasta mixture evenly in the pan. Cover with a second piece of parchment paper and refrigerate for 20 minutes or until cool.

Preheat the oven to 350°F (175°C). Once the pasta mixture has cooled and set, cut out 6 circles with a 2-inch cutter. Place the orzo cakes on a baking sheet sprayed with cooking spray. Bake until crispy and heated through, about 6 minutes.

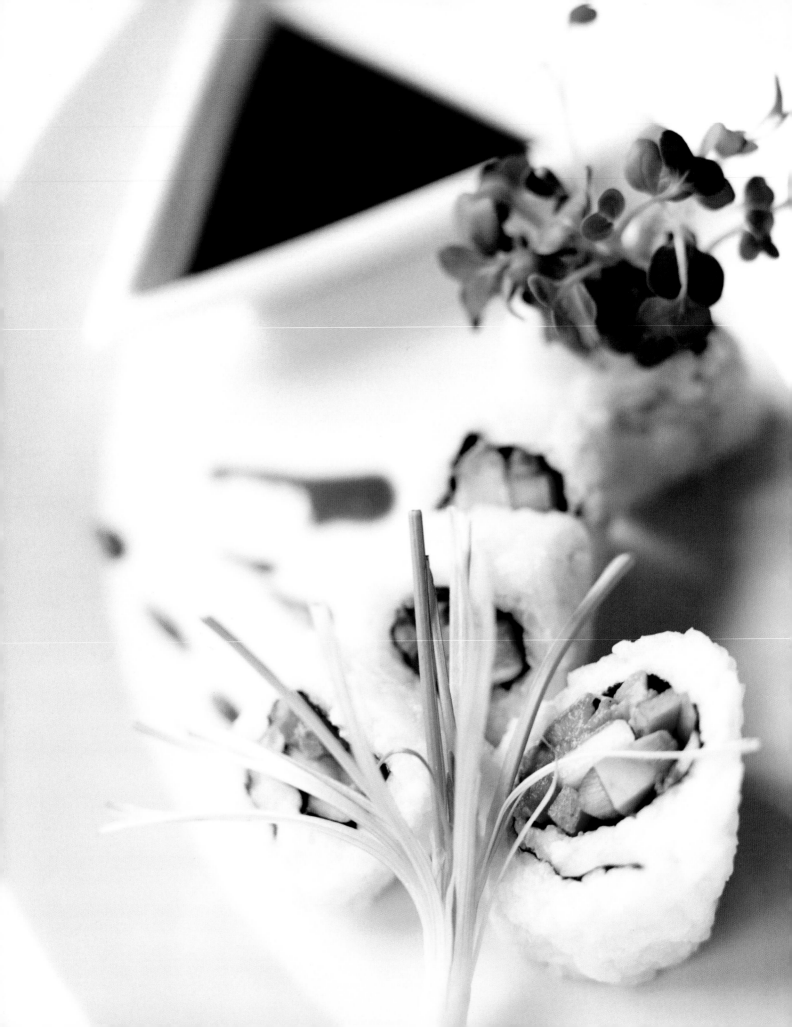

Vegetable Sushi Rolls

Sushi has fast become a favorite food in America. I included this recipe to illustrate how to make the critical rice. Keep in mind that you are limited only by the freshness of the ingredients and your imagination in creating countless other sushi rolls. You will need a sushi mat to shape the rolls—they are very inexpensive and available at Asian grocery stores and most kitchen supply stores.

Ingredients
Makes about 4 servings.

1 cup sushi rice
2 cups water
1 tablespoon seasoned rice wine vinegar
1/2 teaspoon raw cane sugar (Turbinado)
3 sheets toasted nori (seaweed)
1 medium carrot, julienned
1 small cucumber, julienned
1/2 avocado, cut into thin strips
1/2 cup thinly sliced baked tofu

Garnish
Wasabi
Pickled ginger
Tamari (soy) sauce

Preparation

Combine the rice and water in a small saucepan and bring to a boil. Reduce heat to low, cover, and simmer until the rice has absorbed all the water and is a little sticky, 35 to 40 minutes. Transfer the rice to a bowl. Combine the rice wine vinegar and sugar, and stir into the cooked rice. (The rice will be sticky.) Allow the rice to cool in the refrigerator for about 15 minutes.

Lay a sushi mat out on a cutting board and cover with plastic wrap. Place one piece of nori on the mat. Measure out 1 cup of the cooked rice and place on the edge of the nori sheet. Wet your fingers with some warm water and spread the rice out evenly on the nori. Turn over so that nori side is facing up. Place a row of about 8 carrot strips across the nori, 1/2 inch from the bottom edge. Next arrange a layer of about 6 cucumber pieces, then about 3 avocado pieces, and about 4 tofu pieces. Carefully lift up the bottom of the sushi mat and bring it over the rice and vegetables. Tuck the edge of the nori into the rice and begin to roll. Try to keep the roll tight, moving the mat away as you roll. Trim off the edges of the roll with a sharp knife. Repeat with remaining nori, rice, and vegetables to make 3 rolls. Cut each roll into 6 pieces.

Serve the vegetable rolls with wasabi, pickled ginger, and tamari.

Red Rice with Apples and Almonds

Per 1/2 cup:
Calories 90; Protein 2g; Total Fat 1g; Saturated Fat 0g; Carbohydrates 19g; Dietary Fiber 2g; Cholesterol 0mg; Sodium 65mg

While studying and experimenting with whole grains, I found that rice is available in hundreds of varieties. It's a mystery to me why Americans have embraced so few of these delicious alternative complex carbohydrates. The rice used in this recipe is harvested in the Himalayan mountains. Its vibrant maroon color and nutty flavor have made it one of my personal favorites. It is available in specialty markets and health food stores. Introduce yourself to the wide range of flavors that rice offers. See page 326 for grain sources.

Ingredients
Makes 10 servings.

2 1/2 cups Vegetable Stock (see page 152)
1 cup Himalayan red rice
1/2 cup chopped green onion (about 4 onions)
1 cinnamon stick
1 whole star anise
1 cup Granny Smith apple (about 1 apple), chopped, unpeeled
1 tablespoon chopped almonds, toasted
1/4 teaspoon sea salt
1/8 teaspoon freshly ground pepper

Preparation

In a medium saucepan, combine the stock, rice, green onion, cinnamon stick, and star anise, and bring to a boil. Reduce heat to low, cover, and simmer until the rice has started to soften, 20 to 25 minutes.

Remove from the heat and mix in the apple, almonds, salt, and pepper. Cover and let stand for 5 minutes. Discard the cinnamon stick and star anise. Fluff the rice with a fork and serve.

Black-Bean Griddle Patties

Per 1 cake:
Calories 80; Protein 6g; Total Fat 0.5g;
Saturated Fat 0g; Carbohydrates 14g; Dietary
Fiber 5g; Cholesterol 0mg; Sodium 210mg

This recipe was my first attempt at creating a vegetable burger. The high protein content of the black beans and their binding properties make them perfect for the job, combined with colorful vegetables, fresh herbs and spices. These patties make a delicious complement to Cuban or southwestern-style dishes.

Ingredients

Makes 6 cakes.

1/4 teaspoon extra-virgin olive oil
1 3/4 cups cooked or canned black beans
   (15-ounce can), drained
1/4 cup diced red onion
1 teaspoon minced garlic
1/4 cup fresh corn kernels
2 large egg whites
2 teaspoons minced fresh cilantro
1 teaspoon minced fresh oregano
1/4 teaspoon cumin
1/4 teaspoon coriander
1/2 teaspoon sea salt
1/4 teaspoon freshly ground black pepper
1/2 cup cornmeal, for coating the patties

Preparation

Heat a sauté pan over medium-high heat and add the olive oil to lightly coat the bottom of the pan. Add 3/4 cup of the beans, the red onion, garlic, and corn. Cook until the onion has just softened, about 2 minutes. Remove from the heat and set aside.

In a food processor, process the remaining 1 cup of the beans until smooth. Add the egg whites, cilantro, oregano, cumin, coriander, salt, and pepper. Mix the pureed beans with the sautéed beans.

Using 1/4 cup at a time, form the bean mixture into patties and coat with the cornmeal. Heat a griddle over medium-high heat and coat with olive oil spray. Brown the cakes on both sides, about 2 minutes each. Keep in a warm oven until ready to serve.

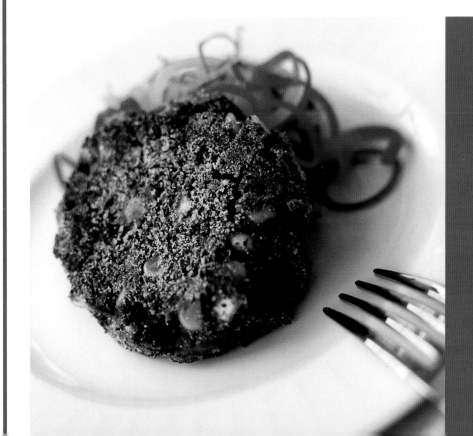

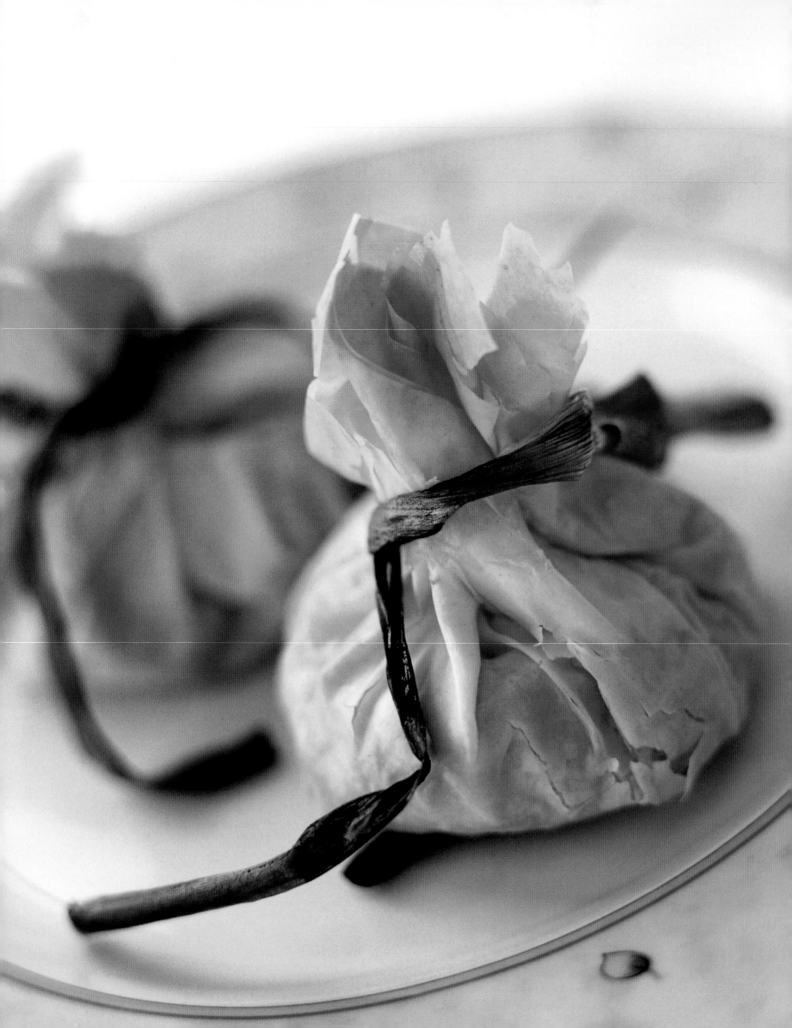

Roasted Vegetable and Lentil Purses

Per serving (1 purse):
Calories 170; Protein 9g; Total Fat 1.5g;
Saturated Fat 0g; Carbohydrates 31g; Dietary
Fiber 10g; Cholesterol 0mg; Sodium 240mg

Roasting root vegetables brings out their natural sweetness. The combination of these vegetables with hearty lentils wrapped in phyllo pastry creates a luscious vegan entrée or a creative complement to any dish. Phyllo dough is available in the frozen foods section of most supermarkets.

Ingredients
Makes 8 servings.

1 cup lentils

1 teaspoon minced fresh garlic

1/2 cup chopped yellow onion (about
   1 medium)

3 1/4 cups Vegetable Stock (see page 152)
   or water

1/2 cup diced, peeled butternut squash
   (1/2 medium)

1/2 cup diced, peeled carrot (1 medium)

1/2 cup diced, peeled parsnip (1 medium)

1/2 cup diced celery (1 medium rib)

1/2 cup diced portobello mushroom, gills
   removed (about 1 medium mushroom)

1/4 teaspoon extra-virgin olive oil

2 tablespoons Fresh Herb Mix (see
   page 39)

1/2 teaspoon sea salt

1/4 teaspoon freshly ground black pepper

2 Roasted Garlic cloves (see page 38),
   minced

6 sheets phyllo dough (about 1/4 of a
   1-lb. box)

8 green onions, blanched and chilled
   in ice water

Preparation

In a small saucepan, combine the lentils, garlic, and yellow onion with 3 cups of the Vegetable Stock and bring to a boil. Reduce heat to low, cover, and simmer until the lentils are softened, 25 to 30 minutes. Remove from the heat.

Meanwhile, preheat the oven to 400°F (205°C).

In a medium bowl, combine the squash, carrot, parsnip, celery, and mushrooms. Toss with the olive oil, 1 tablespoon of the Fresh Herb Mix, 1/4 teaspoon of the salt, and the pepper. Arrange the vegetables on a baking sheet and roast for 7 minutes or until the vegetables are just softened and lightly browned. Remove from the oven and cool on a wire rack.

In a medium bowl, combine 1 cup of the cooked lentils with the roasted vegetables. In a separate bowl, combine the remaining lentils, Roasted Garlic, remaining 1 tablespoon of herbs, and remaining 1/4 cup of stock. Puree with a hand blender (or in a standard blender) until just smooth. Combine the puree with the vegetable mixture and season with the remaining 1/4 teaspoon of salt.

Reduce the oven temperature to 375°F (190°C). Coat a baking sheet with cooking spray.

On a clean cutting board, lay out one sheet of phyllo dough. (Keep remaining sheets covered with a damp cloth to avoid drying out.) Spray with cooking spray to lightly coat the sheet. Lay another sheet over the first one and spray with cooking spray; repeat with one more sheet and cooking spray, to make 3 layers. Cut the stacked phyllo into into 4 rectangles. In the middle of each, place 1/2 cup of the lentil mixture. Gather up the edges and squeeze together to form a "purse." Tie off the top of purse with one of the blanched green onions. Place on the prepared baking sheet. Repeat with remaining phyllo and filling to make a total of 8 bundles.

Bake for 7 to 10 minutes, or until golden brown. The green onion may turn brown on the edges; you can cut these off before you serve the bundles.

Baked Falafel

Falafel is a classic Middle Eastern dish that's typically deep-fried and served with tahini and pita bread. This recipe delivers the original flavor and an improved texture by baking rather than frying. Have fun with this by serving with its traditional accompaniments or build upon its flavor with salad greens, poultry, meats, and even fish.

Ingredients
Makes 5 servings.

Baked Falafel
1 3/4 cups cooked or canned chickpeas
   (15-ounce can), drained
1/4 cup chopped green onion
2 small garlic cloves
1 tablespoon fresh lemon juice
1 teaspoon cumin
1/4 teaspoon coriander
1/2 teaspoon turmeric
1/2 teaspoon sea salt
1/8 teaspoon cayenne pepper
2 tablespoon water
1/3 cup chopped fresh parsley
2 tablespoon unbleached all-purpose flour

Creamy Cucumber Sauce
Makes 1 1/2 cups.

1 cup fat-free plain yogurt
3/4 cup finely chopped cucumber, about
   1/4 of cucumber
3/4 teaspoon minced garlic
1/4 cup seeded and finely chopped tomato
3/4 teaspoon dried dill
1/4 teaspoon sea salt
1/8 teaspoon ground white pepper

Preparation

For the Baked Falafel: Preheat the oven to 375°F (190°C). Coat a baking sheet with cooking spray.

In a food processor, combine all the ingredients except the parsley and flour. Process until a smooth dough is formed. Add the parsley and flour and pulse a few times to mix.

Scoop out the falafel with a tablespoon measure and form into 20 small patties. Place the patties on the prepared baking sheet. Lightly spray the top of the patties with cooking spray.

Bake for 10 minutes. Turn over and bake for 5 minutes more or until golden brown and a little crispy on the outside.

Second serving option: To serve as passed hors d'oeuvres, prepare the falafel as above, but before baking, press a small hole using your index finger into the center of each cake. After removing the cakes from the oven, spoon 1/2 teaspoon of cucumber sauce in the center of each cake and arrange on platter to serve. Garnish with a sprinkle of additional dill.

For the Creamy Cucumber Sauce: Combine all the ingredients in a mixing bowl. Refrigerate for at least 1/2 hour before serving.

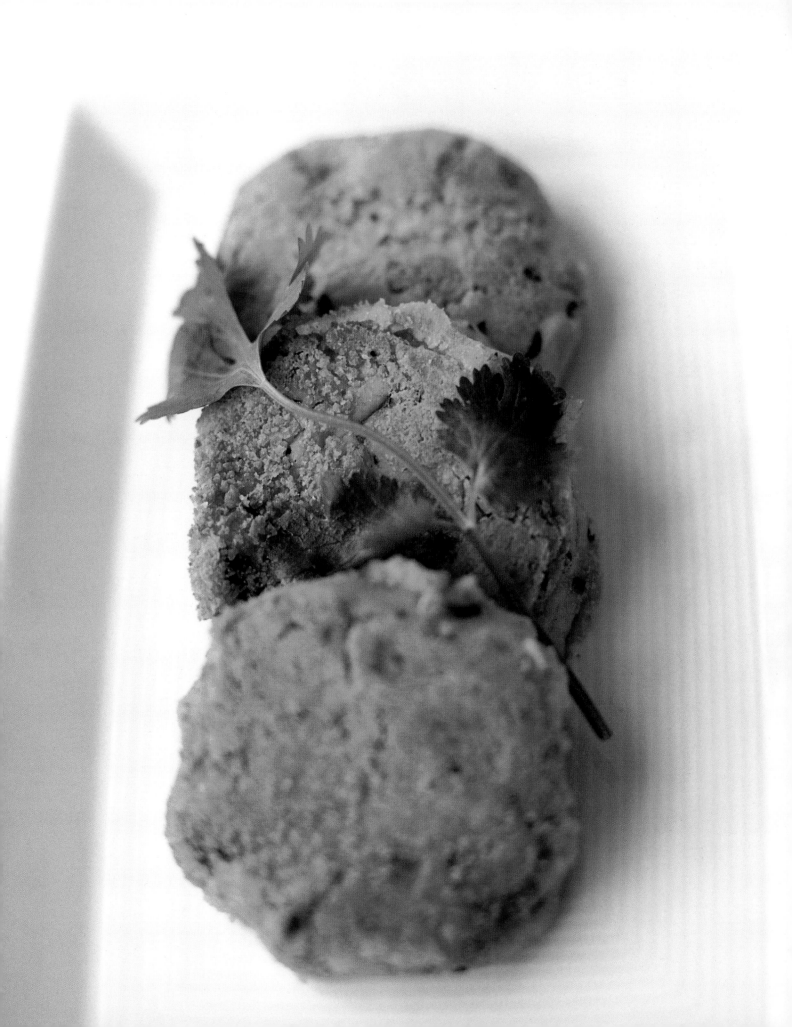

Spinach Risotto with Roquefort Cheese

As in any risotto, the keys to its success are the quality of the rice, a flavorful broth, and a watchful eye. The spinach is quickly cooked and pureed to make a delicious, colorful, and nutritious broth. The risotto is further enhanced by the addition of high-quality arborio rice and Roquefort cheese.

To make it in advance, you can cook the risotto until three-quarters done, cool, and finish when ready to serve. Otherwise, prepare and serve it immediately to avoid overcooking. Nothing is worse than overcooked, gummy risotto; it's hard work gone for naught.

Ingredients

Makes 6 servings.

Spinach Broth

Makes 4 cups.

1/4 teaspoon extra-virgin olive oil
1 cup chopped yellow onion (about
    1 large)
1 teaspoon minced garlic
3 cups spinach leaves, packed
4 cups Vegetable Stock (see page 152)
1/2 teaspoon sea salt
1/4 teaspoon freshly ground black pepper

Spinach Risotto

1/4 teaspoon extra-virgin olive oil
1/2 cup chopped yellow onion (about
    1 medium)
1 teaspoon minced garlic
1 cup arborio rice
3 to 4 cups Spinach Broth (above)
1 tablespoon Roquefort cheese
1/4 teaspoon sea salt
1/8 teaspoon freshly ground black pepper

Preparation

For the Spinach Broth: Heat a medium sauté pan over medium-high heat. Add the olive oil to lightly coat the bottom of the pan. Add the onion and garlic and cook until the onion has just softened, about 2 minutes. Add the spinach and cook, stirring constantly, for 1 minute. Add the Vegetable Stock and bring to a low boil. Season with the sea salt and pepper.

Carefully ladle the spinach mixture into a blender and puree until smooth. Transfer the broth to a saucepan and keep hot. (Makes 4 cups.)

For the Spinach Risotto: Heat a medium saucepan over medium-high heat. Add the olive oil to lightly coat the bottom of the pan. Stir in the onion, garlic, and rice, and cook until the onion has just softened, about 2 minutes.

Stir in 1 cup of the spinach broth and reduce the heat to a simmer. Stir the rice constantly until the liquid is absorbed, then add another 1/2 cup broth. Continue to stir and add broth by 1/2 cups until 3 cups of broth are used; then check for doneness. Risotto should be cooked *al dente*: tender and cooked through, but still with a slight bite to it. Continue to add broth as necessary; the process should take 20-25 minutes.

Crumble the Roquefort cheese into the risotto and stir well to incorporate. (The high quality of the cheese enables you to use less.) Season with the salt and pepper.

Fava Bean, Roasted Garlic, and Truffle Potato Patties

Per 2 patties:
Calories 230; Protein 14g; Total Fat 1g;
Saturated Fat 0g; Carbohydrates 44g; Dietary
Fiber 13g; Cholesterol 0mg; Sodium 250mg

Per 2 salmon patties:
Calories 70; Protein 5g; Total Fat 0.5g;
Saturated Fat 0g; Carbohydrates 11g; Dietary
Fiber 3g; Cholesterol 0mg; Sodium 190 mg

Fava beans are one of my favorite legumes; their interesting flavor speaks to me of exotic comfort. Fava beans are easy to prepare, but are labor intensive. Each pod contains 4 to 6 large, oval beans, which have a thin skin that has to be removed. Try this recipe during the summer months when favas are in season, and you too will be hooked on these luscious beans. The truffle oil can be found in specialty and gourmet food stores.

Ingredients
Makes 5 servings.

1 1/2 cups fresh or frozen, shelled fava
   beans
3 cups chopped, peeled, baked potatoes
   (about 4 medium)
1 teaspoon minced Roasted Garlic (see
   page 38)
1 cup Vegetable Stock (see page 152)
1 teaspoon chopped fresh parsley
1/4 teaspoon truffle oil
1/2 teaspoon sea salt
1/8 teaspoon white pepper

Preparation

Bring 2 cups of water to a low boil in a small saucepan. Add the fava beans and boil for 2 minutes. Remove the beans from the water with a slotted spoon and place into a bowl of ice water to cool. Add 1 1/2 cups of the potatoes to the hot water and boil for 1 minute. Drain well and combine the potatoes with the roasted garlic in a medium bowl. Peel the fava beans and add 3/4 cup to the warm potatoes.

In a mixing bowl, combine the remaining 1 1/2 cups of cold baked potatoes and the remaining 3/4 cup of fava beans. Place a ricer or food mill over the bowl of cold potatoes and fava beans and rice the warm potato mixture into the bowl. You may need to do this in batches depending on the size of your ricer or food mill. Stir in the stock, parsley, truffle oil, salt, and pepper.

Scoop up the potato mixture with a 1/4 cup measure and gently form into 10 patties.

Heat a griddle or nonstick pan over medium-high heat and lightly coat with cooking spray. Add the patties and brown on each side until golden brown, about 3 minutes per side.

Second serving option: Serve with small smoked salmon florets as passed hors d'oeuvre. Use 4 1/2 ounces of smoked salmon. Scoop the potato patties into two tablespoon portions. Cook as directed above. You will have twenty small patties. Divide the salmon into 1/4 ounce portions. You may need to cut the pieces of salmon in half lengthwise. To form the florets, begin folding each piece of salmon into a roll. After it is rolled up, gently fold down the top edges of the salmon to form a flower.

Place one salmon floret on each cooked potato patty. Arrange patties on platter to serve.

Edamame Ragoût

Per serving:
Calories 280; Protein 23g; Total Fat 14g;
Saturated Fat 1.5g; Carbohydrates 22g; Dietary
Fiber 14g; Cholesterol 0mg; Sodium 680mg

Edamame are fresh soybeans often served as an appetizer in sushi restaurants. Green, medium-sized beans with a refreshing, nutty flavor, edamame are an excellent (although underutilized) protein source. This recipe creates a quick and wonderfully delicious stew that's also good for you.

Ingredients
Makes 6 servings.

1/4 teaspoon toasted sesame oil
1 teaspoon minced garlic
1 teaspoon minced fresh ginger
2 cups edamame (shelled green soybeans)
2 cups julienned fresh shiitake mushrooms
1 cup thinly sliced bok choy
1/4 cup chopped green onion
2 tablespoons tamari (soy) sauce
2 tablespoons tahini (sesame seed paste)
1/4 cup Vegetable Stock (see page 152)

Preparation

Heat a medium sauté pan over medium-high heat. Add the toasted sesame oil to lightly coat the bottom of the pan. Add the garlic, ginger, edamame, mushrooms, and bok choy. Cook until the mushrooms are just softened, about 2 minutes. Mix in the green onion, tamari, tahini, and Vegetable Stock. Bring to a low boil and cook for 2 minutes. Remove from heat and serve.

Homemade Tofu

Per serving:
Calories 160; Protein 18g; Total Fat 10g;
Saturated Fat 1.5g; Carbohydrates 5g; Dietary
Fiber 1g; Cholesterol 0mg; Sodium 15mg

Many foodies take pride in knowing how to make items from scratch rather than always relying on the store-bought version. My assistant, Heidi DeCosmo, gave me this tofu recipe. It is time-consuming, but wonderfully gratifying. From this basic recipe, any flavor that you could possibly dream of can be achieved. Stir your choice of herbs and seasonings into the soymilk before you add the lemon juice. Organic soybeans are available in health food stores, or check chapter 13, Pantry Resources.

Ingredients

Makes about 10 servings.

2 1/2 pounds organic soybeans, soaked
   overnight
1 1/4 cups fresh lemon juice or seasoned
   rice wine vinegar

Preparation

Drain the soybeans. In a blender, puree 2 cups of the soybeans with 2 1/2 cups of water until the beans are finely chopped. Pour this mixture into a large stockpot. Repeat this process until all the beans have been pureed.

Place the stockpot over medium heat and bring to a high simmer. Simmer the soybeans for about 45 minutes. The liquid will start to boil up and you will need to cool it quickly by adding 2 or 3 cups of cold water until it subsides. The liquid needs to boil up and be cooled a total of three times.

Line a large colander with cheesecloth and place it in a large stockpot or bowl to collect the liquid. Carefully pour the hot mixture into the colander. *Caution: it will be very hot.* Using the back of a spoon, try to press out as much of the liquid as possible. This liquid is homemade soymilk, which will be used to make the tofu. Reserve the cooked soybeans for use in vegetable burgers, veggie meatballs, or other recipes that call for crumbled tofu.

Slowly drizzle about 1/2 cup of the lemon juice or vinegar into the soymilk and stir gently. You will begin to feel the soymilk coagulating. Be very gentle because you want the curds to stay large and intact. Cover the pot with aluminum foil and let rest for 3 minutes. Repeat the process with more lemon juice, 1/2 cup at a time, until the curds and whey have completely separated and the liquid in the pot is yellow and clear. You may not need all of the lemon juice.

Line a colander with cheesecloth and place over a large pan to collect the whey. Carefully pour the curds and whey into the colander. Cover with cheesecloth and a piece of plastic wrap. Use some clean bricks or large cans to weigh down the tofu. The tofu needs to be pressed for about 45 minutes for firm tofu. Shorten the pressing time if you would like softer tofu.

When the tofu is completely pressed, carefully turn it out onto a plate. Remove the cheesecloth and store the tofu covered with water in an airtight container. You need to change the water each day. The homemade tofu will keep about 5 days in the refrigerator if the water is changed daily.

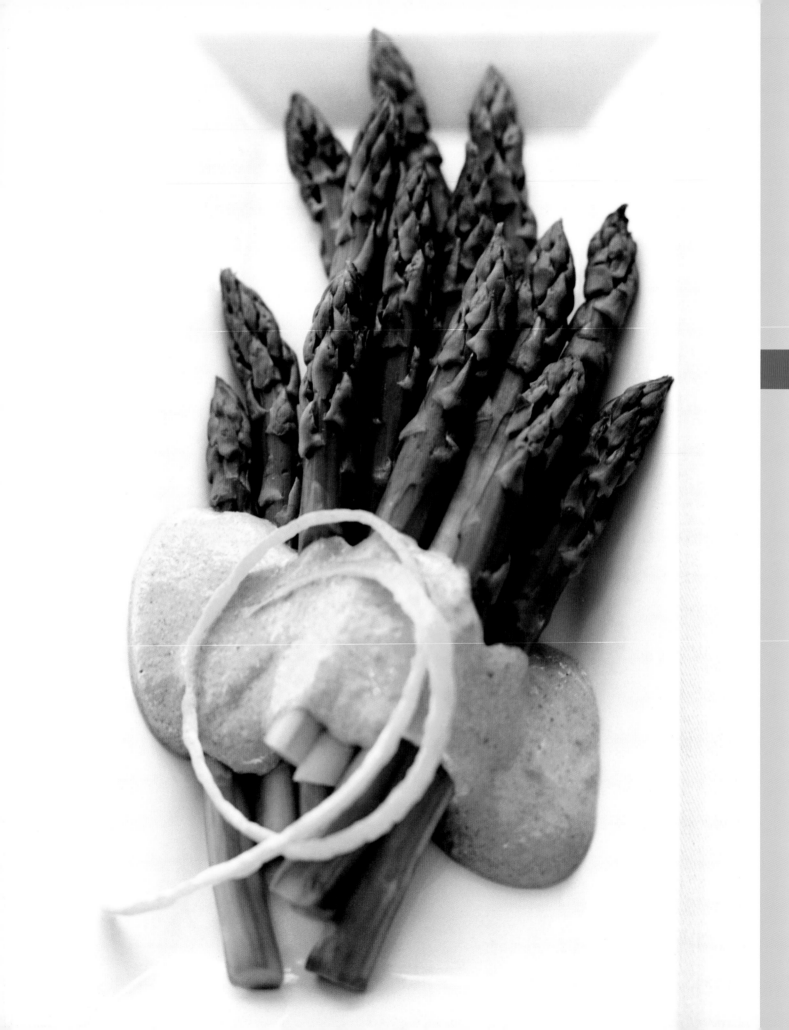

Vibrant Vegetables

Pictured at left: Asparagus with Tarragon Aïoli

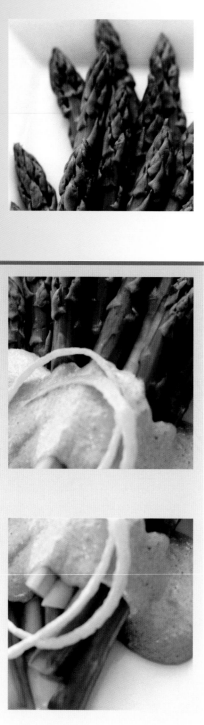

Through *Conscious Cuisine*, it is my goal to teach you to be more conscious of where and how your produce is grown, prepared, and served. Foods that provide sustenance, nourishment, and an abundance of flavor should be used in a more dominant role in our diet commensurate with their nutritional importance. In addition, we must become more active in taking responsibility for ensuring that the food crops we consume and leave for future generations are *sustainable*.

Today, fresh produce is big business. In past decades, the American landscape was fertile with farms large and small. It was common to see farm stands along the side of the road in every region of the United States. Huge outdoor markets were also present in major cities, allowing city dwellers the opportunity to enjoy a wide variety of farm-fresh fruits and vegetables at inexpensive prices.

Fast forwarding to the twenty-first century, much of America's farmland is growing communities of homes and businesses rather than fruits and vegetables. With less fertile land and more cutting-edge technology, the result is brightly colored, perfectly shaped, and flavorless fruits and vegetables.

The era of assuming that fresh produce is grown without the aid of chemicals, radiation, or genetic modification is over. We, the consumers, do have a choice and a voice concerning the integrity of the produce that we purchase. First we must become aware, active, and responsible.

Consciously allow fresh seasonal vegetables to take center stage in your meals, and purchase organically grown produce whenever you can. Revel in the season's luscious vegetables bursting with flavor and nutrition.

Leafy vegetables are excellent sources of beta-carotene, vitamin C, fiber, iron, and calcium.

Flowers, buds, and stalks (i.e. broccoli, cauliflower, celery, and asparagus) are rich in vitamin C, calcium, potassium, and some cancer-fighting compounds.

Seeds and pods (i.e. beans, peas, and corn) are exceptional sources of energy, B vitamins, zinc, potassium, magnesium, calcium, and iron.

Roots, bulbs, and tubers (i.e. onions, turnips, beets, fennel, and potatoes) are good sources of fiber, vitamin C, beta-carotene, and potassium. Onions and garlic have properties that may reduce blood pressure and cholesterol levels.

Fruits and vegetables (i.e. eggplant, squash, peppers, and tomatoes) provide many nutrients and add aromatic flavors that help in creating tantalizing soups, sauces, fillings, and condiments.

Conscious Cuisine teaches you to utilize vegetables as the main component of a meal, rather than as an insubstantial side dish. The focus is on the ingredients that provide the most nutrition and flavor, enabling you to enjoy meals that are balanced with whole grains and reduced portions of proteins.

This chapter will illustrate how to design meals around great-tasting dishes like Carrot and Cardamom Soufflés in Onion Cups; Layered Spinach, Wild Mushroom, and Carrot Mousse; or Curried Cauliflower with Raisins and Cashews, to list a sampling of great vegetable dishes.

Asparagus with Tarragon Aïoli

Per 6 asparagus stalks and 2 tablespoons aïoli:
Calories 40; Protein 4g; Total Fat 0.5g;
Saturated Fat 0g; Carbohydrates 7g; Dietary
Fiber 2g; Cholesterol 0mg; Sodium 190mg

The bright green and white tips of asparagus are cooked quickly and easily in salted boiling water. Serve as a delicious and attractive vegetable dish or appetizer. Photo on page 212.

Ingredients
Makes 4 servings.

1/2 teaspoon sea salt
1 pound green or white asparagus
(24 spears), bottoms trimmed
1/2 cup Tarragon Aïoli (see page 25)

Preparation
If the asparagus is large, use a vegetable peeler to peel the stalks to just below the tips. This will ensure even cooking and remove the outer skin that becomes tough as the asparagus grows.

Bring 2 quarts of water and the salt to a boil in a medium saucepan. Add the asparagus and cook until it is tender, but still firm (a knife will easily pierce the asparagus), 3 to 5 minutes. Remove the asparagus from the water and serve immediately with the aïoli. (You can also chill the asparagus in ice water and serve cold or refrigerate to serve later.)

Roasted Bell Peppers with Broccoli en Papillote

Per serving:
Calories 45; Protein 3g; Total Fat 0g; Saturated Fat 0g; Carbohydrates 9g; Dietary Fiber 3g; Cholesterol 0mg; Sodium 135mg

Fire-roasted bell pepper is a wonderful flavor enhancer for both vegetable and meat dishes. Sealing in foil and baking with fresh broccoli and cauliflower creates a delicious marriage of flavors that retains all of the natural goodness of each vegetable. It is an attractive, convenient way to cook and serve vegetables.

Ingredients
Makes 6 servings.

2 Roasted Red Bell Peppers, (see page 38), peeled, cut into 1-inch strips
1 head broccoli, broken into florets
1 head cauliflower, broken into florets
1/4 teaspoon extra-virgin olive oil
1/2 teaspoon minced garlic
3 teaspoons Fresh Herb Mix (see page 39)
1/4 teaspoon sea salt
1/8 teaspoon freshly ground black pepper

Preparation
Preheat the oven to 400°F (205°C).

Cut six 12-inch squares of foil. Divide the bell peppers, broccoli, and cauliflower, and place on center of each sheet of foil. Season vegetables with equal amounts of olive oil, garlic, herbs, salt, and pepper. Fold over the foil to form a rectangle and seal the edges together. Place the foil packages on baking sheets and bake for 15 minutes.

Serve the vegetables in the foil on a plate and open them at the table.

Glazed Beets

The winter months bring forth a variety of root vegetables at their peak of ripeness. Beets are available in sizes large or small, and my personal favorite is baby beets with their tops. Reserve the delicious green tops to mix with salad greens or cook them as you would spinach. The baby beets range in color from candy-striped to golden to brilliant, deep maroon. Use one of the following glazes to enhance the natural sweetness of the glorious beet.

Per serving with Citrus Glaze:
Calories 60; Protein 2g; Total Fat 0.5g; Saturated Fat 0g; Carbohydrates 15g; Dietary Fiber 2g; Cholesterol 0mg; Sodium 125mg

Per serving with Tamari Glaze:
Calories 60; Protein 3g; Total Fat 0.5g; Saturated Fat 0g; Carbohydrates 13g; Dietary Fiber 2g; Cholesterol 0mg; Sodium 1130mg

Ingredients
Makes 4 servings.

16 baby beets, peeled
1/4 teaspoon extra-virgin olive oil
1/8 teaspoon sea salt
1/8 teaspoon freshly ground black pepper

Citrus Glaze
1 tablespoon freshly grated orange zest
3/4 cup unsweetened orange juice
1/4 cup fresh lemon juice
1 teaspoon honey
1/2 teaspoon minced fresh ginger

Tamari Glaze
3/4 cup unsweetened orange juice
1/4 cup tamari (soy) sauce
1/2 teaspoon minced fresh ginger
1/2 teaspoon minced garlic

Preparation
Preheat the oven 425°F (220°C).

Place the beets on a baking sheet and toss with the olive oil, salt, and pepper. Bake for 15 to 20 minutes or until the beets are just softened.

Make the glaze of your choice. For either glaze, combine all the ingredients in a small saucepan over medium-high heat. Bring to a low boil and boil until the mixture is reduced by half.

Toss the beets with the glaze and serve.

Carrot Cardamom Soufflés in Onion Cups

I was introduced to onion cups and their multitude of uses during culinary school. Although they take little time to prepare, they are seldom seen in restaurants today. The classic preparation of a savory carrot soufflé seasoned with the exotic flavor of cardamom and baked in an onion cup makes for a glorious, show-stopping vegetable presentation that's surpassed only by its deliciousness.

Per serving:
Calories 50; Protein 3g; Total Fat 0g; Saturated Fat 0g; Carbohydrates 9g; Dietary Fiber 2g; Cholesterol 0mg; Sodium 150mg

Ingredients
Makes 12 servings.

3 large yellow onions
4 cups chopped, peeled carrots (about 1 1/4 pounds)
1 teaspoon cardamom
1/2 teaspoon sea salt
1/8 teaspoon white pepper
8 large egg whites

Preparation
Preheat the oven to 375°F (190°C). Coat a 12-cup muffin pan with cooking spray.

For the onion cups: Bring a large saucepan of water and 1 teaspoon sea salt to a boil. Fill a medium mixing bowl with ice and water for an ice-water bath.

Remove the skin from the onions and discard. Cut off 1/4 inch from the root end and 3/4 inch from the top of each onion. Place the onions in the boiling water just long enough for the outer layer of the onion to be cooked, about 2 minutes. Use a slotted spoon to transfer the onions to the ice bath for 30 seconds to stop the cooking process. Remove the onions from the ice bath. Carefully press down on the center of each onion to remove the outer layer. Repeat process to blanch the next outer layer to obtain 12 onion cups. If the onion layer breaks it is still usable. Use the remaining onion for other dishes.

Add the carrots to the boiling water and cook until very soft, about 10 minutes. Drain in a colander.

Place the carrots in a food processor and puree until smooth. Season with the cardamom, salt, and pepper. Transfer the carrot mixture to a medium bowl.

Place the egg whites in a clean bowl and beat with an electric mixer until stiff peaks form, about 3 minutes. Fold the egg whites into the carrot mixture.

Arrange the onion cups in the muffin pan. If there is a tear in the onion, just overlap the edges. Spoon about 1/3 cup of the soufflé mixture into each onion cup. Bake for 15 minutes or until the soufflé has set up and is lightly browned.

Serve as a side dish or a vegetarian entrée.

Variation
Bake the soufflé filling in soufflé cups coated with cooking spray. Use 1/2 cup of filling each and bake for 20 minutes.

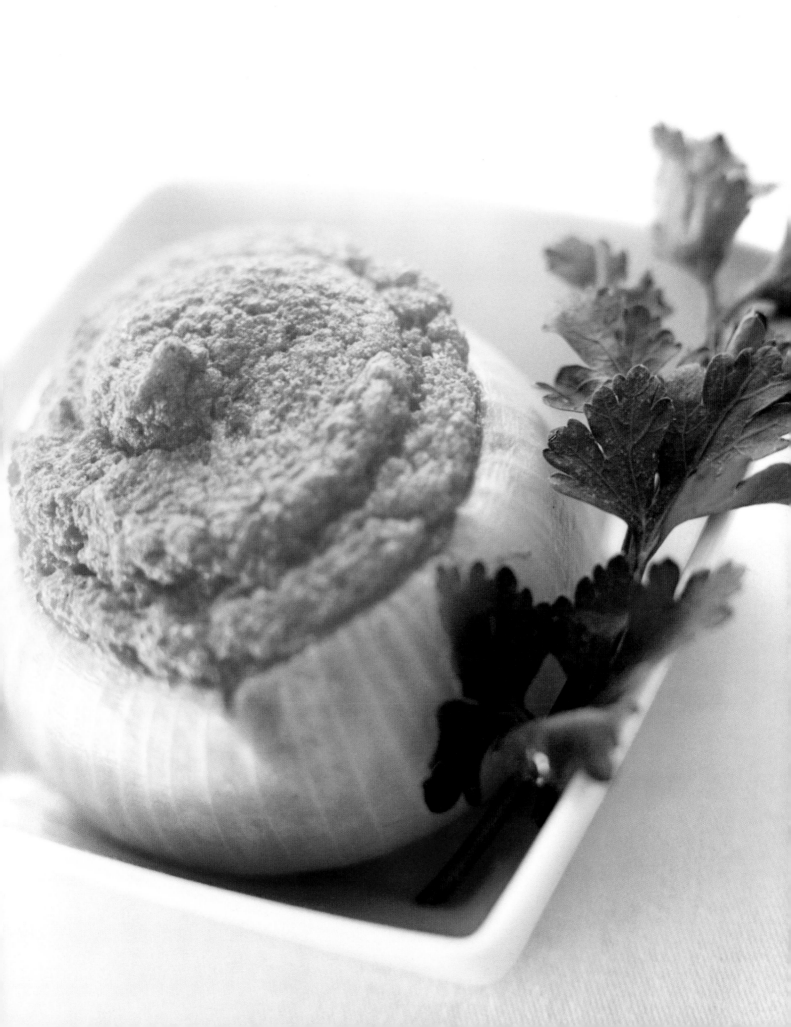

Curried Cauliflower with Raisins and Cashews

Per serving:
Calories 110; Protein 3g; Total Fat 1g;
Saturated Fat 0g; Carbohydrates 24g; Dietary
Fiber 3g; Cholesterol 0mg; Sodium 230mg

Jazz up cauliflower with the delicate flavors of curry and sweet raisins. The color and contrast of textures in this dish will delight cauliflower lovers.

Ingredients

Makes 6 servings.

1 head cauliflower
1 1/2 cups unsweetened apple juice
1 tablespoon curry powder
1/2 teaspoon sea salt
1/2 cup raisins
1 tablespoon chopped cashews

Preparation

Remove the core from the cauliflower and cut into florets.

Combine the apple juice, curry powder, salt, and raisins in a medium saucepan over medium-high heat. Add the cauliflower. Bring to a low boil, cover, and cook for 3 minutes. Carefully remove the lid and stir. Cover again and cook for 3 minutes more. Remove from the heat, stir in the cashews, and serve.

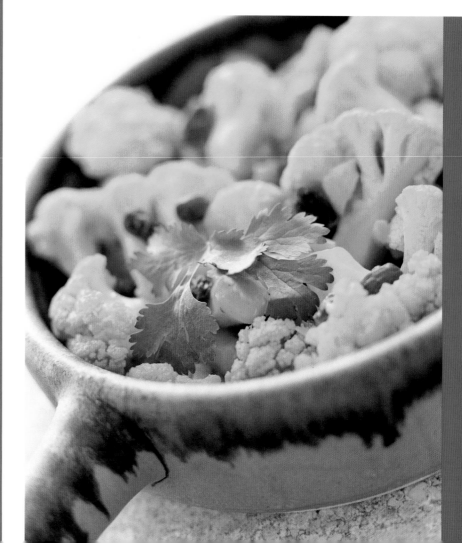

Pumpkin Flan

The warm color and natural sweetness of fall pumpkins make this an attractive and festive treat for fall and winter menus. I often top off the flan cup with cooked black quinoa before unmolding to reveal a two-tone gem of contrasting colors, textures, and flavors.

Per flan:
Calories 60; Protein 5g; Total Fat 1g; Saturated Fat 0g; Carbohydrates 9g; Dietary Fiber 1g; Cholesterol 30mg; Sodium 210mg

Ingredients
Makes 8 flans.

3 cups canned pumpkin puree
1 large egg
3 large egg whites
1 cup fat-free evaporated milk
1/2 teaspoon sea salt
1/2 teaspoon cinnamon
1/2 teaspoon allspice
1/2 teaspoon ginger
1/2 teaspoon cloves
1/2 teaspoon nutmeg
1/4 teaspoon white pepper

Preparation

Preheat the oven to 325°F (165°C). Lightly coat eight 4-ounce ramekins or ovenproof coffee cups with cooking spray. Pour 1 inch of water into a 13 x 9-inch baking pan to use as a water bath.

Place all the ingredients in a blender and process until smooth and incorporated, 2 to 3 minutes.

Spoon 1/2 cup of the pumpkin mixture into each of the prepared cups. Place the filled cups into the water bath. Bake for 25 to 30 minutes or until firm to the touch. Keep warm in the water bath until ready to serve.

The flans can be served in the ramekins, or carefully run a knife around the edge of each cup and turn upside down onto a serving plate to unmold.

Layered Spinach, Wild Mushroom, and Carrot Mousse

As chef entremetier (chef of the vegetable station) of the "old" Park Hyatt Hotel Chicago, I was challenged to prepare light, great-tasting vegetable mousses of various flavors to accompany specialty dishes. The lightness and airiness of the mousse was achieved through the use of heavy cream and whole eggs that were vigorously blended with cooked vegetables. The methodology remains the same, but I have drastically reduced the quantity of cream and eggs to create a mousse that's even more flavorful and has less fat and fewer calories.

Ingredients

Makes 8 mousses.

Carrot Layer

3 cups chopped, peeled carrots (about 5 medium)
1/4 teaspoon sea salt
1/8 teaspoon freshly ground black pepper
4 large egg whites
1/2 cup fat-free milk

Mushroom Layer

1/4 teaspoon extra-virgin olive oil
1/2 cup chopped yellow onion (about 1 medium)
1/2 teaspoon minced Roasted Garlic (see page 38)
4 cups assorted fresh mushrooms (2 portobellos, 6 medium oyster, and 8 medium shiitake)
2 teaspoons Fresh Herb Mix (see page 39)
1/4 teaspoon sea salt
1/8 teaspoon freshly ground black pepper
3 large egg whites
1/2 cup fat-free milk

Preparation

Preheat the oven to 350°F (175°C). Spray eight 4-ounce soufflé ramekins or ovenproof coffee cups with cooking spray; set aside.

For the Carrot Layer: Bring 3 cups of water to a boil in a small saucepan over medium-high heat. Add the carrots, salt, and pepper. Boil until the carrots are soft, 5 to 10 minutes. Drain the carrots in a colander.

Carefully ladle the carrots into a food processor and process until smooth. Add the egg whites and milk. Pulse to mix. Transfer the carrot mixture to a bowl and set aside until ready to assemble the mousse.

For the Mushroom Layer: Heat a sauté pan over medium-high heat and add the olive oil to lightly coat the bottom of the pan. Add the onion, Roasted Garlic, mushrooms, Fresh Herb Mix, salt, and pepper. Cook until the mushrooms are softened, about 3 minutes. Remove from heat. Place in a colander to drain off any excess liquid.

Carefully ladle the mushroom mixture into a food processor and process until smooth. Add the egg whites and milk. Pulse to mix. Transfer the mushroom mixture to a bowl and set aside until ready to assemble the mousse.

For the Spinach Layer: Heat a sauté pan over medium-high heat and add the olive oil to lightly coat the bottom of the pan. Add the onion, garlic, spinach, salt, pepper and nutmeg. Cook until spinach is wilted, about 3 minutes. Remove from heat. Place in a colander to drain off any excess liquid.

Carefully ladle the spinach mixture into a food processor and process until smooth. Add the egg whites and milk. Pulse to mix. Transfer the spinach mixture to a bowl and set aside until ready to assemble the mousse.

To assemble: Spread 2 tablespoons of the carrot mixture over the bottom of each prepared cup. Spread 2 tablespoons of the mushroom mixture over each carrot layer. Spread 2 tablespoons of the spinach mixture over each mushroom layer.

Ingredients continued

Spinach Layer
1/4 teaspoon extra-virgin olive oil
1/2 cup chopped yellow onion (about
    1 medium)
1/2 teaspoon minced fresh garlic
8 cups packed fresh spinach
1/4 teaspoon sea salt
1/8 teaspoon freshly ground black pepper
1/4 teaspoon nutmeg
3 large egg whites
1/4 cup fat-free milk

Add 1/2 inch of water to a 13 x 9-inch baking pan to use as a water bath. Place the mousse cups into the pan. Bake for 30 to 35 minutes or until the mousse has firmed up and is light golden brown. Remove from the oven and place the cups on a cooling rack for 5 minutes. Run a knife around the side of each cup. Turn the cups over onto serving plates to unmold. Cut each circle in half to display the tiered mousse, if desired.

Sautéed Swiss Chard

Per serving:
Calories 50; Protein 5g; Total Fat 1g; Saturated Fat 0g; Carbohydrates 10g; Dietary Fiber 4g; Cholesterol 0mg; Sodium 790mg

This chapter would be incomplete without directions for preparing delicious greens such as Swiss chard, spinach, kale, and bok choy. Each green can be cooked quickly and easily to offer a lift to any meal, while providing a boost of vital nutrients.

Ingredients

Makes 4 servings.

3 bunches Swiss chard, stems removed
1/4 teaspoon extra-virgin olive oil
1/2 teaspoon minced garlic
1 tablespoon tamari (soy) sauce
1/8 teaspoon freshly ground black pepper

Preparation

Rough chop the Swiss chard. Heat a large sauté pan over medium-high heat and add the olive oil to lightly coat the bottom of the pan. Add the Swiss chard, garlic, tamari, and pepper. Cook until the Swiss chard starts to wilt, about 2 minutes. Remove from the heat and serve.

Variations

Substitute 3 bunches of kale, 4 heads of bok choy, or 6 cups of lightly packed spinach for the Swiss chard.

Per serving of kale:
Calories 60; Protein 4g; Total Fat 1g; Saturated Fat 0g; Carbohydrates 10g; Dietary Fiber 2g; Cholesterol 0mg; Sodium 290mg

Per serving of bok choy:
Calories 120; Protein 13g; Total Fat 2g; Saturated Fat 0g; Carbohydrates 19g; Dietary Fiber 8g; Cholesterol 0mg; Sodium 800mg

Per serving of spinach:
Calories 120; Protein 15g; Total Fat 2g; Saturated Fat 0g; Carbohydrates 18g; Dietary Fiber 14g; Cholesterol 0mg; Sodium 650mg

Ratatouille

Per serving:
Calories 40; Protein 1g; Total Fat 0.5g;
Saturated Fat 0g; Carbohydrates 8g; Dietary
Fiber 2g; Cholesterol 0mg; Sodium 200mg

This classic Provençale dish of eggplant, zucchini, and tomatoes is a wonderful marriage of flavors and textures. Ratatouille is versatile, easy to prepare, and packed with the goodness of a rainbow of vegetables. Try it for side dishes and appetizers, as well as a filling for pastas or other vegetables.

Ingredients
Makes 6 servings.

1/4 teaspoon extra-virgin olive oil
1/2 cup diced yellow onion (about
   1 medium)
1/2 cup diced zucchini (about 1 small)
1/2 cup diced yellow squash (about
   1 small)
1/2 cup diced eggplant (about 1/2 small)
1/2 cup diced red bell pepper (about
   1 small)
1/2 cup diced green bell pepper (about
   1 small)
1/2 cup diced portobello mushroom, gills
   removed (about 1 medium mushroom)
1 1/2 cups peeled, chopped, and seeded
   fresh tomatoes (see Chef's Tip, page 186)
   or 1 14 1/2-ounce can
1 tablespoon minced garlic
1 tablespoon balsamic vinegar
1 teaspoon dried thyme
1 teaspoon dried oregano
1 teaspoon dried basil
1/2 teaspoon sea salt
1/4 teaspoon freshly ground black pepper

Preparation
Heat a large sauté pan over medium-high heat and add the olive oil to lightly coat the bottom of the pan. Add all the vegetables and garlic. Sauté until the vegetables have started to soften, about 5 minutes. Add the remaining ingredients and simmer for 10 minutes.

Baked Squash

This simple recipe for baked squash is a delicious and easy way to cook and serve winter squash of any type. Try all three variations—the natural sweetness of the squash is complemented with maple syrup and spices, Parmesan cheese, or even tamari for delightful flavor. I often hollow out kabocha or acorn squash, bake them, and fill them with stews or the lovely Ratatouille (see page 225).

Ingredients
Makes 4 servings.

2 small acorn squash, cut in half, seeds
    removed
4 teaspoons pure maple syrup
1/4 teaspoon cinnamon
1/8 teaspoon nutmeg

Preparation
Preheat the oven to 400°F (205°C).

Place the squash halves, cut side up, on a baking sheet. Drizzle each squash half with 1 teaspoon maple syrup and sprinkle with the cinnamon and nutmeg. Bake for 25 to 30 minutes or until the squash is soft when a knife is inserted.

Variations

Squash with Tamari: Substitute 2 tablespoons tamari (soy) sauce for the maple syrup and spices. Divide the tamari among the 4 squash halves and bake as above.

Squash with Bread Crumbs and Cheese: Substitute bread crumbs and grated Parmesan cheese for the maple syrup and spices. Combine 1/4 cup bread crumbs and 1 tablespoon Parmesan cheese in a bowl. Spray the squash halves with cooking spray and sprinkle with the bread crumb mixture. Bake as above.

Dauphinoise Potatoes

Per serving:
Calories 130; Protein 2g; Total Fat 3g;
Saturated Fat 0g; Carbohydrates 26g; Dietary
Fiber 2g; Cholesterol 0mg; Sodium 230mg

Dauphinoise is a classic potato preparation in which the potatoes are thinly sliced and submerged in a custard of whole eggs and milk or cream before baking; it sometimes includes cheese. It was immensely rewarding to create this version that delivers on its promise of comfort and flavor with far less fat and calories. The blend of rice milk, almonds, and Roasted Garlic creates a nondairy cream sauce that replaces the custard.

Ingredients
Makes 12 servings.

4 cups plain rice milk
1/4 cup blanched almonds
1/4 teaspoon freshly ground black pepper
2 teaspoons minced Roasted Garlic (see
    page 38)
1 teaspoon sea salt
1/4 teaspoon nutmeg
1/4 cup cornstarch
1/4 cup plain rice milk
6 russet potatoes, peeled and thinly sliced

Preparation
Preheat the oven to 375°F (190°C). Lightly coat a 13 x 9-inch baking dish with cooking spray and set aside.

In a blender, combine the rice milk, almonds, pepper, Roasted Garlic, salt, and nutmeg. Process until smooth. Pour the almond mixture into a medium saucepan and bring to a low boil. Combine the cornstarch and 1/4 cup rice milk and whisk into the almond mixture. Cook, stirring, until thickened, about 5 minutes. Remove from the heat.

Place the potatoes in a large mixing bowl and toss with the sauce. Arrange a layer of overlapping potatoes in the prepared baking pan. Repeat with the remaining potatoes and pour any remaining sauce over the top. Bake for 15 to 20 minutes or until the potatoes have just softened.

Remove from the oven and cool for 5 minutes before serving.

Vegetable and Potato Pavé

Per serving:
Calories 250; Protein 6g; Total Fat 2g; Saturated Fat 0g; Carbohydrates 51g; Dietary Fiber 8g; Cholesterol 0mg; Sodium 220mg

Think of this recipe as lasagna without the pasta and tomatoes—the layering is similar to the assembly of a traditional lasagna. The bright colors of butternut squash, mushrooms, spinach, red bell peppers, and potatoes are spectacular, and the combination of flavors is comforting.

Ingredients
Makes 12 servings.

1 tablespoon extra-virgin olive oil

6 cups julienned portobello mushrooms, gills removed (about 8 medium mushrooms)

6 cups julienned fresh shiitake mushrooms (about 1 pound)

15 Yukon Gold potatoes, scrubbed, unpeeled

2 medium butternut squash, peeled, seeded

3 tablespoons potato starch

1/4 cup Fresh Herb Mix (see page 39)

1 teaspoon sea salt

1 teaspoon freshly ground black pepper

8 Roasted Red Bell Peppers (see page 38), peeled and seeded

6 cups packed spinach, stems removed

Preparation

Preheat the oven to 350°F (175°C). Spray a 13 x 9-inch baking dish with cooking spray.

Heat a large sauté pan over medium-high heat and add the olive oil to lightly coat the bottom of the pan. Add the mushrooms and sauté until soft, about 5 minutes.

Cut the potatoes and the butternut squash on a mandoline or with a sharp knife into 1/4-inch-thick slices.

Arrange 1/3 of the potatoes to cover the bottom of the prepared dish in rows, overlapping slightly. Sprinkle with 1 tablespoon of the potato starch and season with 1/3 of the herbs, salt, and pepper. Add a layer of 1/2 of the butternut squash over the potatoes. Add a layer of 1/2 of the roasted peppers.

Spread 1/2 of the cooked mushrooms over the roasted peppers. Layer 1/2 of the spinach over the mushrooms, making sure to arrange it as evenly as possible. Layer another 1/3 of the potatoes over the spinach. Sprinkle the potatoes with 1 tablespoon of the potato starch and 1/3 of the herbs, salt, and pepper. Repeat the process again with the remaining vegetables. Finish with a layer of potatoes, the remaining herbs, salt, pepper, and the remaining 1 tablespoon potato starch. The entire pavé consists of 3 layers of potatoes with 2 sets of vegetable layers in between.

Spray both sides of a piece of parchment paper cut to the size of the pan and place on top of the pavé. Place another baking pan or casserole dish of equal size on top and weigh down with clean bricks or another heavy object that can withstand heat.

Place in the oven and bake for approximately 1 hour or until pavé is soft in the center—check by inserting a small knife into the center. Let the pavé rest for 15 minutes before cutting.

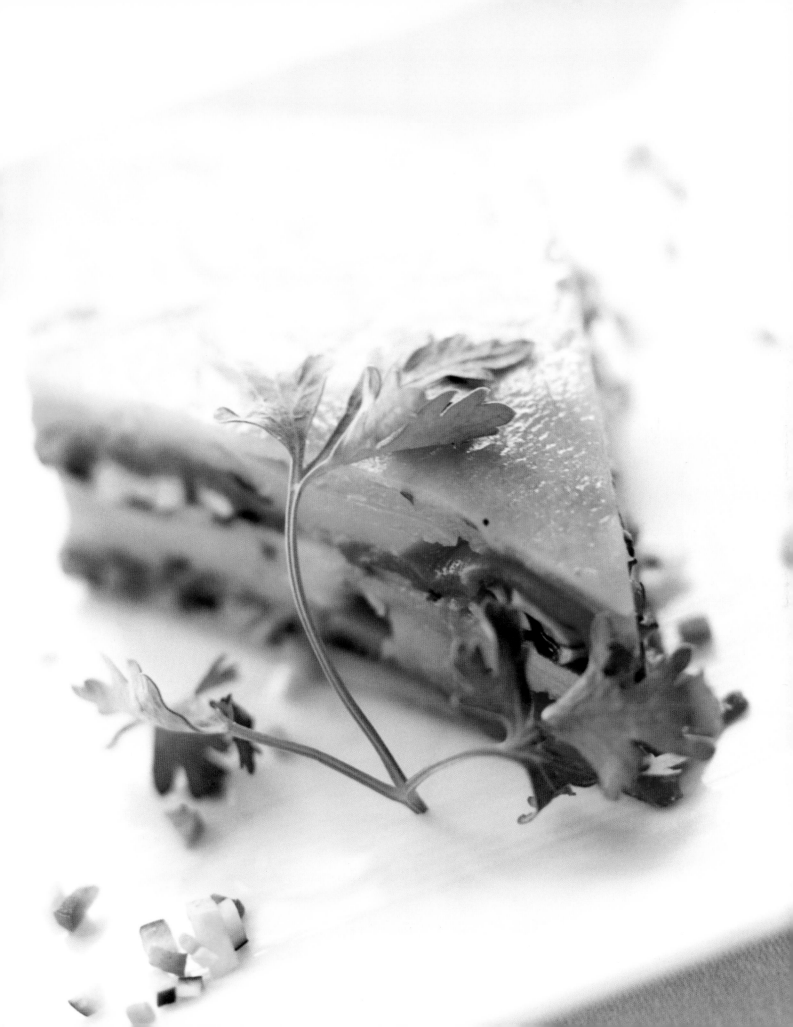

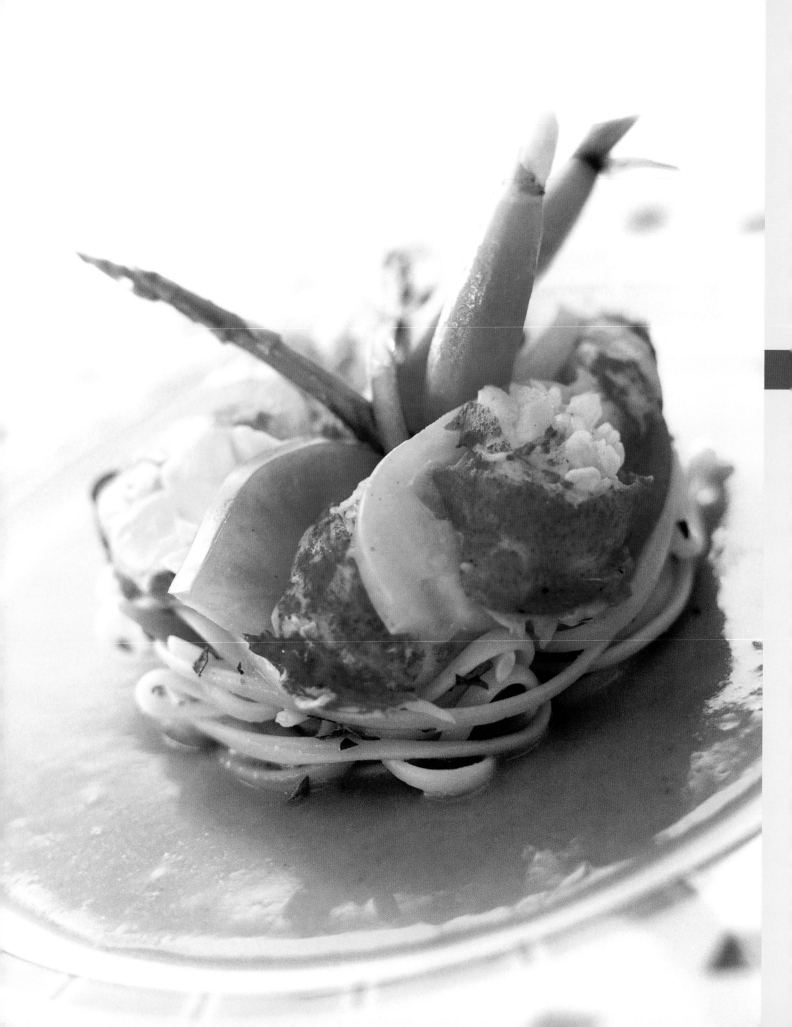

Creative Main Plates

chapter 10

Asian-Style Hot Pot with Sirloin of Beef
Barley Risotto with Wild Mushrooms, Roasted Tenderloin of Beef, and Red Wine Reduction
Red Rice with Apples and Almonds with Roast Loin of Lamb and Tomato-Rosemary Chutney
Chicken Pot-au-Feu
Turkey Osso Buco
Chile Crêpes with Turkey Mole
Asian Slaw with Asian-Marinated Pork Tenderloin
Fried Brown Rice and Sautéed Vegetables with Citrus Five-Spice Marinated Duck Breast
Beet Couscous and Steamed Organic Baby Vegetables with Pan-Seared Orange Roughy and Lemon-Garlic Sauce
Dauphinoise Potatoes, Chile-Crusted Red Snapper, and Yellow Tomato Sauce
Timbale of Soba Noodles with Steamed Vegetable-Wrapped Black Sea Bass and Tamari-Ginger Sauce
Roulade of Salmon Filled with Buckwheat and Wild Rice Stuffing with Beet and Ginger Sauce
Braised Sea Scallops and Gulf Shrimp with Orzo Griddle Cakes in a Saffron-Chive Sauce
Crisp Shrimp and Vegetable Spring Rolls with Edamame Ragoût
Curried Tofu and Napa Cabbage Roulade with Shiitake Mushroom Sauce
Smoked Tofu-Filled Bean Curd Sheet with Shiitake Mushroom Sauce
Tempeh Scaloppini
Grilled Eggplant "Tacos" with Tempeh
Tofu Napoleon with Yellow Tomato Sauce
Baked Kabocha Squash with Seitan
Vegetable Casserole
Roasted Lobster Tails with Linguine and Baby Carrots and English Pea Sauce
Vegetable Tamales with Toasted Fennel and Tomato Sauce

Pictured at left: Roasted Lobster Tails with Linguine and Baby Carrots and English Pea Sauce

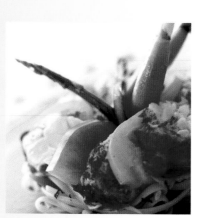

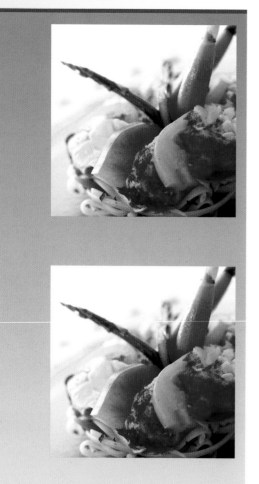

This chapter will illustrate how to prepare a select number of main plates. Through *Conscious Cuisine* you will be shown how main plates are created around wonderfully delicious whole grains and fresh seasonal vegetables, refocusing meal planning around foods that promote good health through balanced nutrition and heightened flavor components. Use these examples as a basis to prepare others on your own.

This chapter includes beautifully presented main plates such as Fried Brown Rice and Sautéed Vegetables with Citrus Five-Spice Marinated Duck Breast. A main plate like Beet Couscous and Steamed Organic Baby Vegetables with Pan-Seared Orange Roughy and Lemon-Garlic Sauce emphasizes how wonderful grains and vegetables can be combined with a protein food to make a balanced meal.

Inventive main plates include Grilled Eggplant Bundles with Tempeh, and Chile Crêpes with Turkey Mole. Various food styles and ethnic cultures are included to illustrate the spectrum of trends and flavors consciously prepared foods can encompass.

Each of these menu items is often featured at Miraval as I travel gastronomically with my staff and guests through the cuisines of the southwestern United States, Italy, the Mediterranean, and Asia. Vegetarian and nouvelle cuisines are also explored within *Conscious Cuisine*.

It is very satisfying to me to serve meals that are prepared with the wellness of Miraval's guests in mind. Our challenge in Miraval's kitchens is to create foods that are delicious, healthful, and rival those prepared in the traditional manner (with all the fat and calories), but so good that no one can tell the difference. Positive proof that we have achieved this goal comes from conversations with and letters from enthusiastic guests who testify that the meals we serve are as good as, or better than, those they cook at home or enjoy in their favorite restaurants.

Asian-Style Hot Pot with Sirloin of Beef

Per serving:
Calories 440; Protein 39g; Total Fat 14g;
Saturated Fat 5g; Carbohydrates 36g; Dietary
Fiber 5g; Cholesterol 95mg; Sodium 390mg

The spicy and exotic flavors of this aromatic broth create a light and refreshing entrée soup. Prepare the broth in large batches and freeze it—it can be used as a sauce on other entrées. Carefully measure the fish sauce, as a small amount will enhance the flavor of the broth, but even a little too much will overpower it. Serve with rice for a delicious, light meal.

Ingredients
Make 4 servings.

1/4 teaspoon extra-virgin olive oil
4 4-ounce beef sirloin medallions
1 teaspoon minced shallots
1 teaspoon minced fresh ginger
1 teaspoon minced fresh lemongrass
1/2 teaspoon fish sauce
2 tablespoons tomato paste
3 cups Veal Stock (see page 158)
1/4 teaspoon sea salt
1/8 teaspoon freshly ground black pepper
8 baby carrots, about 4 ounces
1 tablespoon minced fresh cilantro
1/3 cup chopped green onion
12 snow pea pods
12 broccoli florets
2 cups cooked jasmine or basmati rice

Preparation

Heat a medium saucepan over medium-high heat and add the olive oil to lightly coat the bottom of the pan. Add the beef and sear on all sides until browned, about 5 minutes total. Remove the beef from the pan and set aside.

In the same saucepan, add the shallots, ginger, and lemongrass. Cook until the shallots have just softened, about 1 minute. Stir in the fish sauce and tomato paste and cook for 1 minute. Add the stock and bring to a boil. Stir to loosen the browned bits and sediments on the bottom of the pan. Add the seared beef medallions, salt, pepper, and carrots. Reduce the heat to low and simmer for 20 minutes.

Add the cilantro, green onion, snow peas, and broccoli to the sauce and simmer for about 3 minutes.

To serve: Divide the rice among 4 serving bowls. Cut each beef medallion in half horizontally to make 2 rounds. Arrange the beef rounds on top of the rice, spoon the vegetables and sauce around the beef, and serve.

Barley Risotto with Wild Mushrooms, Roasted Tenderloin of Beef, and Red Wine Reduction

Per serving:
Calories 390; Protein 30g; Total Fat 11g;
Saturated Fat 3.5g; Carbohydrates 34g; Dietary
Fiber 8g; Cholesterol 70mg; Sodium 450mg

Ingredients
Makes 4 servings.

1/2 teaspoon extra-virgin olive oil

4 4-ounce filet mignons (beef tenderloin)

1/2 teaspoon sea salt

1/2 teaspoon freshly ground black pepper

1 tablespoon Fresh Herb Mix (see page 39)

Barley Risotto with Wild Mushrooms (see page 194)

2 cups steamed fresh vegetables, such as asparagus or assorted baby vegetables

4 tablespoons Red Wine Reduction (see page 19)

Prior to developing Conscious Cuisine, I limited my use of barley to beef and barley soup. Remembering this successful flavor combination inspired me to create this dish. If you are as much of a mushroom fan as I am, be sure to use fresh, seasonal wild mushrooms when available. They elevate the flavor of the barley to incredibly delicious heights. Pairing the hearty flavors of barley and wild mushrooms with fresh asparagus and the ultra-lean protein of beef tenderloin makes a feast for the eyes as well as the soul.

Preparation
Preheat the oven to 400°F (205°C).

Heat an ovenproof medium sauté pan over medium-high heat. Add the olive oil to lightly coat the bottom of the pan. Season each filet with the salt, pepper, and herbs. Add the filets to the pan and sear on one side for 2 minutes. Turn and place the pan in the oven to complete the cooking, about 8 minutes for medium-rare.

To serve: Press 1/2 cup of the risotto into a coffee cup, mold, or ring and unmold in the center of a plate. Repeat to make 3 more molds. Remove the filets from the oven and slice each one horizontally into 4 round medallions. Artfully arrange 1/2 cup of the vegetables on each plate. Lean the beef slices against the risotto. Drizzle 1 tablespoon of the wine reduction over the beef, risotto, and vegetables and serve.

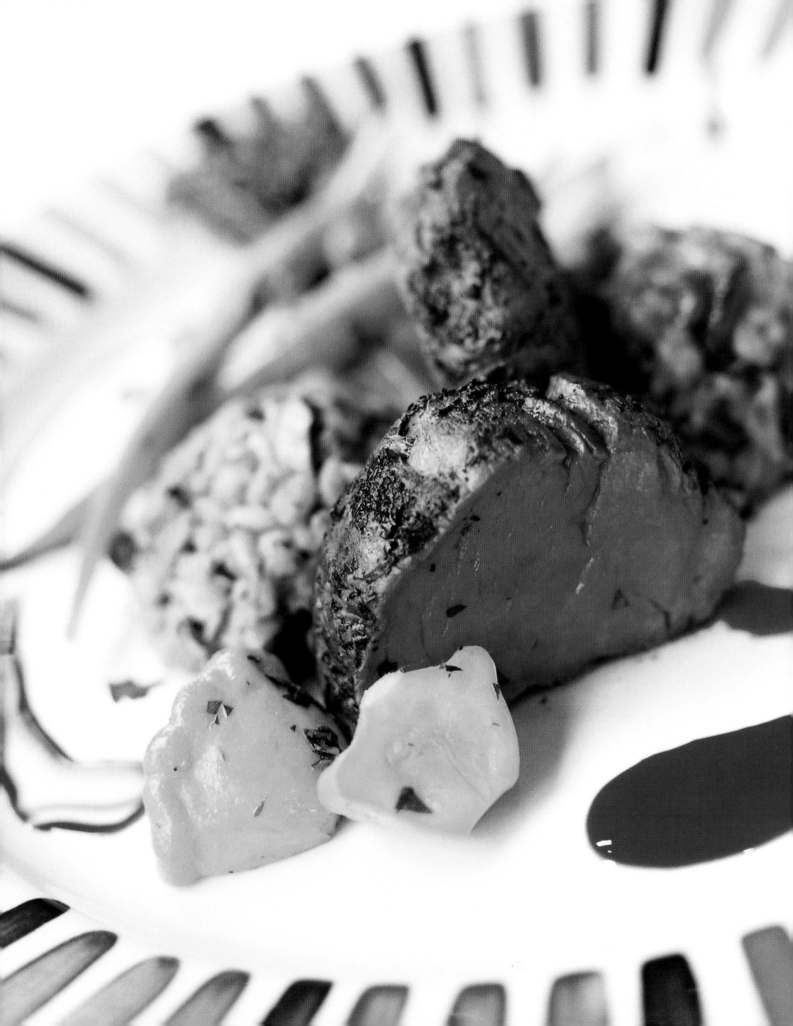

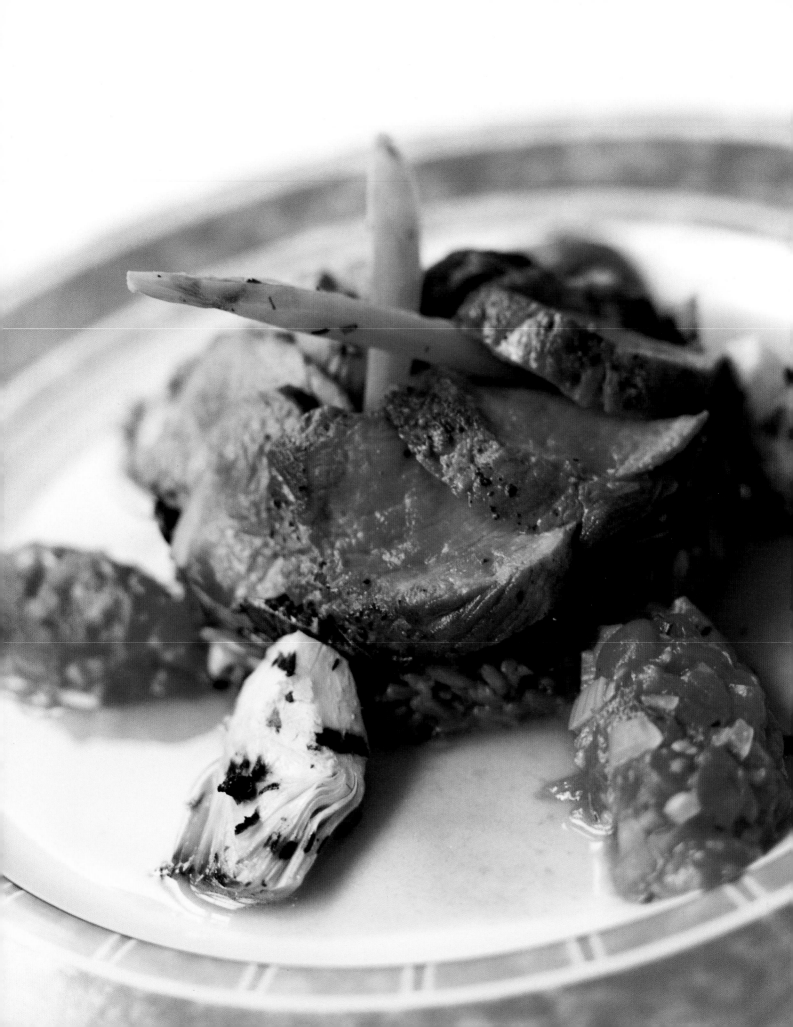

Red Rice with Apples and Almonds with Roast Loin of Lamb and Tomato-Rosemary Chutney

Per serving:
Calories 300; Protein 28g; Total Fat 9g;
Saturated Fat 3.5g; Carbohydrates 27g; Dietary
Fiber 4g; Cholesterol 75mg; Sodium 480mg

The pursuit of health-conscious food unveils the use of uncommon items that are both highly nutritious and great-tasting. I stumbled upon Himalayan red rice about three years ago. I was first struck by its beautiful color and, when I cooked it, its interesting flavor. The addition of tart Granny Smith apples and toasted almonds makes it even more appealing. This dish is complemented with wilted fresh spinach, lamb, and tomato chutney, producing a sophisticated flavor contrast that is a taste sensation.

Ingredients
Makes 4 servings.

1/4 teaspoon extra-virgin olive oil
1 pound whole, boneless lamb loin roast
1/2 teaspoon sea salt
1/4 teaspoon freshly ground black pepper
4 cup packed baby spinach
Tomato-Rosemary Chutney (see page 42)
Red Rice with Apples and Almonds (see
   page 202)

Garnish
Grilled artichoke hearts, optional
Steamed baby carrots, optional

Preparation
Preheat the oven to 375°F (190°C).

Heat a large ovenproof sauté pan over medium-high heat and add the olive oil to lightly coat the bottom of the pan. Season the lamb with a 1/4 teaspoon of the salt and 1/8 teaspoon of the pepper. Place the lamb in the pan and sear for 2 minutes. Place in the oven to finish cooking: 5 minutes for medium rare. Remove from the pan and allow the lamb to rest for about 3 minutes.

Heat a medium sauté pan over medium-high heat and coat the bottom of the pan with cooking spray. Add the baby spinach and season with remaining salt and pepper. Cook, stirring constantly, until the spinach has just softened.

To serve: On each serving plate, place 3 tablespoons of the chutney spaced out around the plate, spoon 1/3 cup red rice in the center of the plate, and arrange 1/4 cup wilted spinach on top of the rice. Cut the lamb into 1/2-inch slices. Divide the lamb among the 4 plates, fanned out into circles on top of the spinach. Garnish with the artichoke hearts and carrots, if using.

Chicken Pot-au-Feu

Per serving:
Calories 290; Protein 37g; Total Fat 2.5g;
Saturated Fat 0.5g; Carbohydrates 25g; Dietary
Fiber 4g; Cholesterol 80mg; Sodium 500mg

This is a classic French dish that dates back centuries. It has innumerable variations, including beef and poultry. A *pot-au-feu* is a complete and balanced meal that provides a richly flavored broth, proteins, vegetables, and carbohydrates. The preparation of a pot-au-feu can be rendered quick and easy by using small cuts of poultry and rough-cut vegetables. It may also be elaborately and elegantly presented by choosing tender, slow-cooking meat and precision-cut vegetables. You'll find that this dish tastes as good as it is good for you.

Ingredients
Makes 4 servings.

8 fingerling potatoes
Olive oil cooking spray
1/2 teaspoon sea salt
1/4 teaspoon freshly ground black pepper
2 teaspoons Fresh Herb Mix (see
    page 39)
1 medium zucchini
4 4-ounce chicken or pheasant breasts,
    skin removed
1/4 teaspoon extra-virgin olive oil
1 leek (white part only), cut in half
    lengthwise, cut into 1/2-inch slices
8 baby carrots
1 cup morel or small crimini mushrooms
1 teaspoon minced garlic
1/2 cup white wine
2 cups Chicken Stock (see page 154)
4 cups chopped Swiss chard

Preparation
Preheat the oven to 400°F (205°C).

Wash the fingerling potatoes, pat dry, and season with olive oil spray and half of the salt, pepper, and fresh herbs. Place the potatoes on a baking sheet and roast for 10 minutes or until soft to the touch.

Slice the zucchini into thirds crosswise; slice each piece into quarters lengthwise. For a classic French presentation, round the angled sides to form twelve oval sticks.

Season the chicken with the remaining 1/4 teaspoon salt, 1/8 teaspoon pepper, and 1 teaspoon herbs. Heat a sauté pan over medium-high heat and add the olive oil to lightly coat the bottom of the pan. Sear the chicken breasts on one side about 2 minutes and turn over. Add the leeks, carrots, mushrooms, zucchini, and garlic. Sauté, stirring constantly, for 1 minute to sear the vegetables. Add the white wine and boil until the wine is reduced by half, about 2 minutes. Stir in the stock and bring to a boil. Reduce heat and simmer until the chicken is cooked through, 7 to 10 minutes. Add the Swiss chard to one side of the pan to braise the greens in the cooking liquid, about 1 minute.

To serve: Place 1/2 cup of the Swiss chard in the center of 4 large soup bowls. Slice each chicken breast on an angle into 5 pieces. Arrange the chicken on top of the Swiss chard. Divide the vegetables among the four bowls and ladle the broth around the vegetables.

Turkey Osso Buco

Per serving:
Calories 620; Protein 38g; Total Fat 6g;
Saturated Fat 1.5g; Carbohydrates 82g; Dietary
Fiber 19g; Cholesterol 95mg; Sodium 1140mg

I love this low-fat version of the Italian classic, *osso buco*, which is made with veal. You will find that this is just as tender and flavorful as its traditional counterpart. It takes about the same amount of time to prepare, but possesses about half of the calories and fat. My dear friend and neighbor, Chef Salvatore Parisi, gave me instructions on how to create this recipe over a friendly game of pool. (Yes, he won the game.) The photo includes Millet-Polenta Quenelles, see page 196.

Ingredients
Makes 4 servings.

1/2 teaspoon extra-virgin olive oil
4 skinless turkey legs
1 teaspoon sea salt
1 teaspoon freshly ground black pepper
2 cups diced yellow onions (about 2 large)
2 cups diced celery (6 medium ribs)
2 cups diced, peeled carrots (4 medium)
1 tablespoon minced garlic
3 cups white wine
2 16-ounce cans diced tomatoes (4 cups)
6-ounce can tomato paste (3/4 cup)
1 teaspoon dried thyme
2 bay leaves
1 teaspoon dried oregano
1 teaspoon dried marjoram
1 teaspoon dried basil
8 cups Vegetable Stock (see page 152)
Millet-Polenta Quenelles (see page 196)

Preparation

Heat a large sauté pan over medium-high heat and add the olive oil to lightly coat the bottom of the pan. Season the turkey with half of the salt and pepper. Add the turkey to the pan and sear on all sides until browned, about 5 minutes. Add the onions, celery, carrots, and garlic. Sauté until the onions are browned, about 5 minutes.

Add the white wine and stir to loosen the browned bits from the bottom of the pan. Bring to an enthusiastic boil, and cook until the wine is reduced to 1/4 of its original volume, about 5 minutes. Add the tomatoes, tomato paste, herbs, and stock. Return to a boil. Reduce heat and simmer uncovered until the turkey is tender and will pull apart with a fork, about 3 hours.

To serve: For each serving, place 2 quenelles on the side of a large soup bowl. Arrange one turkey leg in the middle of the bowl and ladle 1/4 cup of the sauce around.

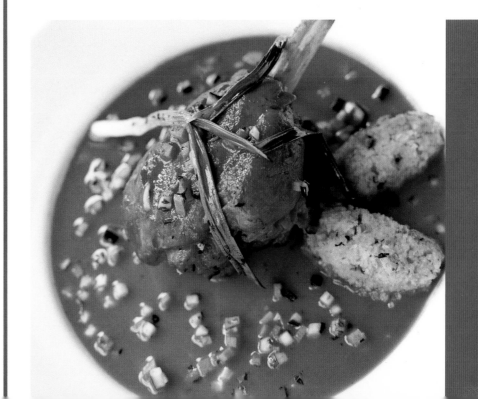

Chile Crêpes with Turkey Mole

Per serving:
Calories 370; Protein 28g; Total Fat 7g;
Saturated Fat 1g; Carbohydrates 51g; Dietary
Fiber 9g; Cholesterol 80mg; Sodium 530mg

I've received critical acclaim for creating a new style of southwestern recipe that pairs the delicious ingredients indigenous to the southwestern United States with the style of cooking that Native Americans and Mexicans have used for centuries. This recipe is derived from the blue corn piki bread of the Hopi people and a traditional Oaxacan mole verde recipe. Ultra-thin crêpes replace the blue corn and juniper ash piki bread. The mole recipe is completely authentic.

Ingredients

Makes 4 servings.

8 crêpes (see page 97) made with 1 teaspoon chile powder in place of the cumin
8 green onions, trimmed
Turkey Mole Filling
Mole Verde
2 teaspoons Sriracha (chile) sauce
4 teaspoons finely chopped red bell pepper

Mole Verde

2 tablespoons shelled pumpkin seeds
3 cups chopped tomatillos (18 medium)
1 teaspoon minced, roasted jalapeño chile (see page 38)
1 1/2 teaspoons minced, roasted poblano chile (see page 38)
1/4 cup diced yellow onion
1/2 teaspoon minced garlic
1 cinnamon stick
2 garlic cloves
1/4 teaspoon cumin
2 cups Vegetable Stock (see page 152)
1/4 cup finely chopped fresh cilantro
1/2 cup packed fresh spinach
2 teaspoons honey

Turkey Mole Filling

8 ounces fresh, boneless, skinless turkey breast, diced
1 cup Mole Verde
1/2 cup Chicken or Turkey Stock (see page 154)
1/4 cup button mushrooms, cut into quarters
2 teaspoons diced red onion
1/2 cup diced tomatillos

Preparation

Fill a small saucepan with water and bring to a boil. Add the green onions and blanch for about 30 seconds. Place in a bowl of ice water to stop the cooking process. Pat the onions dry and set aside.

For the Mole Verde: Preheat the oven to 350°F (175°C). Place the pumpkin seeds on a baking sheet and toast for 3 to 5 minutes or until light brown and puffed. Watch them closely because they can burn easily. Set aside.

Heat a large saucepan over medium-high heat. Add the tomatillos and sear until browned. Stir in the pumpkin seeds, jalapeño, poblano, onion, and garlic.

Place the cinnamon stick, garlic cloves, and cumin in a 10-inch piece of cheesecloth and tie with a 3-inch piece of butcher's twine to make a sachet; add to the tomatillos. Pour the stock over the mixture and bring to a boil. Reduce the heat and simmer for 15 to 20 minutes. Stir in the cilantro. Remove the sachet bag.

Pour the mixture into a blender and add the spinach and honey. Process until smooth. Return the sauce to the pan and keep just simmering until ready to use. Makes 3 cups. Extra sauce will keep for up to 3 days in the refrigerator or up to 1 month in the freezer.

For the Turkey Mole Filling: Heat a wide-bottomed stockpot over medium-high heat. Lightly spray the pot with olive oil spray. Add the turkey breast to the pot and sear on all sides. Stir in 1 cup of the Mole Verde and the 1/2 cup of stock. Reduce the heat to low and simmer until the turkey is fork-tender, about 30 minutes. Stir in the mushrooms, onion, and tomatillos. Simmer for 2 minutes. Remove the turkey mole from the heat. Use immediately or cool the turkey mixture quickly in a shallow pan in the refrigerator until ready to use.

To assemble: Spoon 1/4 cup of the Turkey Mole Filling onto the center of each crêpe. Roll up the crêpes and trim the edges, if desired. Tie each crêpe with a green onion.

To serve: Ladle 1/4 cup of Mole Verde sauce onto each serving plate. Place two crêpes diagonally on each plate and garnish with Sriracha sauce and bell peppers.

Asian Slaw with Asian-Marinated Pork Tenderloin

Per serving:
Calories 270; Protein 34g; Total Fat 6g;
Saturated Fat 2g; Carbohydrates 19g; Dietary
Fiber 2g; Cholesterol 100mg; Sodium 360mg

This slaw recipe is "to die for" and the pork marinade doubles as a terrific sauce for the main dish. Use this marinade on poultry and shrimp dishes to increase your repertoire of fun Asian-style foods.

Ingredients
Makes 6 servings.

Pork
1 1/2- to 2-pound pork tenderloin
Asian Marinade (see page 41)

1/4 teaspoon extra-virgin olive oil

Asian Slaw
1 cup julienned red bell pepper
   (1 medium)
1 cup julienned zucchini (1 medium)
1/2 cup julienned yellow squash
1 cup julienned carrots (2 medium)
1/2 cup julienned fresh shiitake
   mushrooms
1 teaspoon tahini (sesame seed paste)
1 tablespoon tamari (soy) sauce
1 tablespoon seasoned rice wine vinegar
1/2 teaspoon minced garlic
1 teaspoon minced fresh ginger
1/4 teaspoon Sriracha (chile) sauce
1/8 teaspoon ground star anise
1/2 cup unsweetened orange juice

Preparation

For the Pork: Place the pork in a shallow baking pan and coat with the marinade. Marinate for at least 30 minutes or up to 1 hour.

Preheat the oven to 400°F (205°C).

Heat a large ovenproof sauté pan over medium-high heat. Add the olive oil to lightly coat the bottom of the pan. Add the tenderloin and sear on all sides, about 4 minutes total. Place the pan in the preheated oven and roast for 10 minutes to finish cooking.

For the Asian Slaw: Combine all the vegetables in a large bowl. In a small bowl, whisk together the remaining ingredients. Add the dressing to the vegetables and toss to coat. Chill the slaw for at least 30 minutes to allow the flavors to blend.

To serve: Arrange 1/2 cup of slaw on each of 6 plates. Slice the pork thinly and divide among the plates, arranging around the salad.

Fried Brown Rice and Sautéed Vegetables with Citrus Five-Spice Marinated Duck Breast

Per serving:
Calories 430; Protein 37g; Total Fat 10g;
Saturated Fat 2.5g; Carbohydrates 50g; Dietary
Fiber 10g; Cholesterol 85mg; Sodium 620mg

Not long ago, fried rice was everyone's idea of quintessential Asian cuisine. Fortunately, our palates have grown to appreciate a variety of new Asian flavors. I included this nostalgic recipe to illustrate how to enjoy leftover brown rice with a renewed passion. The combination of spices and seasonings creates an awesome sauce or marinade for chicken, seafood, and beef.

Ingredients
Makes 4 servings.

2 cups Asian Marinade (see page 41)
4 4-ounce skinless duck breasts
1/4 teaspoon extra-virgin olive oil
4 bunches baby bok choy
1/4 cup fresh shiitake mushrooms, halved
1 cup julienned carrots (2 medium)
1 tablespoon cornstarch mixed with
   1 tablespoon cold water
2 cups Fried Brown Rice (see page 193)

Garnish
Daikon sprouts, optional

Preparation
Pour 1 cup of marinade over the duck breasts and marinate for 30 minutes.
   Preheat the oven to 325°F (165°C).
   Heat a sauté pan over medium-high heat and add the olive oil to lightly coat the bottom of the pan. Add the duck breasts and sear on one side for about 2 minutes. Place the duck breasts in a baking pan seared-side up and roast for 5 minutes.
   In the same sauté pan, quickly sauté the bok choy, mushrooms, and carrots, about 2 minutes. Remove from the pan and keep warm. Add the remaining 1 cup of marinade to the pan and bring to a boil. Whisk in the cornstarch mixture and cook, stirring, until the sauce is thickened.
   To serve: Place 1/4 cup of the sauce on each plate. Pack 1/2 cup of fried rice at a time into a small mold and turn out onto the center of each plate. Slice the duck breast and arrange around the rice. Arrange one piece of bok choy cut in half, 1/4 cup julienned carrots, and 1 tablespoon shiitake mushrooms on each plate. Garnish with daikon sprouts, if using.

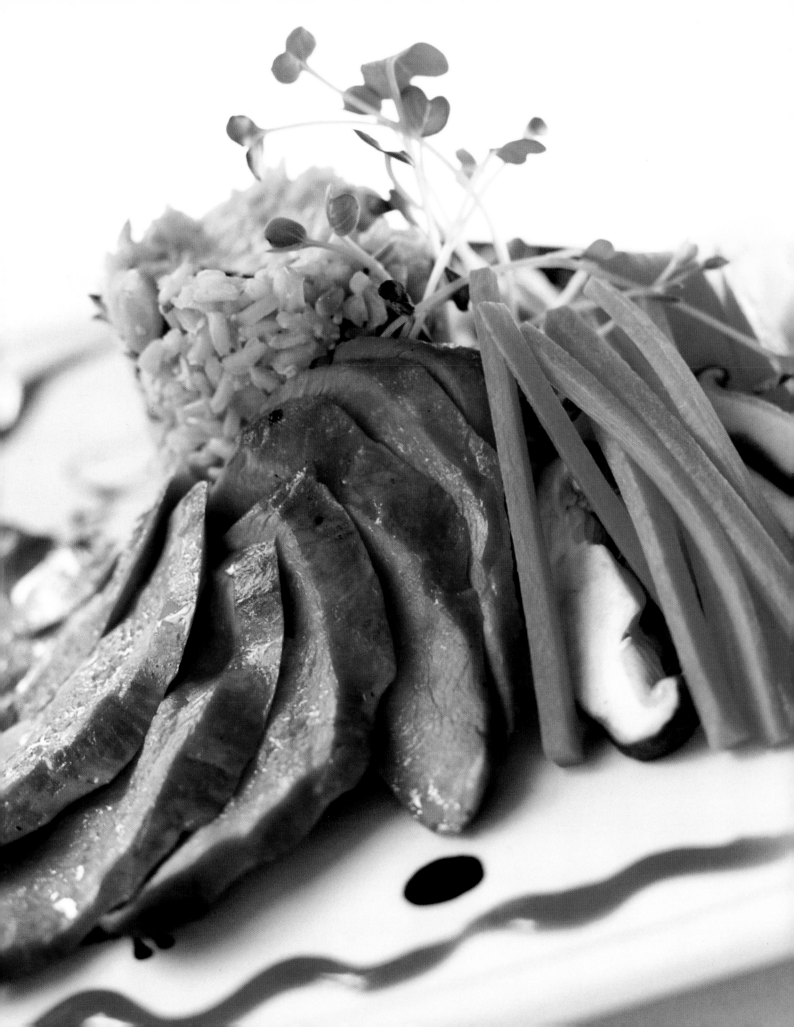

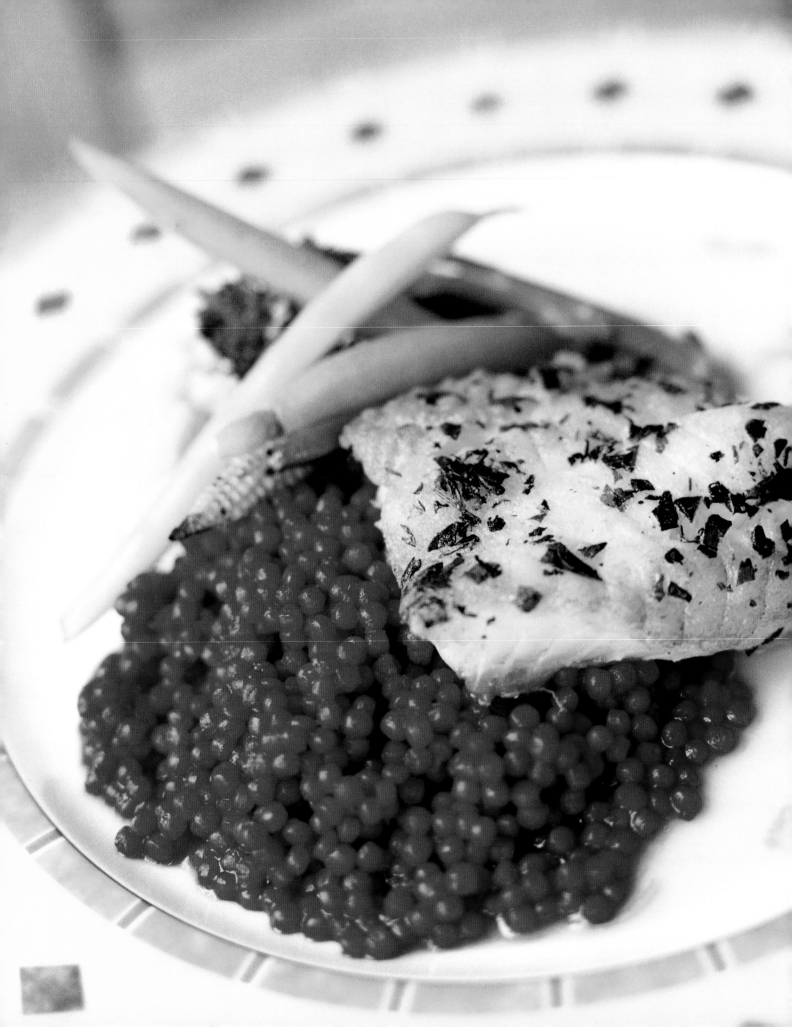

Beet Couscous and Steamed Organic Baby Vegetables with Pan-Seared Orange Roughy and Lemon-Garlic Sauce

Per serving:
Calories 350; Protein 25g; Total Fat 2g;
Saturated Fat 0g; Carbohydrates 55g; Dietary
Fiber 5g; Cholesterol 25mg; Sodium 540mg

The brilliant color and sweet flavor of the beet juice adds a new twist to couscous, providing not only intriguing flavor, but a significant amount of vitamins and nutrients to the dish. It pairs nicely with the light-flavored fish and a zesty sauce such as this simple Lemon-Garlic Sauce.

Ingredients
Makes 4 servings.

1/4 teaspoon extra-virgin olive oil
4 4-ounce orange roughy fillets
2 tablespoons Fresh Herb Mix (see
    page 39)
1/4 teaspoon sea salt
1/8 teaspoon freshly ground black pepper
1 medium zucchini, julienned
1 medium yellow squash, julienned
1 medium carrot, julienned
1/4 cup water
1/4 cup white wine
2 cups Beet Couscous (see page 192)
1/2 cup Lemon-Garlic Sauce (see
    page 24)

Preparation
Heat a large sauté pan over medium-high heat and add the olive oil to lightly coat the bottom of the pan. Season the orange roughy with the herbs, salt, and pepper. Add the orange roughy to the pan and sear on one side for 2 minutes to brown. Turn over and sear the other side for 1 minute. Keeping them in three separate bundles, add the zucchini, yellow squash, and carrots to the pan with the water and wine. Cover and steam for 1 minute.

To serve: Place 1/2 cup of couscous on each plate. Arrange the vegetables along one side of the couscous. Lay the orange roughy along the other edge of the couscous and drizzle 1 to 2 tablespoons of the sauce over the fish.

Dauphinoise Potatoes, Chile-Crusted Red Snapper, and Yellow Tomato Sauce

Pairing this southwestern-style fish entrée with a healthful adaptation of Dauphinoise Potatoes makes a wonderful combination of flavor and comfort. The chile-crumb crust adds zip to the delicate, sweet flavor of the red snapper. This topping is quick and easy to make and also can serve as a great flavor source for chicken or beef dishes.

Ingredients
Makes 4 servings.

1 Roasted Red Bell Pepper (see page 38), finely chopped
1 tablespoon minced green onion
1/2 teaspoon minced garlic
1 tablespoon minced fresh cilantro
1/4 teaspoon freshly ground coriander seeds
1/8 teaspoon chile powder
1/4 teaspoon minced, dried red chile peppers
1/8 teaspoon sea salt
1/8 teaspoon freshly ground black pepper
1/4 teaspoon extra-virgin olive oil
1 1/2 teaspoons fresh lime juice
2 tablespoons dry bread crumbs
1/2 cup white wine
4 4-ounce snapper fillets

Accompaniments
8 baby carrots
4 cups Sautéed Swiss Chard (see page 224)
1/8 teaspoon sea salt
1/8 teaspoon freshly ground black pepper
4 servings Dauphinoise Potatoes (see page 227)
1 cup Yellow Tomato Sauce (see page 22)

Preparation
Preheat the oven to 375°F (190°C).

Combine the vegetables, herbs, spices, oil, lime juice, and bread crumbs in a bowl and mix well. Pour the white wine into a medium baking pan and add the fish. Divide the vegetable mixture among the 4 pieces of fish, patting down to adhere it on top. Bake for 8 minutes or until the fish is just cooked throughout.

For the accompaniments: Bring water to boil in a medium saucepan. Add the baby carrots and blanch for 2 minutes until just softened. Remove the carrots with a slotted spoon and drain. Cook the Swiss chard as directed on page 224. Season the carrots and Swiss chard with the salt and pepper.

To serve: Arrange one portion of Dauphinoise Potatoes on the side of each serving plate. Divide the Swiss chard into 4 equal portions. Press each portion into a small mold and turn out in the center of the plates. Place one piece of snapper on top of the Swiss chard. Arrange the carrots on the plates and pour 1/4 cup of the Yellow Tomato Sauce in a pool in front of the snapper on each plate.

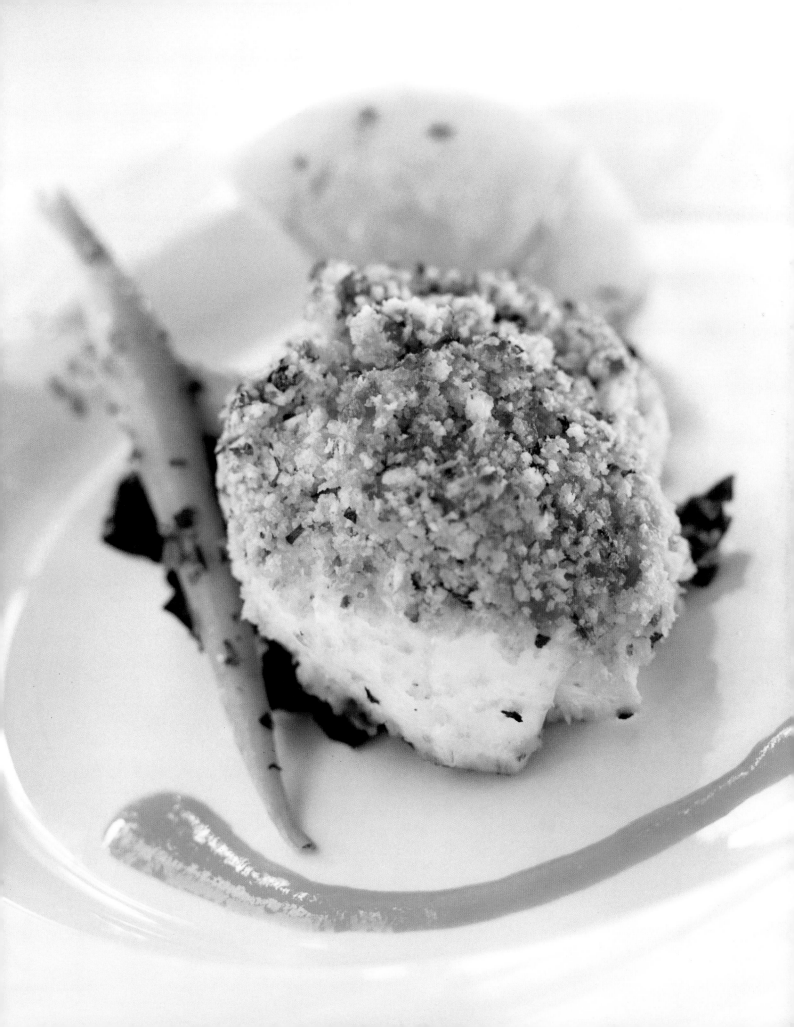

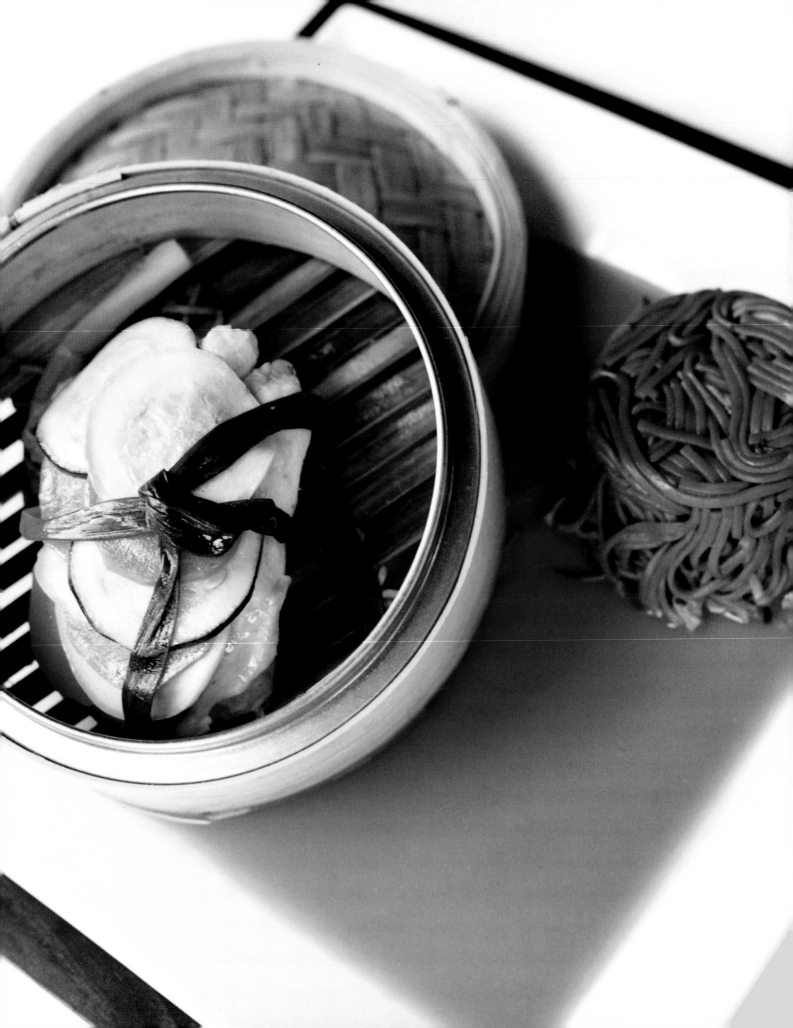

Timbale of Soba Noodles with Steamed Vegetable-Wrapped Black Sea Bass and Tamari-Ginger Sauce

Soba noodles are buckwheat pasta shaped like spaghetti. In this dish, the noodles are tossed with mixed, seasoned vegetables and packed into timbale molds—small, thimble-shaped cups. This presentation serves as a lovely backdrop for the sea bass, which is wrapped with thinly sliced vegetables and steamed. The citrus-based Tamari-Ginger Sauce gives a wonderful zip to this Asian-style main plate.

Ingredients
Makes 4 servings.

Soba Noodles
8-ounce package soba noodles
1/2 teaspoon toasted sesame oil
1/2 cup julienned carrot
1/2 cup shredded napa cabbage
1/2 teaspoon minced garlic
1 teaspoon minced fresh ginger
2 teaspoon tamari (soy) sauce

Sea Bass
4 4-ounce fillets sea bass
1/2 teaspoon sea salt
1/4 teaspoon freshly ground black pepper
1 tablespoon Fresh Herb Mix (see
  page 39)
1/4 cup thinly sliced zucchini
1/4 cup thinly sliced yellow squash
1/4 cup thinly sliced, peeled carrot
4 green onions

1 cup Tamari-Ginger Sauce (see page 26)

Preparation

For the Noodles: Cook the noodles in a large pot of salted, boiling water until *al dente*, about 8 minutes. Drain the noodles and cool until ready to use.

Heat a medium sauté pan over medium-high heat and add the toasted sesame oil to lightly coat the bottom of the pan. Stir in the carrot, cabbage, garlic, and ginger. Sauté for 2 minutes. Stir in the soba noodles and tamari sauce. Place 1/2 cup of the noodles into each of four 4-ounce timbale molds or coffee cups.

For the Sea Bass: Add about 1 inch of water to a large saucepan and bring to a simmer. Season each piece of fish with salt, pepper, and herbs. Arrange the sliced vegetables on the fish in tightly overlapping layers, using the zucchini, carrot, and yellow squash to create a fish-scale pattern. Blanch the green onions in the boiling water for 5 seconds to make them pliable. Cut the root off the green onions. Lay the green onions out on a cutting board and place a piece of fish with vegetables on top. Bring the end of the onion around and tie to help hold the vegetables in place.

Carefully transfer the fish to a steamer insert or bamboo steamer. Place the insert over the simmering water, cover, and steam until fish is just cooked through, 10 to 12 minutes. (Make sure the water does not reach the bottom of the steamer.) Remove the basket from the steamer.

To serve: Unmold the soba noodle timbales on 4 serving plates. Lay the sea bass on the plate against the noodles. Spoon 1/4 cup of Tamari-Ginger Sauce next to the fish on each plate.

Roulade of Salmon Filled with Buckwheat and Wild Rice Stuffing with Beet and Ginger Sauce

Ingredients
Makes 4 servings.

4 4-ounce pieces salmon fillet
1 cup packed fresh spinach
1/4 teaspoon sea salt
1/4 teaspoon freshly ground black pepper
1 tablespoon chopped Fresh Herb Mix
   (see page 39)
1 1/3 cups Buckwheat and Wild Rice
   Stuffing (see page 197)
1 cup Beet and Ginger Sauce (see
   page 32)
4 baby beets, peeled and cooked
1 cup cooked green beans or steamed
   assorted vegetables, such as baby
   squash, asparagus, or baby corn

Roulades are food items that are filled and rolled—a fundamental technique in French cookery. I use roulades in a number of applications, from lobster appetizers to stuffed beef rolls. Typically, you flatten the fish, meat, or chicken by pounding it out with a mallet. The wild rice and buckwheat filling of this roulade is sweetened with dried cherries, creating a delicious, comforting, and complex filling. The dish is complemented beautifully by the flavors of fresh ginger and sweet beets in the sauce.

Preparation
Place each piece of salmon between two sheets of plastic wrap about 8 x 10 inches in size. Gently pound out each salmon fillet to 1/4-inch thickness. Remove the top sheet of plastic and neatly cover each piece of salmon with spinach. Season with salt, pepper, and fresh herbs. Spread 1/3 cup of the Buckwheat and Wild Rice Stuffing near the bottom of each salmon fillet. Lift the bottom sheet of the plastic to fold salmon over the filling. Continue lifting the plastic and roll the salmon into a cylinder. Tuck the far end of the plastic in front of salmon and roll toward you, making a tightly wrapped roulade. Knot each end of the plastic wrap, and poke small holes through the plastic to allow the steam to seep into the salmon. Repeat with remaining fish, seasonings, and stuffing.

Add about 1 inch of water to a large saucepan and bring to a simmer. Arrange the salmon in a steamer insert or bamboo steamer. Place the insert over the simmering water, cover, and steam until the salmon is light pink in color, about 10 minutes. (Make sure the water does not reach the bottom of the steamer.) Remove the salmon from the steamer and cut off one end of the plastic. Carefully push the salmon through the open end and remove it in one piece. Cut each salmon roulade on the bias into five pieces.

To serve: Spoon 1/4 cup of Beet and Ginger Sauce onto each plate. Arrange the salmon pieces on each plate in a circular pattern resembling a flower. Garnish the salmon with an artful arrangement of baby beets and green beans or assorted vegetables.

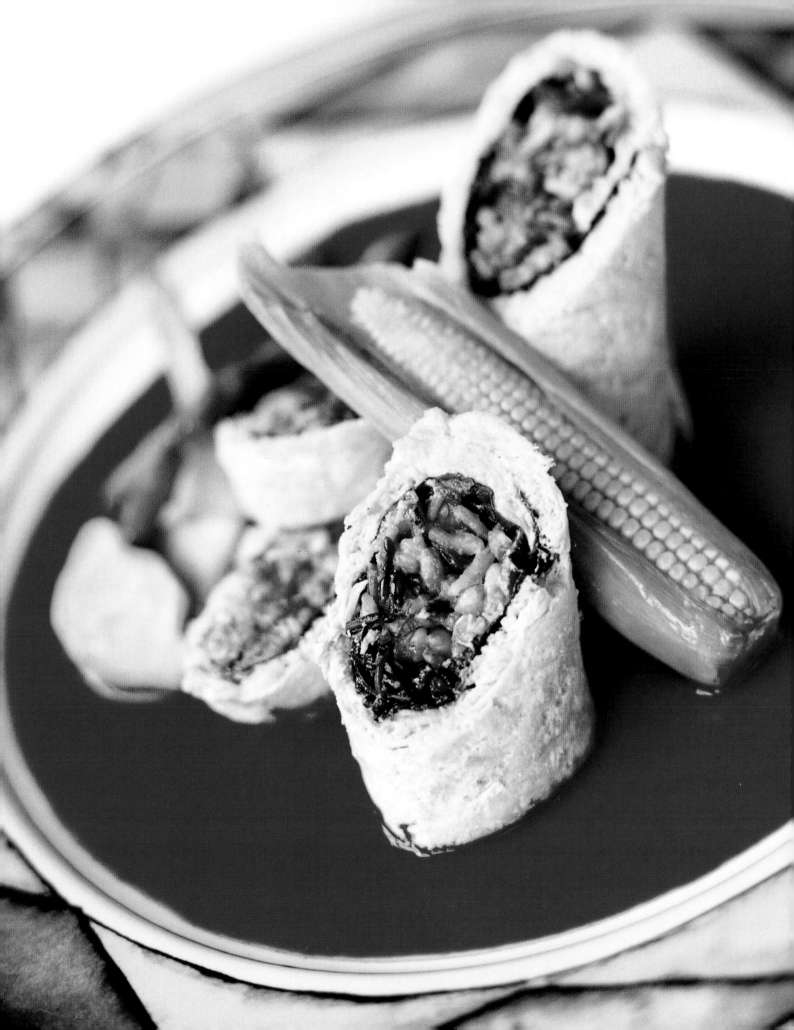

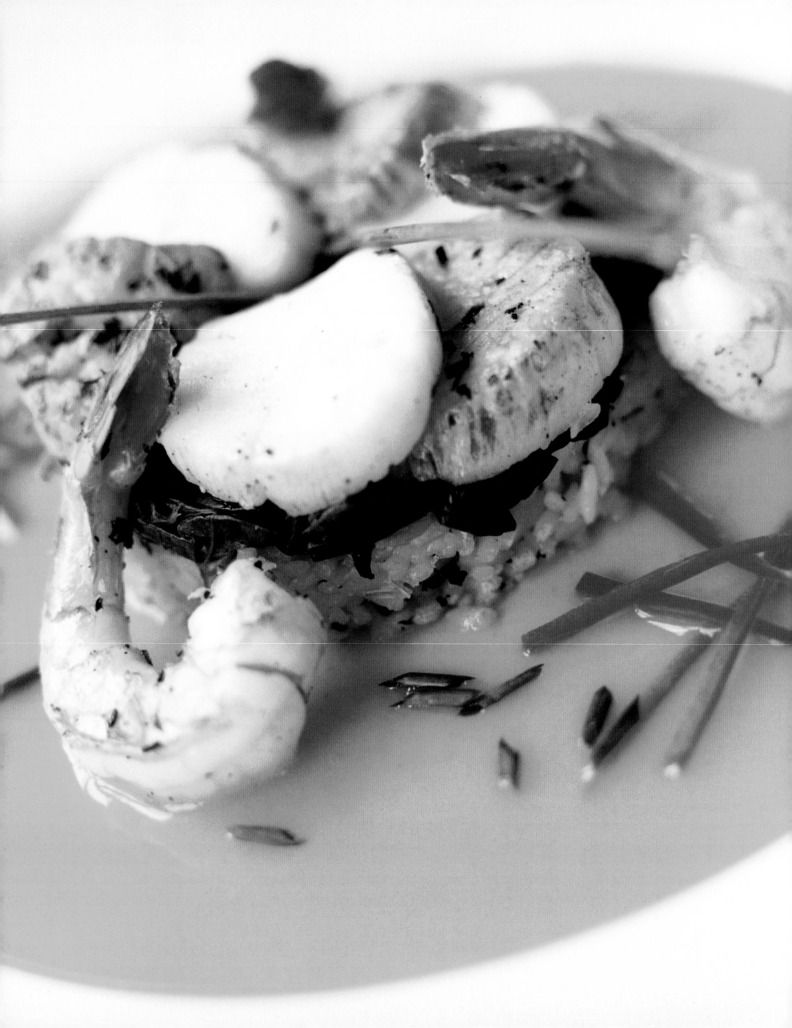

Braised Sea Scallops and Gulf Shrimp with Orzo Griddle Cakes in a Saffron-Chive Sauce

Pairing luscious sea scallops with shrimp is an undeniably opulent combination of flavors and textures. Orzo pasta makes unusual griddle cakes, creating a delicate, visually pleasing platform to showcase the beauty of the seafood. Fresh, seasonal vegetables are essential to this lovely dish.

Ingredients
Makes 4 servings.

4 Orzo Griddle Cakes (see page 199)
1/2 cup Fine Herb Vinaigrette (see
   page 123)
1/2 teaspoon extra-virgin olive oil
12 sea scallops, about 1 ounce each
12 large shrimp, peeled and deveined
1/4 teaspoon sea salt
1/4 teaspoon freshly ground black pepper
1 tablespoon Fresh Herb Mix (see
   page 39)
2 cups steamed spinach
1 1/3 cups Saffron-Chive Sauce (see
   page 31)

Garnish
Minced fresh chives, optional
Julienned red bell peppers, optional

Preparation
Preheat the oven to 425°F (220°C).

Rub both sides of the Orzo Griddle Cakes with the Fine Herb Vinaigrette. Place the cakes on a nonstick baking pan and bake for 5 to 7 minutes.

Heat a medium sauté pan over medium-high heat. Add the olive oil to lightly coat the bottom of the pan. Season the scallops and shrimp with the salt, pepper, and Fresh Herb Mix. Place the scallops and shrimp into the sauté pan and sear on each side for about 1 minute. Turn the scallops and shrimp over, add the sauce, and braise for about 2 minutes. Remove from heat.

To serve: Place one griddle cake in the center of each serving dish. Arrange 1/2 cup of spinach on top of each griddle cake. Slice the scallops in half and place 6 slices around the cake. Lean 3 pieces of shrimp around the scallops. Drizzle each dish with 1/3 cup of the Saffron-Chive Sauce and sprinkle with the chives and red peppers, if using.

Crisp Shrimp and Vegetable Spring Rolls with Edamame Ragoût

Per serving:
Calories 340; Protein 29g; Total Fat 14g;
Saturated Fat 2g; Carbohydrates 31g; Dietary
Fiber 16g; Cholesterol 30mg; Sodium 1300mg

This is a marvelously delicious main plate that begs you to consciously notice the presentation, textures, and Asian-inspired flavors. You will also marvel at how simple it is to prepare and serve this showstopper main dish. Rice paper can be found in Asian food markets; this intriguing ingredient is delicate, yet resilient. Once wet, it is pliable and can be used to wrap foods that are served hot or cold. This is our hot version of spring rolls and a small tribute to the creative use of rice.

Ingredients
Makes 4 servings.

1/2 teaspoon toasted sesame oil
12 large deveined, peeled shrimp
1 cup shredded napa cabbage
1 cup shredded bok choy
1 cup julienned carrots (2 medium)
1 cup julienned fresh shiitake mushrooms
  (about 3 1/2 ounces)
2 tablespoons chopped green onion
1/2 teaspoon minced fresh ginger
1/2 teaspoon minced garlic
2 tablespoons tamari (soy) sauce
1 tablespoon minced fresh cilantro
4 rice paper wrappers
2 cups Edamame Ragoût (see page 210)

Garnish
Sriracha (chile) sauce, optional

Preparation

Preheat the oven to 425°F (220°C). Lightly coat a baking sheet with cooking spray and set aside.

Heat a large sauté pan or wok over medium-high heat. Add the toasted sesame oil to lightly coat the bottom of the pan. Add the shrimp and cook for 1 minute on each side. Remove the shrimp from the pan and set aside. Add the cabbage, bok choy, carrots, mushrooms, green onion, ginger, and garlic to the pan. Stir-fry for 2 minutes to cook lightly. Season the vegetables with the tamari sauce and cilantro. Stir well to incorporate. Remove from the heat and place in a bowl to cool.

Soak the rice paper quickly in a bowl of cold water until just softened, about 30 seconds. Lay the rice paper out on a cutting board and pat dry. Cut each shrimp in half lengthwise. Arrange 6 pieces of shrimp in the center of each piece of rice paper. Top the shrimp with 1/4 cup of the vegetable filling, then fold in the sides and roll up. Place the spring rolls on the prepared baking sheet. Bake for 10 minutes or until the spring rolls are light brown and crispy.

To serve: Spoon 1/2 cup of Edamame Ragoût in the center of each plate. Lay one spring roll on top of the ragout. Drizzle the Sriracha sauce on the side.

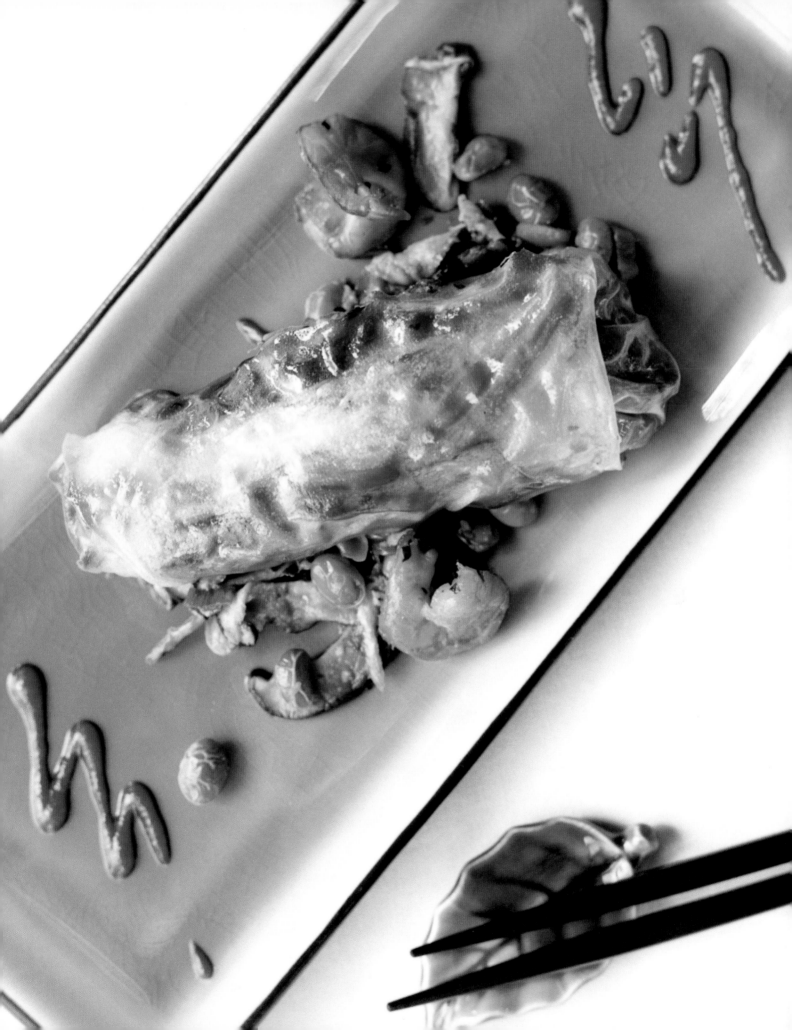

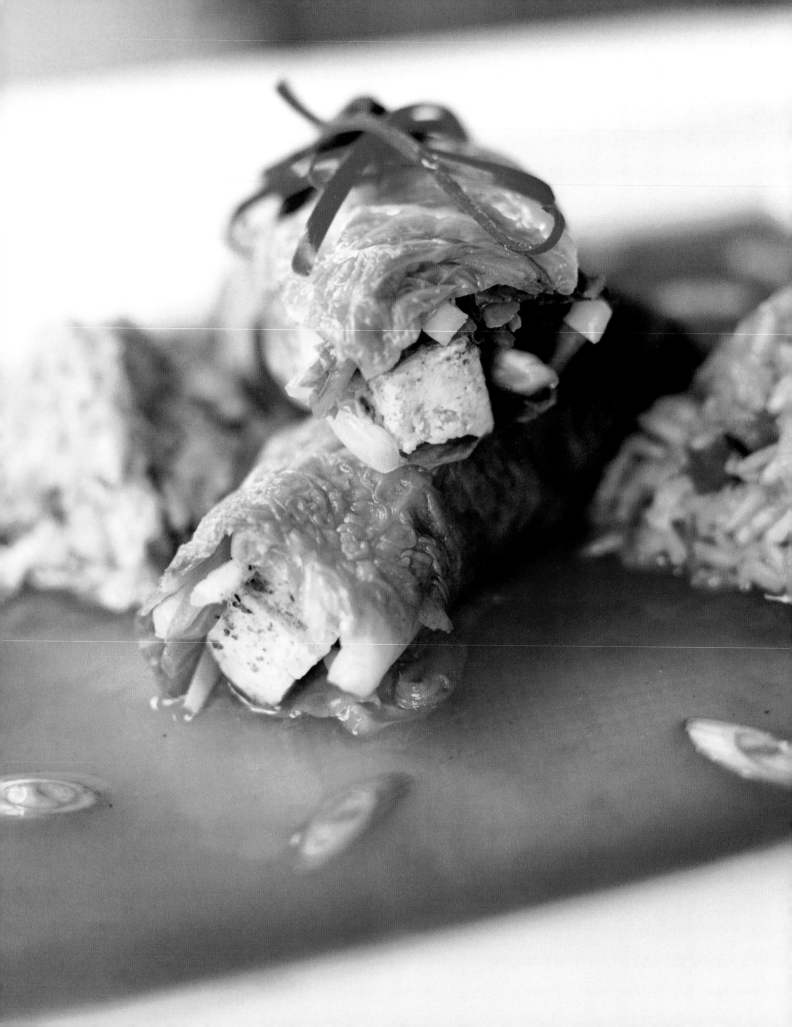

Curried Tofu and Napa Cabbage Roulade with Shiitake Mushroom Sauce

Per serving:
Calories 240; Protein 15g; Total Fat 3g;
Saturated Fat 0g; Carbohydrate 40g; Dietary
Fiber 6g; Cholesterol 0mg; Sodium 380mg

Trust me, it was hard for a chef who grow up in the great midwestern restaurant town of Chicago to embrace tofu.

When I began to prepare health-conscious foods, I tried to enjoy tofu many times to no avail. I then read more, experimented more, and was shown by my trusty assistant, Heidi DeCosmo, how to make fresh tofu. I quickly learned that the difference in enjoying this soy protein is the quality of the tofu.

I have suggested a few brands of tofu that are consistently good (see page 327), or use Heidi's tofu recipe (see page 211).

Ingredients
Makes 4 servings.

8 napa cabbage leaves
1/4 teaspoon toasted sesame oil
1 tablespoon minced garlic
1 tablespoon minced fresh ginger
2 tablespoons finely chopped green onion
1/2 cup julienned carrots
1/2 cup julienned daikon radish
1/2 cup julienned bok choy
1/2 cup julienned zucchini
1/2 cup julienned fresh shiitake
  mushrooms
12-ounce package firm curried tofu, herb
  tofu, or smoked tofu, diced
1 cup Shiitake Mushroom Sauce (see
  page 23)
2 cups cooked brown rice

Garnish
1/4 cup chopped green onions
1/4 cup julienned red bell pepper

Preparation

Fill a medium saucepan with water and bring to a boil. Prepare an ice bath by filling a large bowl half full of cold water and ice. Blanch the cabbage in the boiling water for 30 to 60 seconds. Remove and place in the ice water to stop the cooking process. Set aside.

Heat a medium sauté pan over medium-high heat and add the toasted sesame oil to lightly coat the pan. Add the garlic, ginger, and green onion. Cook 1 minute. Stir in the carrots, daikon, bok choy, zucchini, and shiitake mushrooms. Sauté until the carrots are beginning to soften, about 3 minutes. Remove from the heat and transfer to a mixing bowl. Gently fold in the tofu; stir carefully so the tofu doesn't break up. Set aside.

To assemble: Place one blanched cabbage leaf on a cutting board and scoop 1/4 cup of the vegetable-tofu mixture into the middle. Carefully fold in the sides of the cabbage and roll up to form a roulade. Repeat with remaining pieces of cabbage and filling.

Add about 1 inch of water to a large saucepan and bring to a simmer. Arrange the cabbage roulades in a steamer insert or bamboo steamer. Place the insert over the simmering water, cover, and steam until heated through, 5 to 7 minutes. (Make sure the water does not reach the bottom of the steamer.)

To serve: Ladle 1/4 cup of Shiitake Mushroom Sauce on each serving plate. Divide 1/2 cup of brown rice into two mounds on opposite sides of the sauce. Arrange 2 cabbage roulades between the rice mounds and garnish with the green onions and bell pepper.

Smoked Tofu-Filled Bean Curd Sheets with Shiitake Mushroom Sauce

Per serving:
Calories 150; Protein 2g; Total Fat 3g;
Saturated Fat 1.5g; Carbohydrates 20g; Dietary
Fiber 5g; Cholesterol 0mg; Sodium 1000mg

Fresh bean curd sheets are paper-thin sheets of high-quality bean curd that are rolled into pliable sheets about 18 inches in diameter. Search for this wonderful Chinese culinary work of art in specialty Asian grocery stores; it is well worth the hunt. Their strong, yet light texture, and mellow soy flavor will encourage you to create many other vegetarian masterpieces of your own.

Ingredients
Makes 4 servings.

1/4 teaspoon toasted sesame oil
1 cup smoked tofu, small dice
1 cup carrots, small dice
1/4 cup chopped green onion
1/2 teaspoon minced fresh ginger
1/2 teaspoon minced garlic
1 1/2 cups shredded napa cabbage
2 cups chopped broccoli
2 tablespoons white wine
1 teaspoon minced fresh lemongrass
1 tablespoon chopped fresh cilantro
1/2 cup unsweetened apple juice
3 tablespoons tamari (soy) sauce
1 1/2 teaspoon Sriracha (chile) sauce
2 fresh bean curd sheets
8 green onions, blanched
1 cup Shiitake Mushroom Sauce (see
    page 23)

Garnish
Daikon sprouts, optional

Preparation

Heat a sauté pan over medium-high heat and add the toasted sesame oil to lightly coat the bottom of the pan. Add the smoked tofu, carrots, green onion, ginger, garlic, and napa cabbage. Sauté for 2 minutes. Add the broccoli, wine, herbs, apple juice, and seasonings. Sauté for 3 minutes. Remove from the heat and set aside.

Preheat the oven to 350°F (175°C). Coat a baking sheet with cooking spray.

In a bowl of cold water, moisten the bean curd sheets until just soft and pliable, about 30 seconds. Remove from the water and pat dry. Cut the large sheets into quarters. Place 1 cup of filling in the middle of each piece, and gather up the sides to form a bundle. Tie the tops of the bundles closed using the blanched green onions.

Place on the prepared baking sheet. Bake for 5 minutes or until golden brown.

To serve: Ladle 1/4 cup of Shiitake Mushroom Sauce into the center of each serving plate and top with 2 bundles. Garnish with daikon sprouts, if using.

Tempeh Scaloppini

Tempeh is a fermented vegetarian protein product made from cooked soybeans and other legumes or grains. It's extremely high in protein—almost equal to chicken. Tempeh is at its best when marinated—it easily picks up the characteristics of the marinade. This dish resembles veal scaloppini in texture and flavor.

Ingredients
Makes 4 servings.

Marinade
1/2 cup tamari (soy) sauce
1 1/2 cups unsweetened apple juice
1 cup unsweetened orange juice
2 cloves garlic, minced
2 tablespoons minced fresh rosemary

2 8-ounce packages tempeh
1/2 teaspoon extra-virgin olive oil
1 cup julienned carrots (2 medium)
1 cup julienned zucchini (1 medium)
1 cup julienned yellow squash
2 cups quartered baby button mushrooms
1 teaspoon capers
4 cups cooked angel hair pasta

Preparation

For the marinade: In a small mixing bowl, whisk together the marinade ingredients.

Place the tempeh patties in a shallow baking pan and pour the marinade over the tempeh. Marinate at least 1 hour or up to overnight in the refrigerator (the flavor will intensify if marinated longer). Remove the tempeh from the pan, reserving the marinade for the sauce. Slice each tempeh piece in half lengthwise and again crosswise. You will have 8 slices of tempeh, 2 slices for each serving.

Heat a large, nonstick sauté pan over medium-high heat and add the olive oil to lightly coat the bottom of the pan. Add the tempeh and sear on both sides. Remove from the pan and keep warm in the oven on low. Add the carrots, zucchini, and yellow squash to the pan and sauté for 1 minute. Keep warm in the oven with the tempeh.

Wipe out the sauté pan and place back on the heat. Add the marinade and bring to a boil. Add the mushrooms and simmer for about 3 minutes. Stir in the capers and simmer for 5 minutes more.

To serve: Arrange 1 cup of angel hair pasta in the middle of each plate. Arrange 2 pieces of tempeh on top of the pasta. Divide the vegetables around the pasta. Drizzle with the mushroom sauce.

Grilled Eggplant "Tacos" with Tempeh

I love to experiment using vegetarian food items to create dishes in various styles. I wanted to make a main plate utilizing grilled eggplant slices in the manner of a flour tortilla. In the interests of making a 100 percent vegetable taco, I chose to use tempeh with a spicy marinade to mimic the flavor and texture of traditional taco meat. Combined with a colorful vegetable slaw, this dish delivers all the savory satisfaction you could want.

Ingredients
Make 4 servings.

Eggplant
1 large eggplant, thinly sliced
1/2 cup Fine Herb Vinaigrette (see page 123)

Tempeh Filling
1/4 teaspoon extra-virgin olive oil
1/4 cup chopped yellow onion
1/2 teaspoon minced garlic
1 14-ounce package tempeh, crumbled
1/2 teaspoon chile powder
1/2 teaspoon cumin
1/2 cup tomato juice

Zucchini Slaw
1/2 cup julienned zucchini
1/2 cup julienned jícama
1/2 cup julienned red bell pepper
1/4 cup Fine Herb Vinaigrette

Garnish
Salsa, optional

Preparation

For the Eggplant: Preheat a grill pan or grill to high. Brush the vinaigrette on both sides of each eggplant slice. Grill for 1 minute on each side. Remove from grill pan and cool on a baking sheet. Set aside until ready to fill.

For the Tempeh Filling: Heat a large sauté pan over medium-high heat. Add the olive oil to lightly coat the bottom of the pan. Add the onion and garlic. Cook until the onion has just softened, about 2 minutes. Add the tempeh, chile powder, and cumin. Cook until the tempeh has started to brown, about 3 minutes. Add the tomato juice and simmer for about 5 minutes. Remove from heat.

For the Zucchini Slaw: Toss the finely julienned vegetables with the vinaigrette in a small bowl.

To serve: Spoon 1/3 cup of the slaw into the center of each plate. Holding an eggplant slice in your hand, scoop 2 tablespoons of the tempeh filling into the eggplant "taco" shell. Lay the eggplant bundle on the plate with the side folded over. Repeat with remaining ingredients to make 16 bundles, 4 per serving, arranging the "tacos" around the slaw. Garnish with salsa, if using.

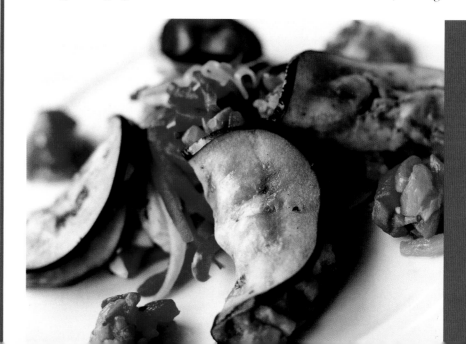

Tofu Napoleon with Yellow Tomato Sauce

The intriguing flavors of roasted garlic and herb tofu inspired me to create this presentation in the style of the classic French Napoleon pastry. Tofu slices are quickly sautéed in olive oil, then carefully stacked with layers of complementary vegetables. The *pièce de résistance* is the delicate Yellow Tomato Sauce.

Ingredients
Makes 4 servings.

8 asparagus spears
8 baby carrots
4 fresh or frozen artichoke hearts, cut in half
2 cups packed fresh spinach
1 Roasted Red Bell Pepper, peeled, julienned (see page 38)
1/4 teaspoon extra-virgin olive oil
2 12-ounce packages Italian seasoned baked tofu, each piece cut in half on the diagonal to form 16 triangles
1 cup Yellow Tomato Sauce (see page 22)

Preparation

Bring water to boil in a medium saucepan. Add the asparagus, carrots, and artichoke hearts. Boil until crisp-tender, about 1 minute. Remove the vegetables with a slotted spoon and add the spinach to the pan. Cook until just wilted, about 1 minute, and drain. Combine the Roasted Red Bell Pepper and spinach in a bowl. Keep the vegetables warm in 250°F (120°C) oven.

Heat a medium sauté pan over medium-high heat and add the olive oil to lightly coat the bottom of the pan. Add the tofu triangles and sear on one side for 1 minute, turn over, and cook about 2 minutes.

To serve: Ladle 1/4 cup of Yellow Tomato Sauce onto each plate. Place 2 tablespoons of the spinach mixture on each plate and top with 2 triangles of tofu arranged pointing out with bases together. Repeat the layers with the tofu triangles pointing the opposite way to form a star. Arrange the asparagus, carrots, and artichoke hearts around the Napoleon.

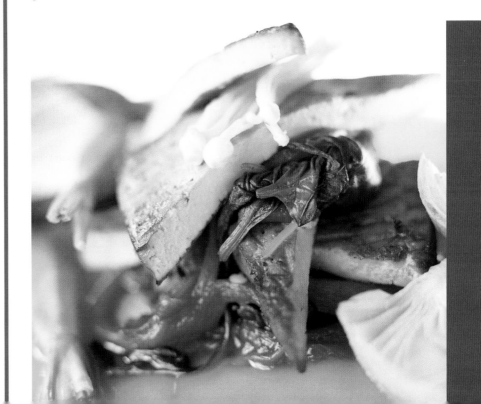

Baked Kabocha Squash with Seitan

Per serving:
Calories 210; Protein 18g; Total Fat 2g;
Saturated Fat 0g; Carbohydrates 34g; Dietary
Fiber 6g; Cholesterol 0mg; Sodium 570mg

Seitan is wheat gluten that is seasoned with tamari and spices then simmered to form a dough. The dough is used in a variety of vegetarian dishes to replace meat in texture, taste, as well as visually. Whether or not you are a vegetarian, you will find that this is a wonderful way to reduce your red meat consumption without relinquishing flavor and enjoyment. Seitan can be found in specialty food stores and health food stores.

Ingredients
Makes 4 servings.

4 small kabocha or acorn squash
4 tablespoons tamari (soy) sauce
1/2 teaspoon extra-virgin olive oil, divided
1 cup chopped seitan
1/4 cup diced yellow onion
1/2 cup diced zucchini (about 1 small)
1/2 cup diced yellow squash (about
    1 small)
1/2 cup diced eggplant (about 1/2 small)
1/4 cup diced red bell pepper
1/4 cup diced green bell pepper
1/2 cup diced portobello mushroom, gills
    removed (about 1 medium mushroom)
1 tablespoon minced garlic
1 cup chopped, seeded, peeled tomatoes
1 teaspoon dried thyme
1 teaspoon dried oregano
1 tablespoon dried basil
1/4 cup chile sauce
1/2 cup tomato juice
1/2 teaspoon sea salt
1/4 teaspoon freshly ground black pepper

Preparation

Preheat the oven to 400°F (205F). Cut around the top of each squash in a zigzag pattern, about 1/2 inch from the top. Remove and reserve the tops. Cut a small piece off the bottom of each squash so it stands upright without wobbling. Remove the seeds and strings and drizzle the inside of each squash with 1 tablespoon of tamari. Oil the outsides of the squash with 1/4 teaspoon of the olive oil to make them shiny. Place the squash, with the lids on the side, on a baking sheet and bake about 20 minutes or until soft.

For the seitan: Heat a large sauté pan over medium-high heat and add the remaining 1/4 teaspoon olive oil to lightly coat the bottom of the pan. Add the seitan and brown lightly for 1 minute. Add the vegetables and cook until the vegetables are just softened, 5 to 7 minutes. Add the herbs and chile sauce and stir to loosen any browned bits from the pan. Stir in the tomato juice and simmer for 2 to 3 minutes. Season with the salt and pepper.

To serve: For each serving, place one squash on an entrée plate; fill with the seitan vegetable mixture and top with the lid off-center as a garnish.

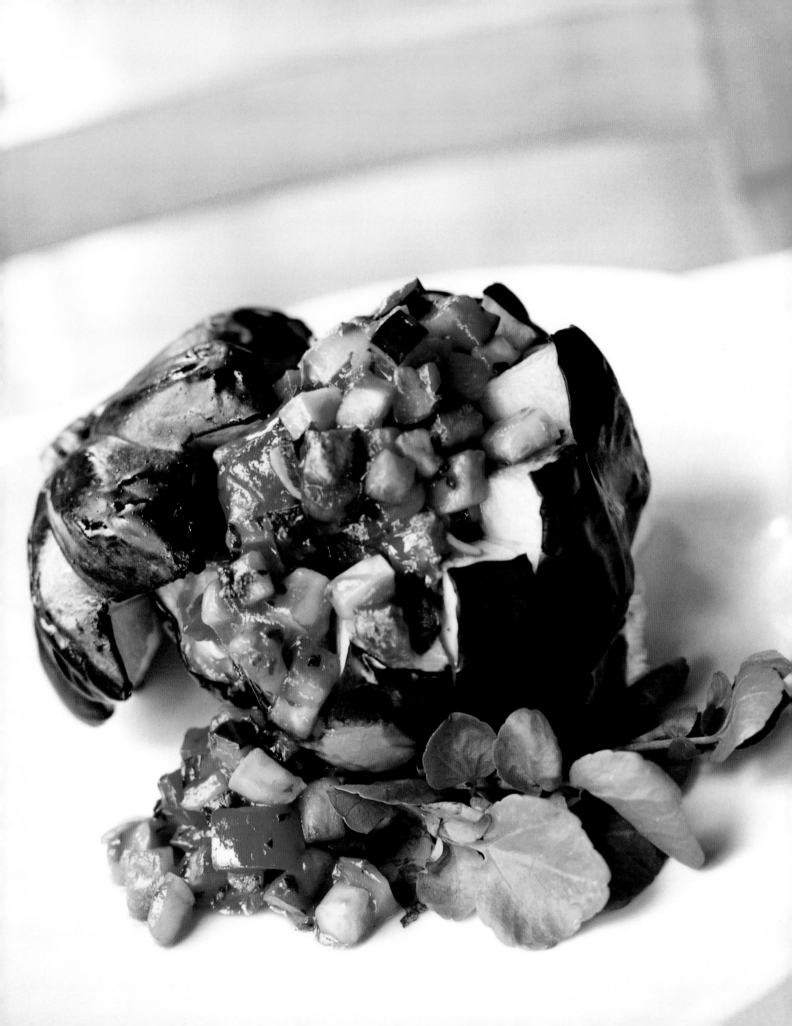

Vegetable Casserole

Per serving:
Calories 350; Protein 21g; Total Fat 3.5g;
Saturated Fat 1g; Carbohydrates 69g; Dietary
Fiber 23g; Cholesterol 0mg; Sodium 300mg

The warm and comforting flavors of eggplant Parmesan inspired this dish. The challenge, as with other consciously prepared dishes, is either to mimic the flavor of old favorites while reducing excess fats and calories or to remind the diner of old favorites with a new twist. This is the latter approach, with a white bean spread replacing the tomato sauce. The beans add moisture to the bottom of the casserole while providing protein for balanced nutrition. The beautiful layers of fresh squash, eggplant, mushrooms, and tomato slices create a delightful combination of flavors and colors. Freshly grated Parmigiano Reggiano cheese sprinkled over each dish before serving awakens the senses to the good things within.

Ingredients

Makes 2 servings.

2 small Japanese eggplants

2 small zucchini

2 small yellow squash

4 medium portobello mushrooms, gills removed, sliced 1/4 inch thick

2 tablespoons Fine Herb Vinaigrette (see page 123)

1/2 cup Spinach, White Bean, and Tofu Spread (see page 311)

2 medium tomatoes, sliced 1/4 inch thick

2 tablespoons dry bread crumbs

1 1/2 teaspoon grated Parmesan cheese

2 teaspoons Fresh Herb Mix (see page 39)

1 teaspoon Balsamic Reduction (see page 19)

Preparation

Heat the oven to 400°F (205°C).

Use a mandoline or sharp knife to cut the eggplant, zucchini, and yellow squash into 1/4-inch diagonal slices. In a medium bowl, toss the eggplant, zucchini, yellow squash, and mushrooms with the Fine Herb Vinaigrette. Transfer the vegetables to a baking sheet and spread out evenly. Roast for 3 minutes.

Layer the bottoms of 2 individual casserole dishes or a 13 x 9-inch baking pan with the eggplant slices. Spread the eggplant with half of the tofu spread. Layer the tomatoes on top of the spread. For the next layer, alternately overlap half of the zucchini and yellow squash slices. Spread the remaining tofu spread on top of the squash. Layer the mushrooms over the tofu spread and finish with another layer of overlapping squash.

Combine the bread crumbs, cheese, and Fresh Herb Mix in a small bowl. Sprinkle the bread crumb mixture over top of the casseroles. Bake for 15 minutes or until vegetables are heated through.

Drizzle each casserole with 1/2 teaspoon of Balsamic Reduction.

Roasted Lobster Tails with Linguine and Baby Carrots and English Pea Sauce

Lobster is low in cholesterol and calories, and is an excellent source of protein, iron, and B vitamins. Unfortunately, most Americans submerge this sweet, tender crustacean in butter, raising the cholesterol to unhealthy levels. This recipe instructs you to roast the tail in its shell, which provides a burst of additional flavor. (Lobster shells provide most of the flavor for lobster bisque or sauce.) You will love the beautiful color and contrasting flavor that the English Pea Sauce contributes. Photo on page 230.

Ingredients
Makes 4 servings.

8 bamboo skewers, soaked
4 6-ounce lobster tails with shells
1 teaspoon extra-virgin olive oil
1/2 teaspoon sea salt
1/4 teaspoon freshly ground black pepper
1 tablespoon Fresh Herb Mix (see
*   page 39)*
2 cups cooked linguine
4 Roma tomatoes, thinly sliced
8 chives
8 baby carrots, steamed
1 cup English Pea Sauce (see page 21)

Preparation
Preheat the oven to 400°F (205°C). Push two skewers lengthwise through each lobster tail to prevent them from curling up. Rub the lobster tails with the olive oil and sprinkle with the salt, pepper, and herbs. Place the lobster tails in a baking pan and roast for 12 minutes. Remove the tails from the pan and place on a cutting board. Using a pair of kitchen shears, cut through the bottom shells and remove the lobster meat. Slice each tail into 5 slices.

Toss the linguine in the lobster pan to soak up the juices.

To serve: Place 1/2 cup of the linguine on each plate. Alternating lobster and tomato slices, arrange them on top of the linguine. Add 2 chives and 2 baby carrots on top of the lobster. Ladle 1/4 cup of sauce onto each plate.

Vegetable Tamales with Toasted Fennel and Tomato Sauce

Freshly prepared tamales filled with red chile beef, chicken, or green chile and cheese are staples in Mexico and a holiday favorite in the southwestern region of the United States. Follow my approach to assemble the tamales; it is designed to allow you to shape them quickly, creating tamales which are uniform in size and shape. Dried corn husks, traditionally used for wrapping the tamales before steaming, are used here to create an attractive presentation. They are available in the international foods section of many supermarkets.

Ingredients

Makes 8 servings.

Masa

4 cups fresh masa, masa harina, or fine
    cornmeal
1/2 cup Vegetable Stock (see page 152) or
    vegetable stock base (see page 326)
2 teaspoons baking powder
1/2 teaspoon sea salt
2 teaspoons finely chopped fresh cilantro

Tamale Filling

1/2 teaspoon extra-virgin olive oil
1/2 cup zucchini, small dice
1/2 cup yellow squash, small dice
1/2 cup yellow onion, small dice
1 cup bell pepper, small dice
1/2 cup portobello mushroom, small dice
1 cup tomatoes, small dice
1/2 cup corn kernels
1/2 cup eggplant, small dice
1 teaspoon minced garlic
3 1/2 cups cooked or canned black beans
    or pinto beans, drained (2 15-ounce
    cans), divided
1 1/2 teaspoons chile powder
1/4 teaspoon cayenne powder
2 teaspoons chopped fresh cilantro
1 cup tomato juice

Preparation

For the Masa: Using an electric mixer, whip the masa and stock until the masa becomes light and fluffy, about 5 minutes. (If using masa harina, additional stock may be needed.) Add the baking powder, salt, and cilantro. Stir to combine. Set aside.

For the Tamale Filling: Heat a large sauté pan over medium-high heat. Add the olive oil to lightly coat the bottom of the pan. Add the vegetables and garlic. Cook until the onion has just softened, about 5 minutes. Mix in 1 cup of the black beans (reserve remaining beans for the salsa), the chile powder, cayenne, cilantro, and tomato juice. Simmer for 10 minutes.

For the Black Bean Salsa: Heat a small saucepan over medium heat and spray with olive oil. Add the onion and sauté until the onion is just softened, 2 minutes. Stir in the tomatoes, cilantro, cayenne, and 2 1/2 cups black beans. Heat about 2 minutes. Set aside until ready to serve; reheat just before serving.

To assemble the tamales: On a cutting board, lay out a large sheet of plastic wrap (about 12 inches long). Use a spatula to spread out 1 cup of the masa in a thin rectangle, 10 inches long and 4 inches wide. This should be about 1/8 inch thick.

Place 1 1/2 cups of the filling along one long side of the masa rectangle in a long, thin row. Carefully peel the end of the masa off the plastic wrap and begin rolling it up to form a long tube. Wrap the masa tube with plastic wrap, with at least 2 inches of plastic wrap on each end. Twist the ends of the plastic wrap to make a firm, secure roll, and knot on each end. Repeat to make a total of 4 rolls.

Add about 2 inches of water to a large saucepan and bring to a boil. Arrange the tamales in a steamer insert or bamboo steamer. Place the insert over the boiling water, cover, and steam until the masa has cooked and is firm to the touch, 20 minutes. (Make sure the water does not reach the bottom of the steamer.) Remove pan from the stove. Cool for 5 minutes. Trim

Black Bean Salsa

1/2 cup finely chopped red onion
2 cups chopped fresh tomatoes (about 2
   medium)
4 tablespoons finely chopped fresh cilantro
1/2 teaspoon cayenne pepper
2 1/2 cups black beans reserved from the
   filling

Garnish

10 dried corn husks, optional
2 cups Toasted Fennel and Tomato Sauce
   (see page 35)
Sautéed baby zucchini and yellow squash,
   optional

the end of the plastic wrap off one end of each tamale. Push the tamales through the open ends. Cut each tamale into 2 equal pieces.

Meanwhile, soak 10 corn husks in water for 5 minutes. Tear 2 of the husks into 4 thin strips each. Use the strips to tie off the top of the other 8 husks into a bow.

To serve: Ladle 1/4 cup of Toasted Fennel Sauce onto each plate. Lay one of the husks in middle of each plate and place one tamale in the husk. Place 2 tablespoons of black bean salsa on each plate. Garnish with zucchini and yellow squash, if using.

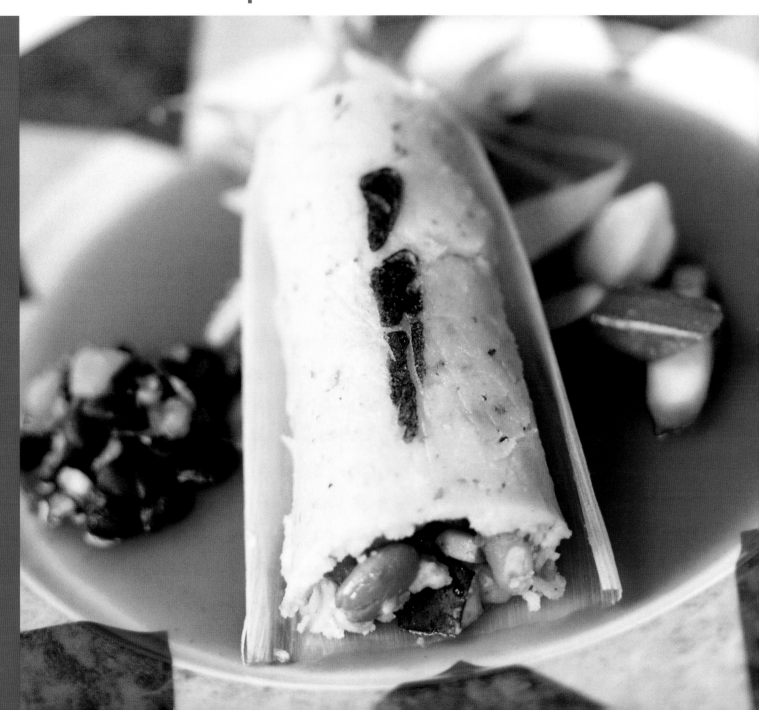

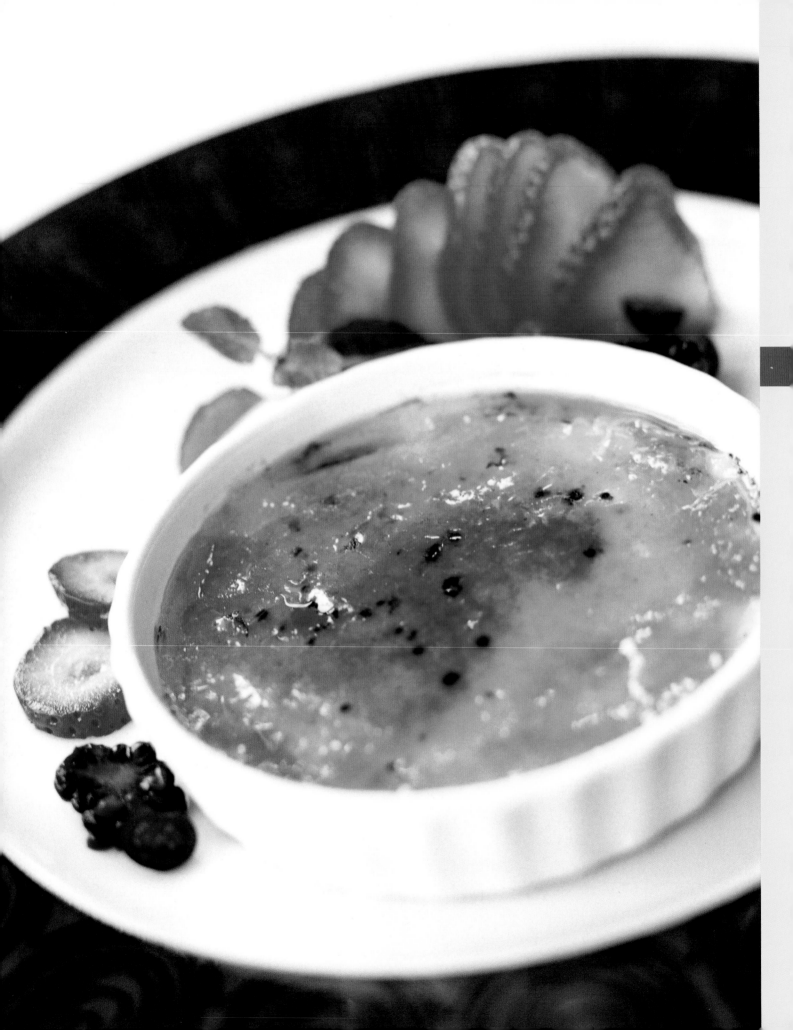

Delectable Desserts

chapter 11

Lavender Crème Brûlée
Chocolate-Banana Bread Pudding
Kahlúa Flan
Fresh Berry Napoleons with Strawberry-White Chocolate Mousse
Sour Apple Consommé with Mango-Ginger Sorbet and Mixed Berry Sorbet
Mango-Ginger Sorbet
Mixed Berry Sorbet
Tiramisu
Tropical Fruit Compote
Espresso Cake
Chocolate Truffles
Pineapple Upside-Down Cake
Cream Puffs with Low-Fat Pastry Cream
Lemon Mousse Cake
Warm Pineapple and Mango Tart
Peach Ricotta Tarts
Cheesecake Creativity
Tequila-Lime Cheesecake
Chocolate Taco with Fresh Fruit Salsa
Strawberry-White Chocolate Mousse
White Chocolate Mousse
Vanilla Bean Tapioca
Berry Consommé
Chilled Chocolate Soufflé with Berry Consommé

Pictured at left: Lavender Crème Brûlée

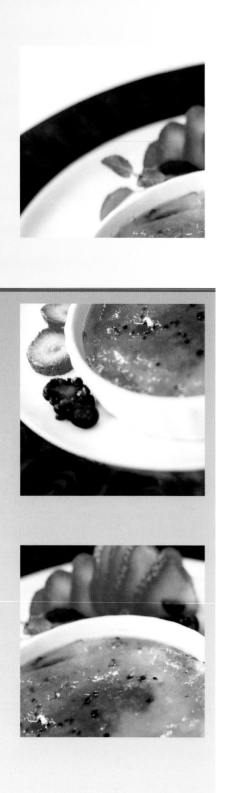

When it came time to create desserts that have considerably less fat and fewer calories than the traditional treats, I developed and stuck by these three rules.

Rule One: Artificial ingredients, such as sweeteners, margarines, or creams, cannot be good for you in comparison to natural ingredients and will not be used. Whole and natural food products present the safest and surest way of obtaining balanced health and nutrition. If I cannot pronounce it or if I need a chemistry book to define it, then I shouldn't be using it. To reduce calories, I rely on natural sweeteners that are least processed, such as raw cane sugar, honey, and fruit syrups. I have found that the use of these ingredients allows me to reduce the amount of sugar that is normally found in traditional recipes.

Rule Two: Being a chocoholic myself, I insist that chocolate should taste like chocolate. Just say no to carob. Chocolate desserts must be decadent or they are not worth serving. A viable solution in Conscious Cuisine is to keep favorite recipes intact and then reduce their portion sizes. That's far better than serving a dessert that's low in fat and calories and lacking in flavor.

Rule Three: Dessert, by its definition, should be a treat that deserves to be eaten. It doesn't matter how low in fat or calories a dessert may be; if it fails to deliver delectable flavors or to satisfy the senses, it isn't worth eating.

With these rules in mind, I've created desserts utilizing the best ingredients available. Many times I rely on the vibrant flavors of fresh seasonal fruits and berries, enhancing their natural sweetness with vanilla beans, mint, or other luscious ingredients. Fruits and berries are relatively low in calories, and are available in a myriad of shapes, sizes, colors, and flavors, allowing us thousands of creative uses. Fruits and berries provide excellent choices for snacks and desserts, while supplying us with a healthful dose of vitamins and other nutrients:

- Apples and pears are a great source of fiber.
- Stone fruits (i.e. peaches) are packed with luscious sweet juices and vitamins.
- Berries are not only gorgeously attractive, they are also good sources of fiber and vitamins.
- Citrus fruits are good sources of vitamin C and other nutrients.
- Melons, rich in vitamin C and beta-carotene, have a delightful flavor.
- Frozen fruits are processed without cooking, so they lose few if any nutrients, which makes them ideal to purchase and use when their fresh season has past. Freezing allows us to continue to enjoy the delicious flavors of fruits year 'round in wonderful smoothies, pies, and sauces.
- Canned fruit packed in water or unsweetened juices is a good choice when fresh or frozen fruit is unavailable. Nutrients are retained and calories are considerably lower than fruit packed in heavy syrup.
- Drying fruit preserves summer jewels. Drying reduces the fruit's water content, increasing the fruit's supply of vitamins and minerals proportionally. It also concentrates its sugar and caloric content. Because of their sticky, chewy consistency and high concentration of natural sugars, dried fruits are an ideal substitute for processed sugars in many dessert recipes.

Once I identify where the high-fat ingredients are in a recipe, it's a conscious choice and challenge to replace or reduce these ingredients without losing the integrity of the dessert. An example of this is the use of mashed bananas or prune puree, which offer sweetness and body while reducing the sugars and oils needed. I dramatically reduce the amount of egg yolks and shortening to decrease the high fat content of desserts, leaving just enough in the recipe to provide richness, color, and sufficient binding components.

Reducing or eliminating the high-fat and calorie-laden ingredients in old favorites, such as tiramisu, crème brûlée, Napoleons, and even cheesecakes, results in boldly flavored, delectable, and healthy desserts, which are served in responsible, sensibly sized portions.

Lavender Crème Brûlée

Per serving:
Calories 50; Protein 5g; Total Fat 2g; Saturated Fat 0.5g; Carbohydrates 5g; Dietary Fiber 0g; Cholesterol 55mg; Sodium 60mg

Ingredients

Makes 12 servings.

1/2 vanilla bean, split in half lengthwise
1 1/4 cups low-fat milk
1 1/4 cups fat-free milk
1 1/2 teaspoons dried lavender flowers
3 large eggs
4 large egg whites
1/3 cup raw cane sugar plus 6 teaspoons for topping

Crème brûlée is without a doubt one of my favorite desserts. I was once assigned the difficult task of comparing crème brûlée from five of New York City's finest restaurants and reporting the subtle differences that I found back to the director of operations of the Princess Hotel. The real task was to assure him that this kid from Chicago understood the difference between good and great. I think Mr. Esposito will agree that this version of the French classic will hold its own with the great ones. Dried lavender flowers are available in health food stores or can be ordered from the supplier listed in chapter 13, Pantry Resources. Photo on page 268.

Preparation

Scrape the seeds from the vanilla bean pod. In a medium saucepan, combine the vanilla bean pod and seeds, the milks, and the lavender flowers. Bring to a simmer over low heat. Remove from the heat, cover, and steep for 30 minutes.

Preheat the oven to 325°F (165°C). Return the pan to medium heat and bring the milk mixture back to a low boil.

Combine the eggs, egg whites, and sugar in a bowl. Slowly whisk the hot milk into the egg mixture, stirring constantly until all the milk has been added. Strain the custard through a fine mesh strainer or a colander lined with cheesecloth.

Pour 1/2 cup of custard into each of 12 ramekins and place them in a baking pan. Add enough hot water to the baking pan to bring the water halfway up the sides of the ramekins. Bake for 50 minutes or until the custard is set. Cover and refrigerate until well chilled (1 to 2 hours).

When ready to serve, preheat the broiler. Place the ramekins of chilled custard on a baking sheet. Sprinkle 1/2 teaspoon raw cane sugar in each ramekin and broil quickly until the sugar is caramelized, 1 or 2 minutes. Watch carefully to avoid burning. Let cool at room temperature for 5 to 10 minutes before serving.

Chocolate-Banana Bread Pudding

I grew up with bread pudding. My mom would sometimes save the scraps and ends of each loaf of bread to make a delicious treat at the end of the week for our family. Making this into a conscious dessert meant two things had to change. First, the quality of bread had to be better. This was accomplished with the use of banana bread, providing substance, nutrients, and flavor. Second, the custard part of the pudding needed work. Fats and calories were diminished by the use of more health-conscious ingredients. These revisions created a dessert that Mom would be proud of and happy to eat.

Ingredients

Makes 12 servings.

Banana Bread

2 ripe bananas, mashed
1 large egg white
1/2 cup prune puree
   or unsweetened applesauce
1 teaspoon canola oil
1/2 cup raw cane sugar (Turbinado)
1 cup whole-wheat pastry flour
1/2 cup unbleached all purpose flour
1 teaspoon baking soda

Custard

2 cups fat-free milk
1/2 cup raw cane sugar (Turbinado)
1/2 teaspoon pure vanilla extract
3 large eggs
4 large egg whites
1/4 cup Wax Orchards Fudge Fantasy (see
   page 326) or other chocolate sauce
1 teaspoon cinnamon

1 ripe banana, diced

Preparation

For the Banana Bread: Preheat the oven to 350°F (175°C). Lightly coat the bottom of a loaf pan with cooking spray.

In a medium mixing bowl, beat together the bananas, egg white, prune puree, oil, and sugar. In a small mixing bowl, combine the flours and baking soda. Mix the dry ingredients into the wet ingredients; the batter will be thick. Pour the batter into the prepared pan. Bake for 35 to 40 minutes or until a knife inserted in the middle comes out clean.

For the Custard: Combine the milk and sugar in a small saucepan over medium heat. Meanwhile, in a large bowl, combine the vanilla, eggs, egg whites, chocolate sauce, and cinnamon. When the milk begins to bubble around the sides of the pan, remove from the heat. Slowly whisk the hot milk into the egg mixture, stirring constantly until all the milk is added.

To assemble: Turn the oven down to 325°F (165°C). Lightly coat the bottom and sides of 12 baking cups (muffin pans or soufflé cups) with cooking spray.

Dice the banana bread and place in a large bowl. Add the diced banana and custard and mix well. Allow the mixture to soak for at least 10 minutes for the bread to begin absorbing the custard.

Spoon into the prepared cups and place the cups in a baking pan. Add enough hot water to the baking pan to bring the water halfway up the sides of the cups. Bake the puddings for 45 to 50 minutes or until firmed up and lightly browned.

Kahlúa Flan

My pastry chef and good friend Jessica Smith offered me a taste of this wonderful flan early one morning. I quickly responded with, "It's great—but does it meet our guidelines?" She confidently and proudly replied, "Yes." You see, Jessie can easily make a great-tasting flan, and the dramatic reduction from the original recipe with 300 calories and 9 grams of fat to her new version with 200 calories and 2.5 grams of fat was a proud moment, indeed. The photo at the right shows Kahlúa Flan with Menlo strips.

Ingredients

Makes 9 servings.

1 1/4 cups granulated sugar
1/2 cup water
1 vanilla bean, split in half lengthwise
1 1/4 cups fat-free milk
1 1/2 cups 2-percent milk
1/2 cup half-and-half
2 cinnamon sticks
1 large egg
6 large egg whites
1/3 cup raw cane sugar (Turbinado)
1 1/2 tablespoons Kahlúa
1/2 tablespoon molasses

Preparation

Lightly coat nine 1/2-cup ramekins with cooking spray. Combine the granulated sugar and water in a saucepan and cook over medium heat, stirring constantly, until the sugar is dissolved. Bring to a boil and cook until the sugar turns amber in color, 10 to 15 minutes. Remove from the heat. Immediately pour the caramelized sugar into the prepared ramekins. Set aside.

Scrape the seeds from the vanilla bean pod. In a medium saucepan, combine the vanilla bean pod and seeds, the milks, half-and-half, and cinnamon sticks. Bring to a simmer over low heat. Remove from the heat, cover, and steep for 30 minutes.

Preheat the oven to 325°F (165°C). Return the pan to medium heat and bring the milk mixture back to a low boil.

Combine the egg, egg whites, sugar, Kahlúa, and molasses in a bowl. Slowly whisk the hot milk into the egg mixture, stirring constantly until all the milk has been added. Strain the custard through a fine mesh strainer or a colander lined with cheesecloth.

Pour the custard into the prepared ramekins and place them in a baking pan. Add enough hot water to the baking pan to bring the water halfway up the sides of the ramekins. Bake for 1 hour or until the custard has set up and is slightly firm to the touch. Remove from the water bath and chill.

To serve: Run a hot knife around the inside edges of the ramekins and invert the flans onto serving plates.

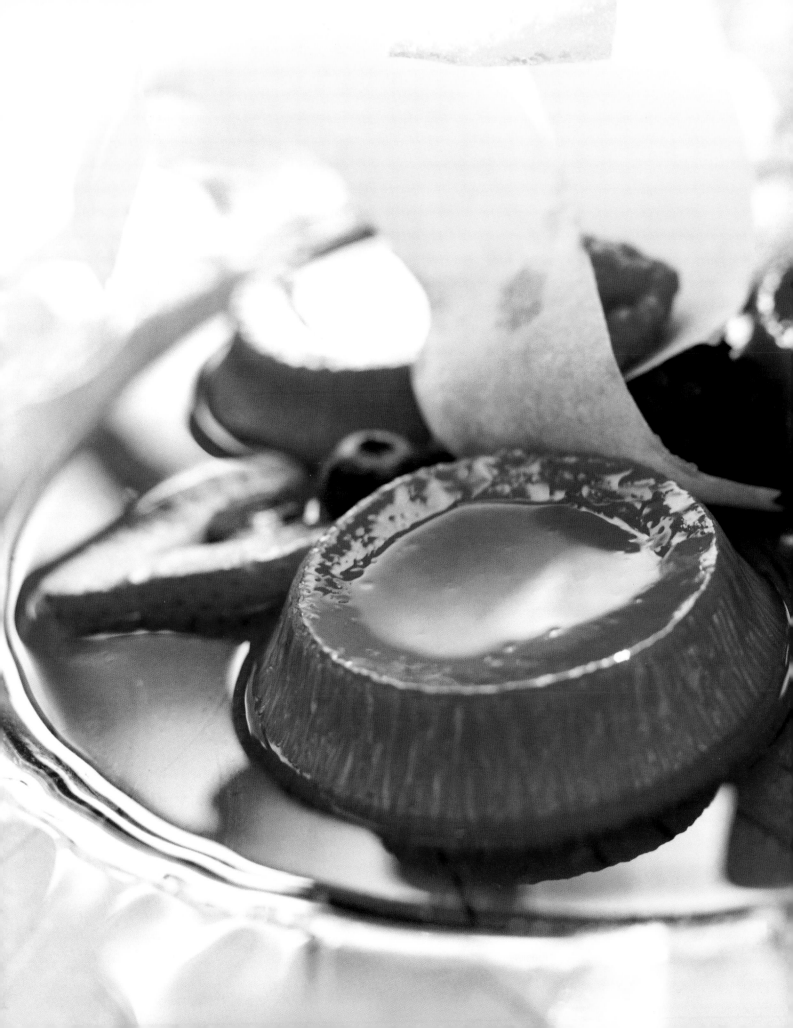

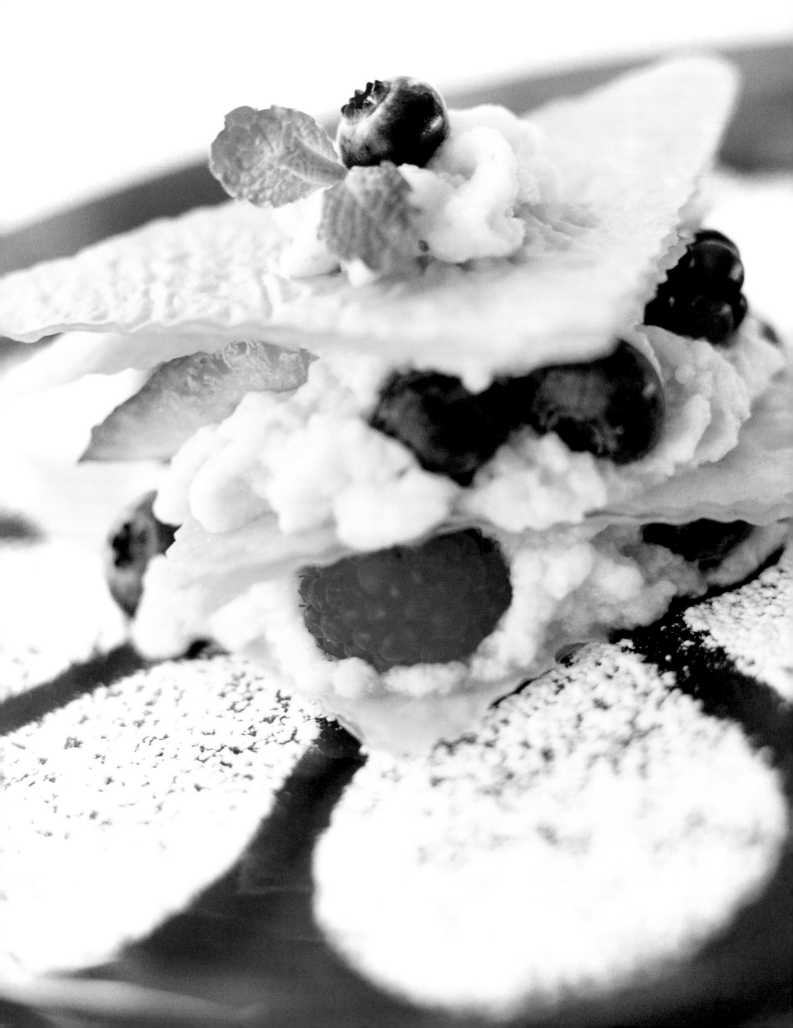

Fresh Berry Napoleons with Strawberry-White Chocolate Mousse

Per Napoleon:
Calories 90: Protein 3g; Total Fat 3.5g;
Saturated Fat 1.5g; Carbohydrates 15g; Dietary
Fiber 3g; Cholesterol 0mg; Sodium 35mg

The traditional layered Napoleon, with its successful contrast of crisp pastry and rich cream, has been revered and interpreted in numerous ways. This version relies heavily on the sweetness of fresh seasonal berries. Rich, buttery puff pastry is replaced with crisp phyllo pastry, offering beautiful, crisp layers and delicate flavor from a mist of hazelnut oil.

Ingredients
Makes 4 Napoleons.

2 to 4 sheets phyllo dough (extra to allow for breakage)
Hazelnut oil spray or cooking spray
1 1/2 teaspoons raw cane sugar (Turbinado), for sprinkling
1/2 cup Strawberry-White Chocolate Mousse (see page 300)
1/2 cup fresh blackberries
1/2 cup fresh raspberries
1/2 cup fresh blueberries

Garnish
Powdered sugar or unsweetened cocoa powder

Preparation
Preheat oven to 350°F (175°C). Line a baking sheet with parchment paper.

Place 1 sheet of phyllo dough on a clean cutting board. Spray with hazelnut oil and sprinkle with 1/2 teaspoon of sugar. Place a second layer of dough on top, spray with oil and sprinkle with sugar. Fold the sheet in half lengthwise. Spray the top with oil, and sprinkle with sugar. Cut the layered sheet in half lengthwise and each half into 6 rectangles or diamonds. You should have 12 layered pieces. Place these pieces on the prepared baking sheet. (You may want to repeat with two more sheets because the phyllo dough is delicate and some of the rectangles may break.)

Cover with another piece of parchment paper. Put another baking sheet on top to help the phyllo dough layers bake together so they will not break as easily. Bake for 12 to 15 minutes or until golden brown and crispy. Cool and store in an airtight container until ready to use.

To assemble: Fill a pastry bag fitted with a small star tip with the mousse. Place 1 phyllo rectangle or diamond on a serving plate. Pipe a small, zig-zag line onto the rectangle, using about 1 tablespoon of mousse. Arrange 3 of each kind of berry on the mousse. Repeat with another layer of phyllo, mousse, and berries, and top with a third phyllo piece. Dust with cocoa or powdered sugar to garnish.

Sour Apple Consommé with Mango-Ginger Sorbet and Mixed Berry Sorbet

Per 1/4 cup consommé:
Calories 35; Protein 0g; Total Fat 0g; Saturated Fat 0g; Carbohydrates 9g; Dietary Fiber less than 1 gram; Cholesterol 0mg; Sodium 5mg

Per serving with 1/4 cup consommé and 1/4 cup of each sorbet:
Calories 110; Protein 1g; Total Fat 0g; Saturated Fat 0g; Carbohydrates 29g; Dietary Fiber 4g; Cholesterol 0mg; Sodium 10mg

Clear, intensely flavored apple consommé is a wonderful flavor complement to small scoops of colorful, cool, and delicious sorbets. The simple sugar syrup used to make most sorbets is replaced here by natural fruit juice. The recipes can be halved.

Ingredients
Makes 16 servings.

4 cups unsweetened apple juice
5 lemon tea bags
2 lemons, sliced
2 cinnamon sticks
1 teaspoon minced fresh ginger
1/8 teaspoon cracked black pepper
1/8 teaspoon anise seeds
Mango-Ginger Sorbet (see page 279)
Mixed Berry Sorbet (see page 279)

Preparation
Bring the apple juice to a low boil in a medium saucepan. Add tea bags, lemons, cinnamon sticks, and spices. Remove from heat and steep for 15 minutes. Strain and chill.

To serve: Pour 1/4 cup of consommé into a martini glass or decorative dessert dish. Add 1/4 cup scoops of each sorbet.

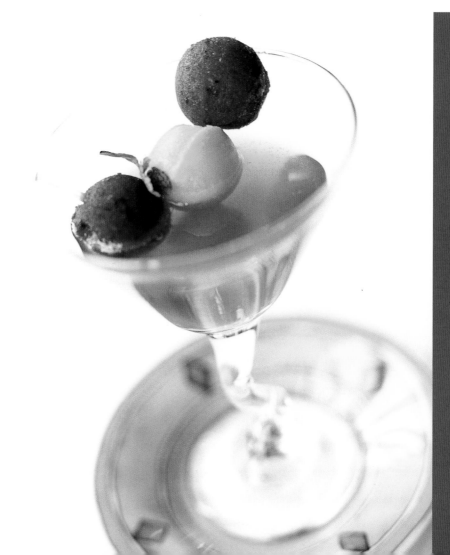

Mango-Ginger Sorbet

Mangoes are an exorbitantly delicious fruit when eaten at the peak of their ripeness. The fruit is lusciously sweet and sticky, with exotic flavor and vibrant color.

This recipe captures the goodness of mango in a smooth sorbet heightened with grated ginger. If you don't have an ice cream freezer, simply freeze the mixture in a shallow stainless steel or glass pan. Scrape the sorbet crystals from the pan with a fork for *granita*. Photo on page 278.

Ingredients
Makes 1 quart.

3-inch piece of fresh ginger
3 1/2 cups pureed mangoes (about 2 medium)
1/4 cup orange liqueur
1 cup papaya juice
1/3 cup water

Preparation
Peel and grate the ginger; squeeze handfuls of the grated ginger to yield 2 tablespoons of ginger juice. Combine the ginger juice with the remaining ingredients in a mixing bowl. Pour into an ice cream freezer and process according to the manufacturer's instructions.

Mixed Berry Sorbet

Created by the Chinese and introduced to the Italians in the seventeenth century, sorbets have played a creative role in dining for centuries. Made from fruits, herbs, and even liqueurs, sorbets are served when a cool and refreshingly light dessert is wanted. At formal dinners, sorbet is frequently served between courses as an *intermezzo*—a pause to cleanse the palate. Photo on page 278.

Ingredients
Makes 1 quart.

1 pint hulled fresh or frozen strawberries
1 pint fresh or frozen blueberries
1 pint fresh or frozen raspberries
1/2 cup Wax Orchards Fruit Sweet (see page 326) or corn syrup
Juice of 1/2 lemon
2 tablespoons red wine
1/2 cup cold water

Preparation
Combine the berries, syrup, and lemon juice in a mixing bowl. Cover and refrigerate for at least 1 hour. When ready to freeze, add the red wine and water. Puree the berry mixture in a blender. Pour into an ice cream freezer and process according to the manufacturer's instructions.

Tiramisu

Per serving:
Calories 220; Protein 13g; Total Fat 7g;
Saturated Fat 5g; Carbohydrate 25g; Dietary
Fiber 0g; Cholesterol 25mg; Sodium 370mg

This decadent, Italian-style dessert lives up to its name as "a pick-me-up." In this version, the richness of Mascarpone and ricotta cheese is replaced with fat-free cottage cheese and reduced-fat cream cheese. The combination of espresso and liquors creates a sensational dessert that deserves to be enjoyed any time.

Ingredients
Makes 16 servings.

Cake
10 large egg whites
1 pinch cream of tartar
2/3 cup raw cane sugar (Turbinado)
1 cup unbleached all-purpose flour, sifted

Filling
3 cups fat-free cottage cheese, pureed in
    food processor until smooth
2 1/2 cups reduced-fat cream cheese
1 1/4 cups raw cane sugar (Turbinado)
1/3 cup fat-free milk
1 package unflavored gelatin powder (1
    tablespoon)
2 tablespoons dark rum
2 tablespoons Marsala wine
2 teaspoons Kahlúa

Espresso Syrup
2 tablespoons Wax Orchards Fruit Sweet
    (see page 326) or corn syrup
1/2 cup espresso
2 tablespoons Kahlua

2 tablespoons unsweetened cocoa powder

Preparation

For the Cake: Preheat the oven to 375°F (190°C). Lightly spray a 10-inch springform pan with cooking spray.

Using an electric mixer, beat the egg whites with the cream of tartar until frothy. Gradually add the sugar and continue beating until stiff peaks form. Gently fold the flour into the egg white mixture.

Spoon the batter into the prepared cake pan. Bake for 8 to 10 minutes or until a wooden pick inserted in the center comes out clean. Cool in the pan on a wire rack for 5 minutes; release the spring of the baking pan to prevent the cake from sticking to the sides of the pan and cool completely.

For the Filling: In a large bowl, beat together the cottage cheese, cream cheese, and sugar with an electric mixer.

Pour the milk into a small saucepan and sprinkle the gelatin on top. Let stand for about 2 minutes. Stir over medium heat until the gelatin has dissolved completely, about 2 minutes. Quickly stir the milk mixture into the cream cheese mixture. Fold in the rum, Marsala, and Kahlúa.

For the Espresso Syrup: Combine all the ingredients in a small bowl.

To assemble: Slice the cake in half horizontally. Place one layer in the bottom of the springform pan. Brush with half of the espresso syrup.

Smooth half of the filling onto the cake. Place the second cake layer on the filling. Brush with the remaining espresso syrup. Top with the remaining filling. Refrigerate for at least 4 hours to allow the gelatin to set up.

Dust the top of the cake with cocoa powder before serving.

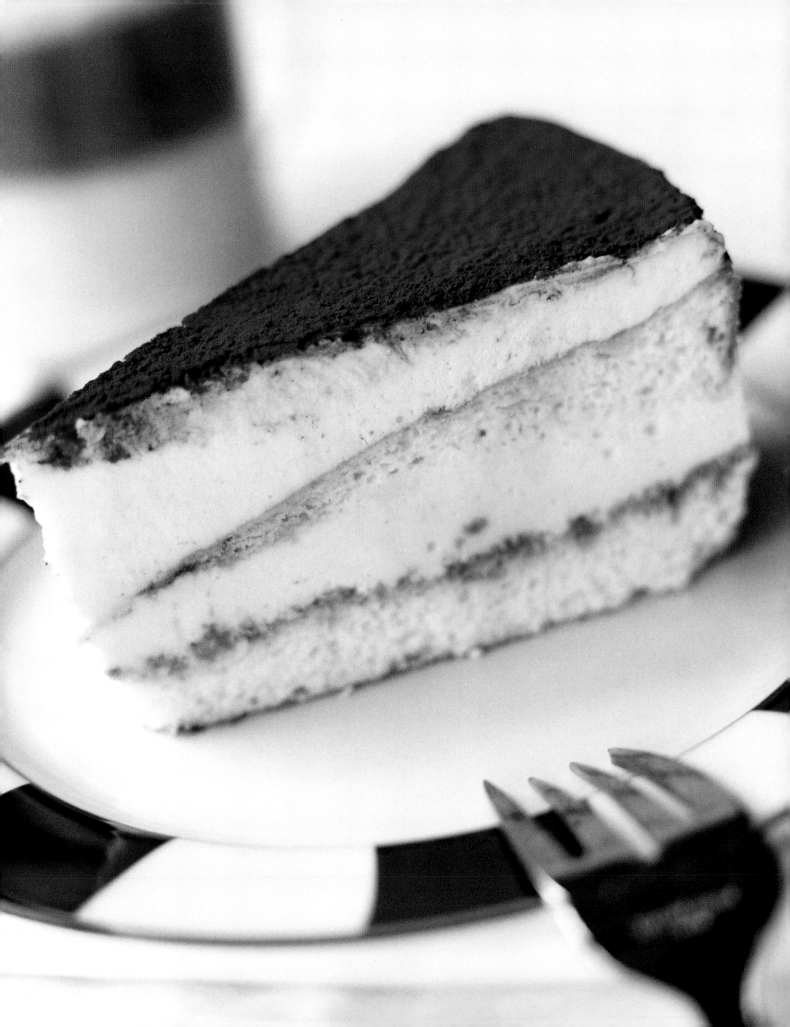

Tropical Fruit Compote

This is wonderful compote to add to your repertoire. It's great on countless dishes from Vanilla Bean Tapioca to ice creams, cakes, or waffles. The marriage of sweet and tart flavors in this aromatic mixture will bring the cool breezes of the tropics to your kitchen.

Ingredients
Make 8 servings.

1/2 vanilla bean, split in half lengthwise
1 cup unsweetened pineapple juice
2 tablespoons unsweetened orange juice
1 star anise
1 cinnamon stick
2 teaspoons cornstarch
2 teaspoons unsweetened orange juice
1/4 cup chopped pineapple
1/2 cup chopped mangoes
1/4 cup diagonally sliced banana
1 star fruit (carambola), thinly sliced

Preparation

Scrape the seeds from the vanilla bean pod and combine them with the pineapple juice, orange juice, star anise, and cinnamon stick in a medium saucepan over medium heat. (The remaining pod can be put to another use such as flavoring vanilla sugar, see page xix.) Bring to a low boil, reduce heat, and simmer for 15 minutes.

Combine the cornstarch and orange juice, and whisk into the hot juices. Cook, stirring constantly, until the sauce has thickened and coats the back of a spoon, about 5 minutes. Remove pan from heat and stir in the fruit.

Let cool completely. Transfer to a container with an airtight lid. The compote will keep for up to 5 days in the refrigerator. Remove the star anise and cinnamon stick before serving.

Espresso Cake

Per serving
Calories 80; Protein 3g; Total Fat 0.5g;
Saturated Fat 0g; Carbohydrates 18g; Dietary
Fiber 2g; Cholesterol 0mg; Sodium 105mg

The combination of chocolate and coffee is a wonderful marriage of bitter and sweet flavors. The sweetness of the prunes adds moisture, body, and character to this cake, making it a wonderful treat in place of brownies or fudge. It can also be used to make remarkable low-fat Chocolate Truffles (see page 285). Photo on page 284.

Ingredients
Makes 14 servings.

2/3 cup whole-wheat pastry flour
1/4 cup unbleached all-purpose flour
1 cup raw cane sugar (Turbinado)
2/3 cup unsweetened cocoa powder
1 1/2 teaspoons baking powder
1/4 teaspoon baking soda
1/4 teaspoon salt
1/2 cup pureed prunes
    or unsweetened applesauce
3 large egg whites
1 teaspoon pure vanilla extract
1 cup coffee

Preparation
Preheat the oven to 350°F (175°C). Spray a 9-inch cake pan with cooking spray and dust with additional cocoa powder; set aside.

In a medium bowl, combine the flours, sugar, cocoa, baking powder, baking soda, and salt; set aside. In another bowl, combine the prune puree, egg whites, vanilla, and coffee. Mix the wet ingredients into the dry ingredients and pour into the prepared cake pan.

Bake for 20 to 25 minutes or until a toothpick inserted in the middle of the cake comes out clean. Cool the cake in the pan on a wire rack for 10 minutes. Run a knife around the edge of the cake and invert onto a wire rack to cool completely. Cut into 14 wedges to serve.

Variations
Serve with fat-free frozen yogurt, Wax Orchards Fudge Fantasy Sauce (see page 326), or raspberry sauce and powdered sugar.

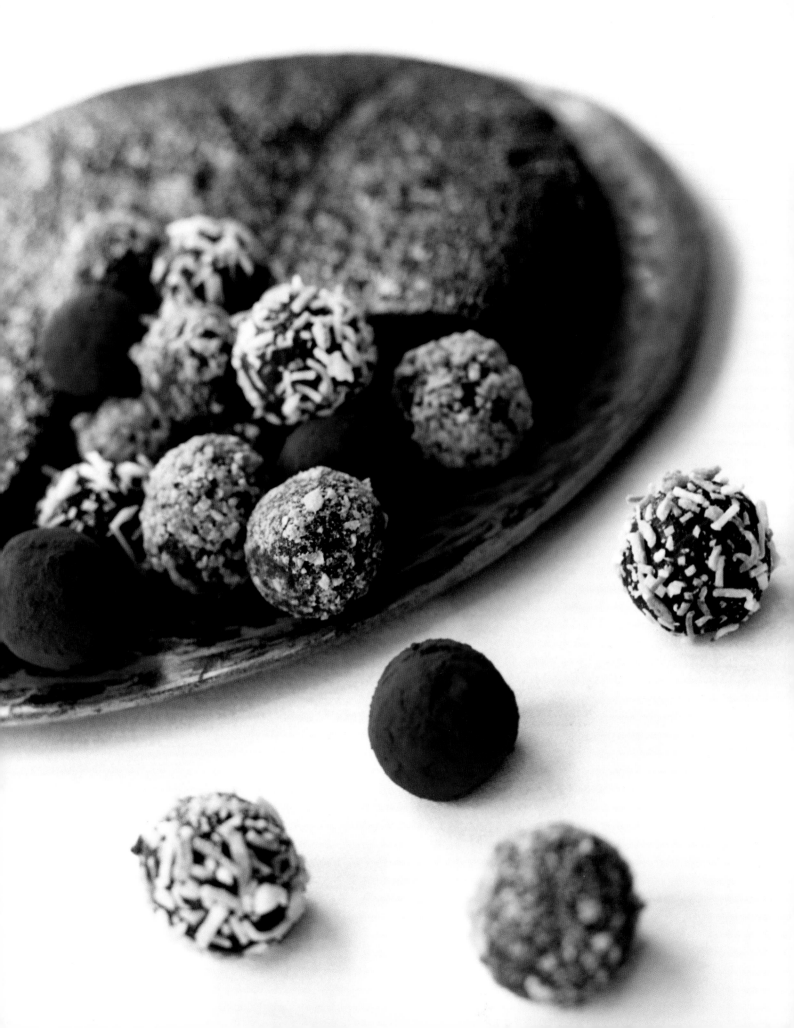

Chocolate Truffles

Ingredients
Makes 50 truffles.

1 baked Espresso Cake (see page 283)
1/4 cup part-skim ricotta cheese or nonfat
  plain yogurt

Coatings
Unsweetened cocoa powder
*Finely chopped nuts (walnuts, pecans,
  pistachios)*
Finely chopped toasted coconut

There's not much you can substitute for the rich chocolate ganache used to make fancy chocolate truffles. But this surprising recipe provides the deep chocolate flavor and satisfaction associated with chocolate truffles without the use of ganache. It's cleverly made with the use of Espresso Cake and ricotta cheese. Yes, ricotta cheese—the cheese binds the cake crumbs together, enabling you to make delectable small morsels with a delicious mocha flavor. The photo at the left shows Espresso Cake (see page 283) and assorted truffles.

Preparation
Allow the cake to cool to room temperature. Cut the cake into small cubes and place in a mixer bowl. Add the ricotta cheese and blend to a smooth consistency (use a paddle attachment, if possible). Chill the mixture before shaping into balls.

Scoop out 1 tablespoon at a time and roll into balls. Roll in cocoa powder, finely chopped nuts, or toasted coconut.

Per 1 truffle rolled in 1/2 teaspoon finely chopped nuts:
Calories 30; Protein 1g; Total Fat 1g; Saturated Fat 0g; Carbohydrates 6g; Dietary Fiber 0g; Cholesterol 0mg; Sodium 30mg

Per 1 truffle rolled in 1/2 teaspoon finely chopped coconut:
Calories 30; Protein 1g; Total Fat 0.5g; Saturated Fat 0g; Carbohydrates 5g; Dietary Fiber 0g; Cholesterol 0mg; Sodium 35mg

Pineapple Upside-Down Cake

Per serving:
Calories 200; Protein 4g; Total Fat 2g;
Saturated Fat 1g; Carbohydrates 42g; Dietary
Fiber 1g; Cholesterol 30mg; Sodium 230mg

A meal of comfort foods is not complete without a satisfying, home-style dessert. If you haven't had a pineapple upside-down cake in a while, try this recipe and reminisce of times past while caring for the waistline of the present.

Ingredients
Makes 8 servings.

1/4 cup honey
8 pineapple rings
1 tablespoon unsalted butter
2 tablespoons prune puree
    or unsweetened applesauce
3/4 cup raw cane sugar (Turbinado)
1 large egg
1 teaspoon pure vanilla extract
1 1/2 cups unbleached all-purpose flour
1 1/2 teaspoon baking powder
1/2 teaspoon baking soda
1/2 teaspoon cinnamon
1/4 sea salt
3/4 cup low-fat buttermilk

Preparation

Preheat the oven to 350°F (175°C). Coat a 10-inch, round cake pan or eight individual angel food or muffin pans with cooking spray. Heat the honey and pour it into prepared cake pan. Arrange the pineapple rings in the honey.

Beat together the butter, prune puree, and sugar until creamy, 4 minutes with an electric mixer on medium speed. Add the egg and vanilla; mix well.

Combine the flour, baking powder, baking soda, cinnamon, and salt; stir well. Add the flour mixture to creamed mixture alternately with the buttermilk, beginning and ending with the flour mixture; mix well after each addition.

Spoon the batter evenly over the pineapple. Bake for 35 to 40 minutes or until a wooden pick inserted in the center comes out clean. (Bake individual cakes for 25 to 30 minutes.) Let cool in the pan for 5 minutes.

To serve, run a knife around the edges and invert the cake onto serving plate. Cut into 8 slices.

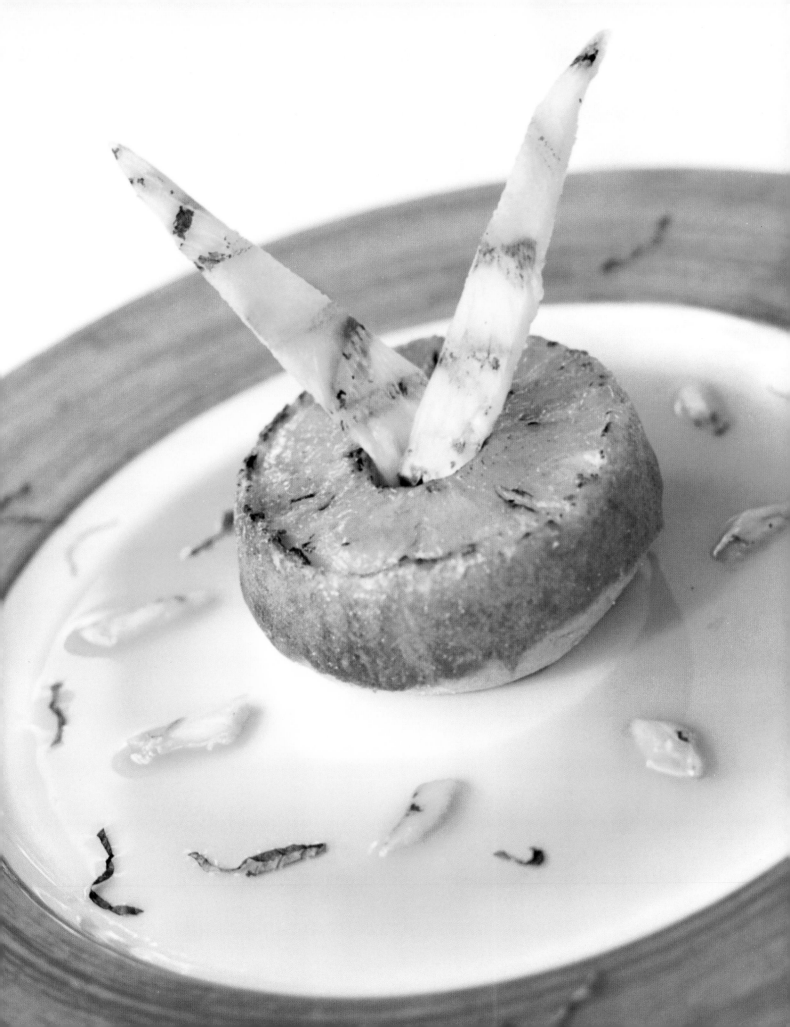

Cream Puffs with Low-Fat Pastry Cream

Per filled cream puff:
Calories 90; Protein 3g; Total Fat 3.5g; Saturated Fat 2g; Carbohydrates 13g; Dietary Fiber 1g; Cholesterol 50mg; Sodium 55mg

Ingredients
Makes 36 cream puffs.

Pâte à Choux
2 1/4 cups water
1/3 cup unsalted butter
1/2 teaspoon sea salt
1 tablespoon raw cane sugar (Turbinado)
2 cups unbleached all-purpose flour
5 large eggs

Pastry Cream
1/3 cup cornstarch
2 large egg yolks
4 cups fat-free milk
1 vanilla bean, split in half lengthwise
1 cup raw cane sugar (Turbinado)
2 tablespoons unsalted butter

Glaze
1/2 cup water
1/4 cup Wax Orchards Fruit Sweet (see page 326) or corn syrup
3/4 cup raw cane sugar (Turbinado)
1 cup unsweetened cocoa powder

I have included this recipe to introduce this marvelous, low-fat pastry cream. Fat-free milk replaces the cream, and only two egg yolks are used to provide color and richness. Cornstarch provides the binding properties needed when using fewer egg yolks. The result is a pastry cream that is ideal to pipe inside light and airy *pâte à choux*, which are especially delicious when coated with a chocolate glaze that uses fruit syrup and high-quality unsweetened cocoa powder instead of melted, semisweet chocolate.

Preparation

Preheat the oven to 350°F (175°C). Line a baking sheet with parchment paper.

For the Pâte à Choux: In a saucepan over medium heat, combine the water, butter, salt, and sugar. Bring to a boil. Add the flour all at once to the water, stirring constantly. Reduce the heat to medium. Cook, stirring constantly with a wooden spoon, until the batter comes away from the sides of the pan, 3 to 5 minutes. (This is a very thick batter.) Remove from the stove and begin beating in the eggs, one at a time. The batter will become stiff and shiny. Carefully place the batter in a pastry bag fitted with a large star tip. If the batter is too warm, wrap the pastry bag with a towel. Pipe the dough in 2-inch mounds on the prepared baking sheet. Bake for 20 to 25 minutes, or until the puffs have risen and are golden brown. (Do not open the oven door for at least 20 minutes.)

For the Pastry Cream: In a mixing bowl, combine the cornstarch, egg yolks, and 1/4 cup of the milk; set aside. Scrape the seeds from the vanilla bean pod and combine them with the remaining 3 3/4 cups of milk, sugar, and butter in a medium saucepan. (The remaining pod can be put to another use such as flavoring vanilla sugar, see page xix.) Bring to a boil over medium-high heat. Slowly whisk the hot milk into the egg mixture, stirring constantly. Return the egg mixture to the saucepan and cook over medium heat, stirring constantly, until the pastry cream is thick, about 5 minutes. Strain through a fine mesh strainer or a colander lined with cheesecloth. Pour the pastry cream into a bowl; cover with a piece of plastic wrap directly on the surface of the cream. Chill for at least 1 hour. Makes 3 cups.

For the Glaze: Combine the water, Fruit Sweet, and sugar in a medium saucepan over medium heat. Bring the mixture to a boil. Remove the saucepan from the stove and whisk in the cocoa powder. Strain the sauce through a fine mesh strainer or a colander lined with cheesecloth. Chill well before serving. Makes 1 3/4 cups.

To assemble: Fit a pastry bag with a plain, round tip and fill with the pastry cream. Cut a small slit in the side of each cream puff. Carefully insert the tip of the pastry bag into the cream puff and squeeze gently to fill the puff. Dip the top of each cream puff in the chocolate glaze. Place the finished cream puffs on a baking sheet lined with parchment paper. Allow the chocolate to harden. Serve the cream puffs as soon as the chocolate glaze is firm.

Lemon Mousse Cake

Per serving:
Calories 100; Protein 7g; Total Fat 2.5g;
Saturated Fat 1g; Carbohydrates 12g; Dietary
Fiber 0g; Cholesterol 60mg; Sodium 160mg

Many residents of Arizona grow bountiful citrus trees in their yards. The trees usually bear more fruit than the owners—or their neighbors—can use. This light and delicious cake was created to help make use of the spring crop of fresh citrus. Try this cake with key lime or orange juice to make other delectable desserts.

Ingredients

Makes 16 servings.

Lemon Cake
1 cup unbleached all-purpose flour
4 large eggs, separated
1/2 cup raw cane sugar (Turbinado)
1/2 teaspoon grated lemon zest

Lemon Mousse
1 1/2 cups fat-free cottage cheese
1 cup reduced-fat cream cheese (8 ounces), softened
3/4 cup raw cane sugar (Turbinado)
2 tablespoons cold water
1 package unflavored gelatin powder (1 tablespoon)
1/4 cup lemon juice
1/2 teaspoon grated lemon zest

Preparation

For the Lemon Cake: Preheat the oven to 350°F (175°C). Coat a 10-inch springform pan with cooking spray and dust with flour; set aside.

Sift the flour into a mixing bowl. In a separate bowl, whisk the egg yolks with 1/4 cup of the sugar until the mixture is light yellow in color.

In a clean bowl, beat the egg whites with an electric mixer until frothy. Gradually add the remaining 1/4 cup of sugar and continue beating until stiff peaks form. Fold the egg whites into the egg yolk mixture. Gently fold the flour into the batter. Fold in the lemon zest.

Pour the batter into the prepared pan. Bake for 25 to 30 minutes or until a knife inserted in the center comes out clean. Cool in the pan on a wire rack for 5 minutes; release the sides of the pan and cool completely.

For the Lemon Mousse: Puree the cottage cheese in a food processor until smooth. Add the cream cheese and sugar. Process until combined.

Pour the water into a small saucepan and sprinkle the gelatin on top. Let stand for about 2 minutes. Stir in the lemon juice and lemon zest. Stir over medium heat until the gelatin has dissolved completely, about 2 minutes. Fold the gelatin into the cream cheese mixture.

To assemble: Cut the cake in half horizontally. Place one piece of the cake in the bottom of the springform pan. Pour half of the soft mousse mixture onto the cake. Place the other half of the cake over the mousse. Pour the remaining mousse onto the cake. Chill for at least 2 hours to allow the gelatin to set up.

Warm Pineapple and Mango Tart

Per serving:
Calories 270; Protein 7g; Total Fat 3g;
Saturated Fat 0.5g; Carbohydrates 55g; Dietary
Fiber 7g; Cholesterol 0g; Sodium 5mg

This recipe received the Best of 2000 award from the *Food and Wine Radio Network*. This daily radio show highlights the best of food and wine and those who make it happen throughout the United States. The show's host, Jennifer English, was wowed by the bold flavors and simple preparation of this wonderful summer dessert.

The crust is an interesting use of oats and is bound with Wax Orchards Fruit Sweet Syrup, a syrup of reduced fruit juices.

Ingredients
Makes 6 servings.

Filling
1 vanilla bean, split in half lengthwise
2 cups diced pineapple (1 small)
2 mangoes, peeled and cut into small dice
1/4 cup Wax Orchards Fruit Sweet (see page 326) or corn syrup

Crust
3 cups rolled oats
1/4 cup Wax Orchards Fruit Sweet or corn syrup

Preparation
Preheat the oven to 350°F (175°C).

For the Filling: Scrape the seeds from the vanilla bean pod and combine them with the pineapple, mangoes, and Fruit Sweet in a mixing bowl; set aside. (The remaining pod can be put to another use such as flavoring vanilla sugar, see page xix.)

For the Crust: In another mixing bowl, stir together the oats and syrup until the oats are coated. (The oats should stick together when pressed with your fingers.)

Place 6 4-inch pastry rings or tart pans on a baking sheet and coat with cooking spray. (Or coat an 8-inch cake pan with cooking spray.)

Using about 2 tablespoons of the oat mixture per ring, press it into the rings to form a bottom crust. Spoon 1/2 cup of the fruit mixture into each ring and press down with the back of the spoon to remove any air bubbles. Sprinkle 2 tablespoons of the remaining oat mixture on top of the fruit to form the top crust.

If using a cake pan, press half of the oat mixture into the bottom of the pan. Pour the fruit mixture over the oats and press down with the back of the spoon to remove any air bubbles. Sprinkle the remaining oat mixture on top of the fruit to form the top crust.

Bake for 12 minutes, or until the oats are golden brown. (The 8-inch tart may take longer.)

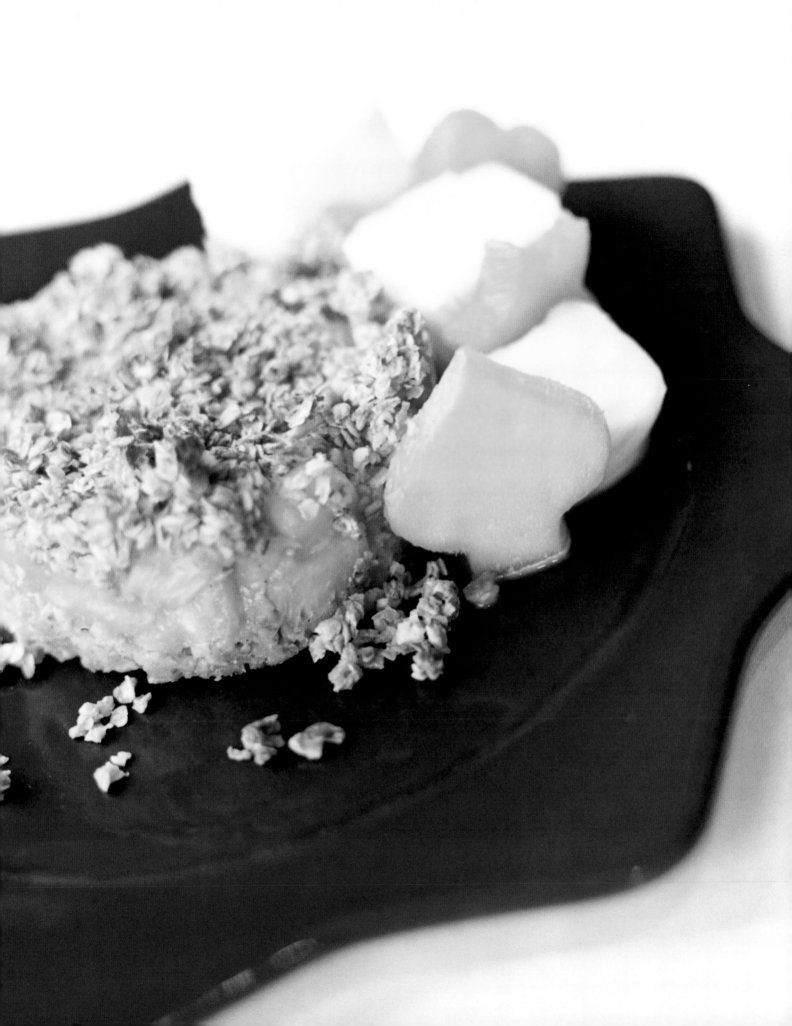

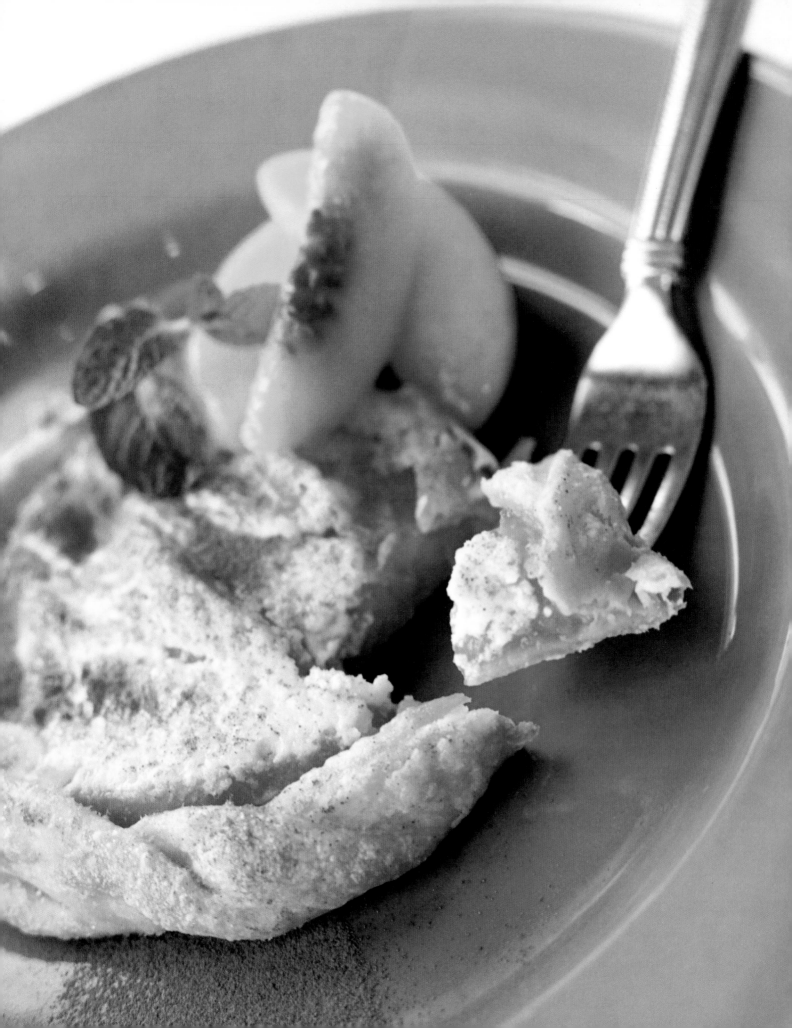

Peach Ricotta Tarts

Per tart:
Calories 210; Protein 8g; Total Fat 6g;
Saturated Fat 4g; Carbohydrates 31g; Dietary
Fiber 3g; Cholesterol 40mg; Sodium 210mg

I love this dessert—but please don't tell anyone it has half the calories and fat of traditional tarts because they will never believe you. Replace the peaches with any ultra-ripe fruit. I love the neat individual portions that allow you to free-form the dough to enclose the fruit. Serve warm with frozen vanilla bean yogurt.

Ingredients
Makes 8 tarts.

Peach Filling
1 vanilla bean, split in half lengthwise
3 cups sliced fresh or thawed frozen
* peaches (about 1 1/2 pounds)*
1 tablespoon honey
1 teaspoon fresh lemon juice
1/2 cup fat-free ricotta cheese
2 tablespoons raw cane sugar (Turbinado),
* plus additional for sprinkling*
1 teaspoon brandy
1 large egg
1 large egg white
1/2 teaspoon cinnamon

Dough
3 tablespoons fat-free sour cream
1/3 cup ice water
1 cup unbleached all-purpose flour
1/3 cup cornmeal
1 teaspoon raw cane sugar (Turbinado)
1/2 teaspoon sea salt
4 tablespoons reduced-fat cream cheese
3 tablespoons cold, unsalted butter, cut
* into small pieces*

Preparation

For the Peach Filling: Scrape the seeds from the vanilla bean pod and combine them with the peaches, honey, and lemon juice in a medium bowl. (The remaining pod can be put to another use such as flavoring vanilla sugar, see page xix.) Cover and let stand for 1 hour. In a separate bowl, combine the ricotta, sugar, brandy, egg, egg white, and cinnamon. Whisk until smooth and refrigerate until needed.

For the Dough: Combine the sour cream and water in a small bowl. Mix well and set aside. In another bowl, combine the flour, cornmeal, sugar, and salt. Add the cream cheese and butter, and work in with a pastry blender or 2 knives until the dough is crumbly. Add the sour cream mixture. Mix just until a dough forms. Roll the dough into a log and cut the log into 8 equal portions. Let the dough rest for 1 hour in the refrigerator.

Preheat oven to 375°F (190°C). Coat a baking sheet with cooking spray.

To assemble: On a floured board, roll out each dough portion into a 6- to 7-inch circle. Place the circles on the prepared baking sheet. Place 1/4 cup of the peach filling in the center of each circle. Spoon 1 tablespoon of the ricotta mixture onto the peaches. Fold in the edges of the dough to form a small, free-form tart. Sprinkle with a little additional sugar.

Bake for 15 to 20 minutes or until lightly browned. Serve warm.

Cheesecake Creativity

Per serving of basic cheesecake:
Calories 210; Protein 13g; Total Fat 5g;
Saturated Fat 2g; Carbohydrates 28g; Dietary
Fiber less than 1 gram; Cholesterol 30mg;
Sodium 530mg

Ingredients
Makes 12 servings.

2 cups graham cracker crumbs
1/4 cup unsweetened applesauce
3 cups fat-free cottage cheese
1 1/2 cups reduced-fat cream cheese
   (12 ounces), softened
1 large egg
5 large egg whites
1 1/2 cups raw cane sugar (Turbinado)
1 1/2 teaspoons pure vanilla extract
1/8 teaspoon sea salt

There are two ways to prepare cheesecake. One is the refrigerated method, which relies on gelatin to bind the ingredients together, and the other is the baked method—as shown below—which relies on eggs to bind the cheese. The use of reduced-fat cream cheese cuts down on fat and calories simply, without altering the flavor of the cake. I also substituted fat-free cottage cheese for the ricotta or mascarpone cheese that is traditionally used. The unsweetened applesauce is used to reduce the amount of sugar needed, and egg whites replace most of the egg yolks. Try this rendition of cheesecake; its flavor and richness will prove that favorite treats can be enjoyed without excess fat and calories.

Preparation
Preheat the oven to 325°F (165°C). Lightly coat a 9-inch springform pan with cooking spray. Cover the outside of the pan bottom with aluminum foil. Combine the graham cracker crumbs and unsweetened applesauce in a small bowl. Press the crumbs into the bottom of the springform pan; set aside.

Puree the cottage cheese in a food processor until smooth. Add the cream cheese, egg, egg whites, sugar, vanilla, and salt. Process until smooth, about 2 minutes. Pour the batter into the prepared pan.

Place the pan in a larger baking pan and fill the baking pan with 1/2 inch of water. Bake for 1 to 1 1/2 hours, or until the cake has set and is firm to the touch. Cool completely before serving. Cut into wedges with a sharp warm knife.

Variations
Sprinkle 1 cup chocolate chips onto the batter before baking. Or arrange 1 pint sliced fresh strawberries, 2 pints fresh raspberries, or mixed fruits on top of the cooled cheesecake. Heat 1/2 cup orange marmalade in a small saucepan until melted. Using a pastry brush, brush the marmalade over the fruit.

Per serving with chocolate chips:
Calories 310; Protein 14g; Total Fat 9g; Saturated Fat 4.5g; Carbohydrates 46g; Dietary
Fiber 1g; Cholesterol 30mg; Sodium 540mg

Per serving with strawberries:
Calories 250; Protein 13g; Total Fat 5g; Saturated Fat 2g; Carbohydrates 39g; Dietary
Fiber 1g; Cholesterol 30mg; Sodium 540mg

Per serving with raspberries:
Calories 270; Protein 13g; Total Fat 5g; Saturated Fat 2g; Carbohydrates 42g; Dietary
Fiber 3g; Cholesterol 30mg; Sodium 540mg

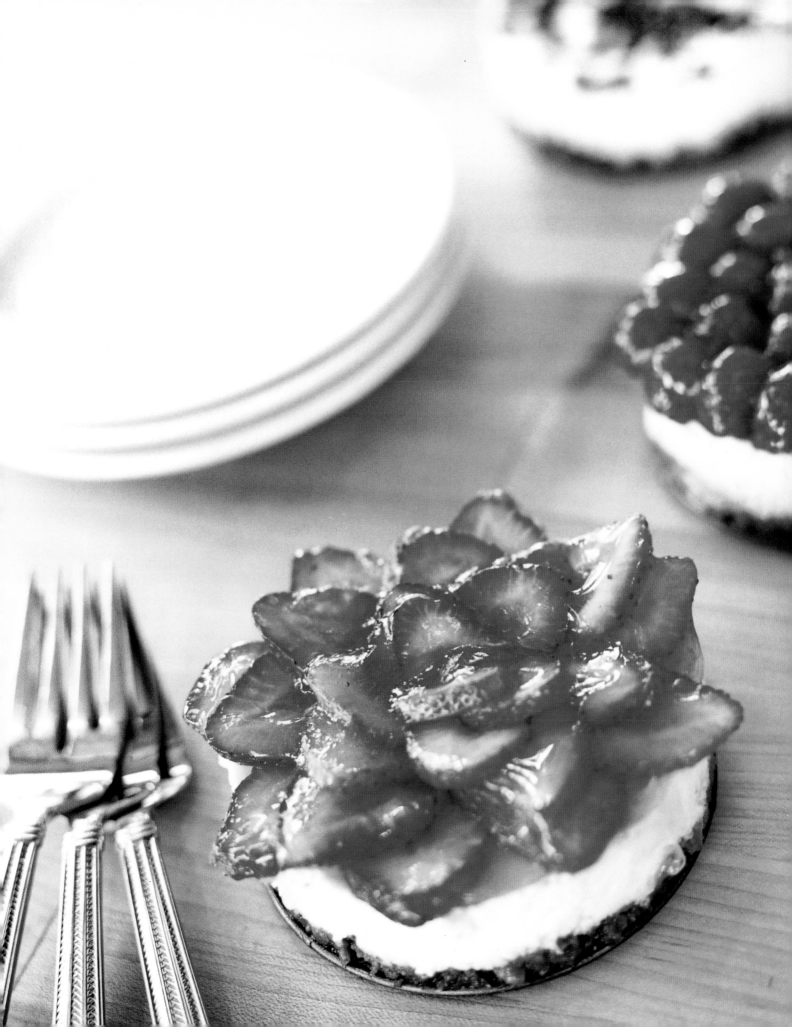

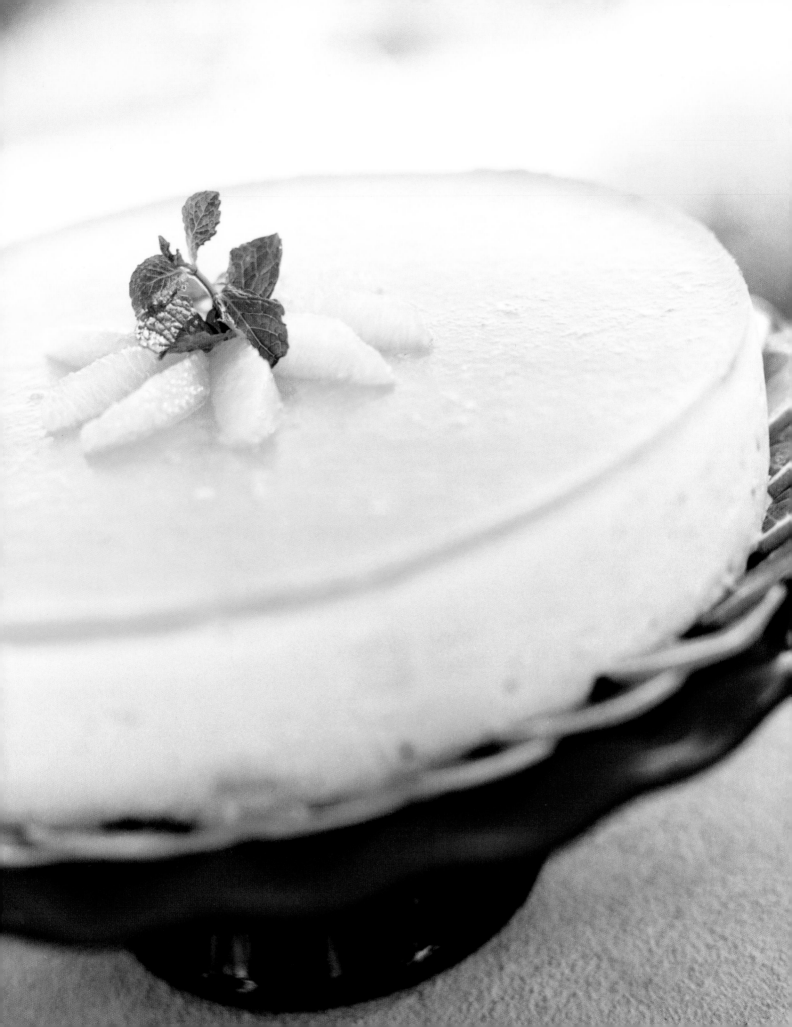

Tequila-Lime Cheesecake

This recipe utilizes the refrigerator method of preparing cheesecake. The combination of tequila and lime has soothed the raging heat of the Southwest for some time now and has inspired me to create this desert-cooling dessert.

Ingredients

Makes 16 servings.

Cheesecake

2 cups graham cracker crumbs
1/4 cup unsweetened applesauce
3 cups fat-free cottage cheese
1 1/2 cups reduced-fat cream cheese
   (12 ounces), softened
2 cups raw cane sugar (Turbinado)
1 teaspoon grated orange zest
1 teaspoon grated lemon zest
1 teaspoon grated lime zest
1/4 cup key lime juice
1 cup unsweetened orange juice
2 packages unflavored gelatin powder
   (2 tablespoons)
1 tablespoon tequila

Tequila-Lime Glaze

1/4 cup raw cane sugar (Turbinado)
1 teaspoon grated lime zest
1 teaspoon grated lemon zest
1/2 cup key lime juice
1/4 cup fresh lemon juice
1/2 cup unsweetened orange juice
1 package unflavored gelatin powder
   (1 tablespoon)
1/4 cup tequila

Preparation

For the Cheesecake: Combine the graham cracker crumbs and unsweetened applesauce in a small bowl. Press the crumbs into the bottom of a 10-inch springform pan; set aside.

Puree the cottage cheese in a food processor until smooth. Add the cream cheese, sugar, zests, and lime juice. Process until combined, about 2 minutes. The mixture should be light and fluffy. Pour the orange juice into a small saucepan and sprinkle the gelatin on top. Let stand for about 2 minutes. Stir over medium heat until the gelatin has dissolved completely, about 2 minutes. Stir in the tequila. Add softened gelatin to cream cheese mixture and mix well.

Pour the cream cheese mixture onto the prepared crust. Smooth out the top. Cover and refrigerate for 2 hours to allow the gelatin to set up.

For the Tequila-Lime Glaze: Combine all the ingredients in a small saucepan. Let stand for about 2 minutes. Stir over medium heat until the gelatin has dissolved completely, about 2 minutes. Remove from heat and let cool for about 30 minutes at room temperature so the glaze will not melt the cheesecake. Remove the cheesecake from the refrigerator and slowly pour the glaze over the top. Chill until the glaze is set, at least 4 hours.

Chocolate Taco with Fresh Fruit Salsa

Per taco with mousse and salsa:
Calories 110; Protein 3g; Total Fat 5g;
Saturated Fat 3g; Carbohydrates 14g; Dietary
Fiber 1g; Cholesterol 0mg; Sodium 15mg

Per taco with frozen yogurt and salsa:
Calories 60; Protein 2g; Total Fat 2g; Saturated
Fat 1g; Carbohydrates 11g; Dietary Fiber 0g;
Cholesterol 0mg; Sodium 15mg

Ingredients
Makes 8 tacos.

Taco Shells
*1/3 cup (2 ounces) semisweet chocolate
chips*
*1/2 teaspoon Wax Orchards Fruit Sweet
(see page 326) or corn syrup*

Fresh Fruit Salsa
Makes 2 1/2 cups.

8 medium strawberries, finely chopped
1/4 cup raspberries
1/4 cup blueberries
1 kiwifruit, peeled and finely chopped
1 tablespoon minced fresh mint
1 tablespoon minced fresh cilantro
2 tablespoons unsweetened orange juice

*1/2 recipe Berry Consommé (see
page 303), optional*
*1 cup White Chocolate Mousse (see
page 301) or 1 cup frozen, fat-free
yogurt of your choice*
1 cup Fresh Fruit Salsa

Garnish
8 strawberry fans
8 mint sprigs

This dessert was originally created in 1988 when I worked as chef de cuisine of the Arizona Kitchen at the Wigwam Resort. It instantly became a hit. The dessert was presented with a kaleidoscope of sweet sauces featuring ingredients indigenous to the Southwest.

This is my new version of the chocolate taco; I reduced the portion size, made the mousse more consciously, and highlighted the fruit salsa as an essential ingredient. Once again, it's a hit.

Preparation
To form the Taco Shells: Empty one shelf in your refrigerator or freezer. On the shelf, place two tin cans spaced out to support a long wooden spoon or dowel. Place the wooden spoon on the cans. This will be the mold that makes the taco shell.

Cut a circle 4 inches in diameter from a piece of thin cardboard. (The bottom of a 28-ounce can of tomatoes is the perfect size.) Draw a 3-inch circle within the first circle, (1/2 inch from the edge). Cut out the center circle to make a cardboard frame to form your taco shell. (You can also cut the center out of a plastic lid.)

Place the chocolate chips in a small stainless steel bowl or the top of a double boiler. Place the bowl over a pan of simmering water. Stir until the chips are just beginning to melt, remove from the heat, and continue stirring until the chips are completely melted. Add the Fruit Sweet and stir until just combined. Do not overmix.

Cut a piece of waxed paper about 6 inches square and place it on a baking sheet. Place the cardboard circle on the waxed paper. Spoon 2 tablespoons of chocolate into the center of the circle. Use a rubber spatula to spread the chocolate to fill the circle. Remove the cardboard. Drape the chocolate circle and waxed paper over the set-up wooden spoon with the waxed paper side down. You may need to hold the paper together for a few minutes while the chocolate sets up. (If you have room in your refrigerator or freezer, make 3 chocolate shells at a time.)

Allow the chocolate shell to set about 10 minutes. You can then place the shell on a baking sheet and place in the freezer. Repeat the process until you have 8 shells. Keep the shells in the freezer until ready to fill and serve.

For Fruit Salsa: Combine all the ingredients in a small bowl. Cover and store in the refrigerator for up to 2 days.

To serve: Spread 1/4 cup of the Berry Consommé, if using, on a dessert plate. Place a chocolate shell on the plate. Spoon, or use a pastry bag to pipe, 2 tablespoons of the mousse into the shell. Spoon 2 tablespoons of the salsa on the edge of each taco. Garnish with a strawberry fan and a mint sprig. Repeat with the remaining shells, mousse, and salsa. Serve immediately.

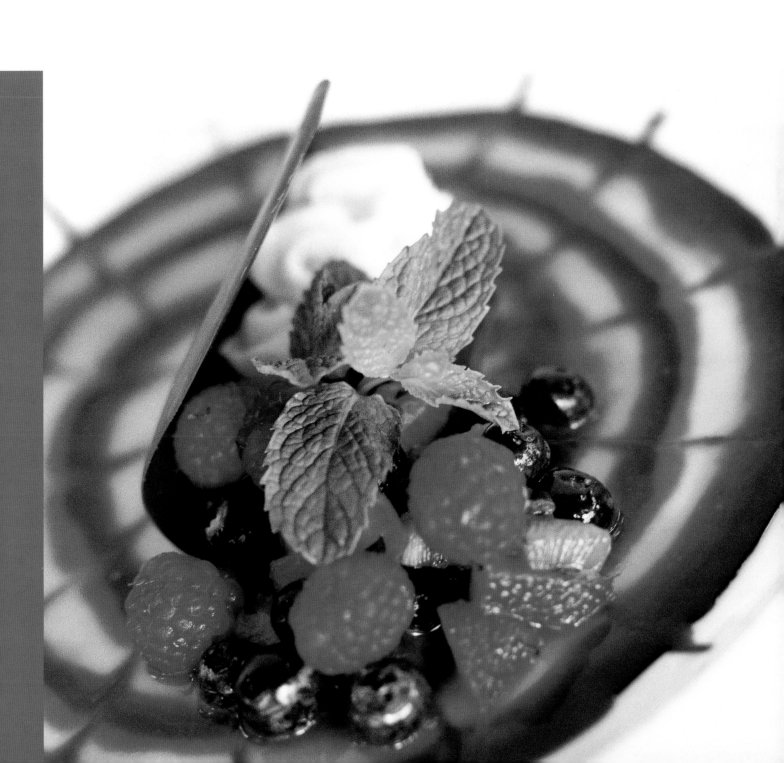

Strawberry-White Chocolate Mousse

Conscious Cuisine encourages us to use fresh fruits when they are in season and vibrantly sweet and luscious. This recipe relies heavily on the use of fresh strawberries captured at the peak of the summer season. You can preserve these summer jewels in your freezer and combine them with creamy white chocolate for a sweet taste of the summer all year long. Use this mousse with fruit to make a beautiful parfait, or as a light and delicious filling for cakes or tarts.

Ingredients

Makes 2 1/2 cups.

1 cup white chocolate chips
2/3 cup plain or vanilla fat-free yogurt,
    excess liquid drained off
1/2 teaspoon pure vanilla extract
1/4 cup raw cane sugar (Turbinado)
1/3 cup pureed strawberries (about
    7 medium pureed in a blender)
1/2 cup fat-free milk
1 package unflavored gelatin powder
    (1 tablespoon)
1/2 cup pasteurized large egg whites
    (available in the dairy or freezer section
    of the grocery store)
1/2 teaspoon cream of tartar

Preparation

Place the white chocolate in the top of a double boiler or stainless steel bowl. Place over simmering water and heat until the chocolate has just melted. Set aside.

In a small bowl, whisk together the yogurt, vanilla, sugar, and strawberry puree. Pour the milk into a small saucepan and sprinkle the gelatin on top. Let stand for about 2 minutes. Stir over medium heat until the gelatin has dissolved completely, about 2 minutes.

Whisk the melted white chocolate and yogurt mixture together. Stir in the milk mixture and set aside.

Combine the egg whites and cream of tartar in a bowl. Beat with an electric mixer on high speed until stiff peaks form, about 2 minutes. Fold the whipped egg whites into the chocolate-yogurt mixture. Chill for at least 1 hour prior to serving to allow the gelatin to set up.

White Chocolate Mousse

Forget the zabaglione and whipped cream—this white chocolate mousse tastes as good or better than others made with high-fat ingredients. You can really taste the chocolate, and that's what it's all about.

Ingredients

Makes 2 1/4 cups.

1 cup white chocolate chips or chunks
1/2 cup plain or vanilla fat-free yogurt,
    excess liquid drained off
1/2 cup low-fat buttermilk
1/2 teaspoon pure vanilla extract
1/2 cup raw cane sugar (Turbinado),
    divided
1/4 cup fat-free milk
1 package unflavored gelatin powder
    (1 tablespoon)
1/2 cup pasteurized large egg whites
    (available in the dairy or freezer section
    of the grocery store)
1/2 teaspoon cream of tartar

Preparation

Place the chocolate in a small stainless steel bowl or the top of a double boiler. Place the bowl over simmering water. Stir until the chocolate is just beginning to melt, remove from the heat, and continue stirring until the chocolate is completely melted. Set aside.

In a mixing bowl, whisk together the yogurt, buttermilk, vanilla, and 1/4 cup of the sugar. Set aside.

Pour the milk into a small saucepan and sprinkle the gelatin on top. Let stand for about 2 minutes. Stir over medium heat until the gelatin has dissolved completely, about 2 minutes.

Stir the melted chocolate into the yogurt mixture. Stir in the milk mixture and set aside.

Place the egg whites and cream of tartar in a mixing bowl and beat with an electric mixer on high speed until medium peaks form. Add the remaining 1/4 cup sugar and beat until stiff peaks form. Fold the beaten egg whites into the chocolate-yogurt mixture.

Cover and chill to allow the gelatin to set up, at least 1 hour.

Vanilla Bean Tapioca

Per 1/2 cup of tapioca:
Calories 110; Protein 5g; Total Fat 0.5g;
Saturated Fat 0g; Carbohydrates 20g; Dietary
Fiber 0g; Cholesterol 30mg; Sodium 75mg

Per 1/2 cup of tapioca with 1/4 cup compote:
Calories 150; Protein 6g; Total Fat 1g;
Saturated Fat 0g; Carbohydrates 30g; Dietary
Fiber 1g; Cholesterol 30mg; Sodium 75mg

Ingredients
Makes 8 servings.

1/2 cup plus 2 tablespoons medium pearl
    tapioca
1/2 cup cold water
1/2 vanilla bean, split in half lengthwise
1 cinnamon stick
4 cups fat-free milk
1/3 cup raw cane sugar (Turbinado) or
    granulated sugar
1 large egg
2 cups Tropical Fruit Compote (see
    page 282), optional

While searching for dessert ideas for guests who are wheat (gluten) intolerant, I remembered using tapioca in school as a thickening agent, as well as for tapioca pudding. Tapioca is available in a flour form, but I prefer the tiny white pearls. When cooked with vanilla beans, milk, and sugar, it has the consistency and flavor of custard with attractive little pearls throughout. I often serve a timbale of tapioca with the Tropical Fruit Compote. The mango puree, star anise, pineapple, and bananas make this dessert sensation a culinary excursion to the tropics—not only for those searching for a wheat-free alternative.

Preparation
In the top of a double boiler or in a stainless steel mixing bowl, soak the tapioca pearls in the cold water until the tapioca soaks up the all of the water, about 10 minutes.

Scrape the seeds from the vanilla bean pod. Stir the vanilla bean pod and seeds, cinnamon stick, 3 1/2 cups of the milk, and sugar into the tapioca. Place the mixture over slowly boiling water. Reduce the heat to medium and cook, stirring constantly, about 10 minutes.

In a mixing bowl, whisk the egg with the remaining 1/2 cup of milk. Whisk 1 cup of the hot tapioca mixture into the beaten egg. Slowly whisk the egg mixture back into the remaining hot tapioca. Cook, stirring constantly, until the tapioca pearls are clear, about 15 minutes. Remove the vanilla bean pod.

Remove from the heat and transfer the tapioca to a shallow dish. Cover with plastic wrap directly on the pudding's surface and chill. The pudding will keep for up to 5 days in an airtight container in the refrigerator.

To serve, spoon 2 tablespoons of Tropical Fruit Compote into each of eight glass dessert dishes, add 1/2 cup tapioca, and top with 2 more tablespoons of compote.

Berry Consommé

This wonderfully refreshing berry consommé serves brilliantly as a compliment for the Chilled Chocolate Soufflé on page 304.

Ingredients

Makes 4 cups.

1 pint fresh or frozen raspberries
1 quart fresh or frozen strawberries
1 pint fresh or frozen blackberries
2 cups water
1/2 cup Wax Orchards Fruit Sweet (see page 326) or corn syrup
3 tablespoons cherry brandy

Preparation

Combine the berries and water in a medium saucepan. Bring to a boil, reduce heat, and simmer for 10 minutes. Strain the mixture through a fine mesh strainer or a colander lined with cheesecloth. Reserve the berries for other desserts, if desired.

Stir in the fruit syrup and brandy. Cover and chill before serving.

Chilled Chocolate Soufflé with Berry Consommé

There are two basic types of soufflés: savory soufflés, which are served as an appetizer or entrée, and sweet soufflés, which are served as desserts. This sweet, frozen soufflé offers an elegant finish to a meal. This chocolate soufflé is elevated to new heights of complex flavor by serving with the Berry Consommé. A traditional chilled soufflé has about 460 calories and 35 grams of fat per serving, compared with our lighter version at 230 calories and 10 grams of fat.

Ingredients
Makes 6 servings.

Chocolate Soufflé
3/4 cup semisweet chocolate chips or chunks
1/4 cup water
1 1/2 teaspoons unflavored gelatin powder
1/2 cup plain, fat-free yogurt, excess liquid drained off
5 large egg whites
1/2 teaspoon cream of tartar
1/4 cup raw cane sugar (Turbinado)

Glaze
3/4 cup semisweet chocolate chips or chunks

1/2 recipe Berry Consommé (see page 303)

Garnish
Fresh berries
Mint sprigs

Preparation

For the Chocolate Soufflé: Place the chocolate in a small stainless steel bowl or the top of a double boiler. Place the bowl over simmering water. Stir until the chocolate is just beginning to melt, remove from the heat, and continue stirring until the chocolate is completely melted. Set aside.

Pour the water into a small saucepan and sprinkle the gelatin on top. Let stand for about 2 minutes. Stir over medium heat until the gelatin has dissolved completely, about 2 minutes. Stir the dissolved gelatin into the chocolate mixture. Mix the yogurt into the chocolate mixture.

Using an electric mixer, beat the egg whites and cream of tartar on high speed until soft peaks form. Gradually add the sugar and beat until medium peaks form. Fold the beaten egg whites into the chocolate mixture.

Place six 1/2-cup aluminum molds (or pieces of 2-inch PVC pipe cut into 2 1/2-inch lengths) on a baking sheet lined with parchment paper. Spray the molds with cooking spray. Ladle the chocolate mixture into the molds and level off the tops. Place in the freezer overnight.

For the Glaze: Place the chocolate in a small, stainless steel bowl or the top of a double boiler. Place the bowl over simmering water. Stir until the chocolate is just beginning to melt, remove from the heat, and continue stirring until the chocolate is completely melted.

Remove the soufflés from the freezer and run a knife around the inside edges of the molds. Carefully push the soufflés out of the molds. Use a spatula to place them on a baking rack set over a baking sheet.

Carefully pour enough chocolate glaze over each soufflé to cover. You can scoop the chocolate off the baking sheet and reheat if you need additional chocolate to coat all the soufflés. Return the soufflés to the refrigerator to set.

To serve: Spoon 1/3 cup of the Berry Consommé into each individual dessert dish. Add a soufflé and garnish with berries and mint sprigs.

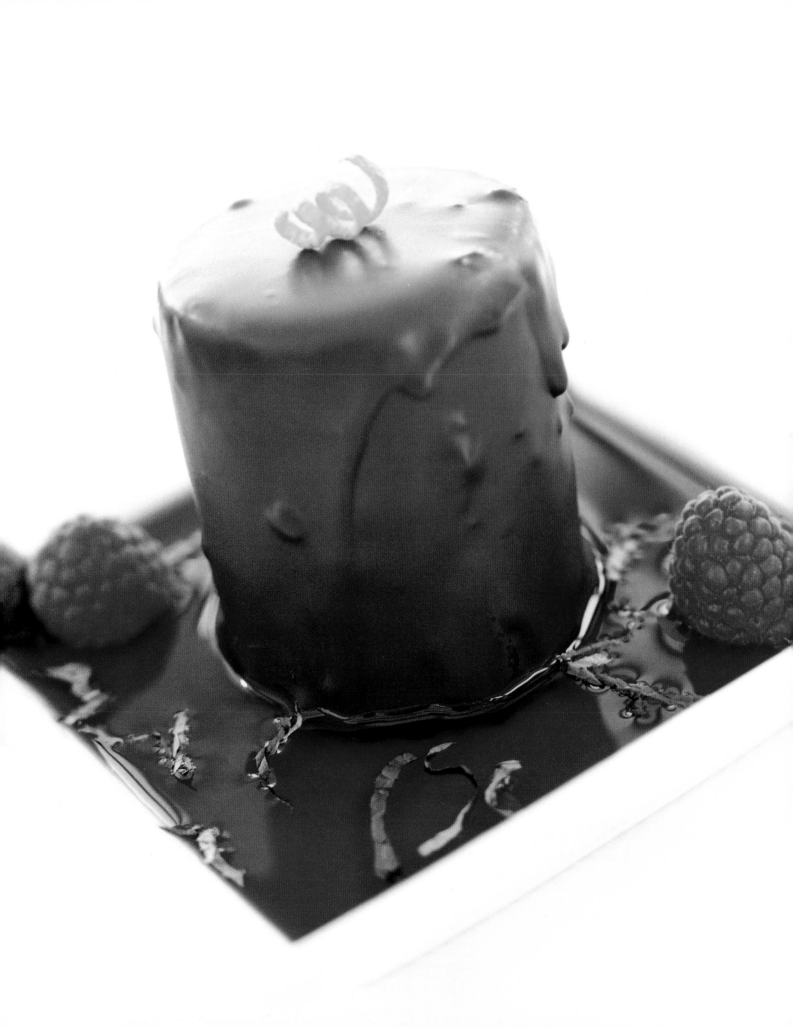

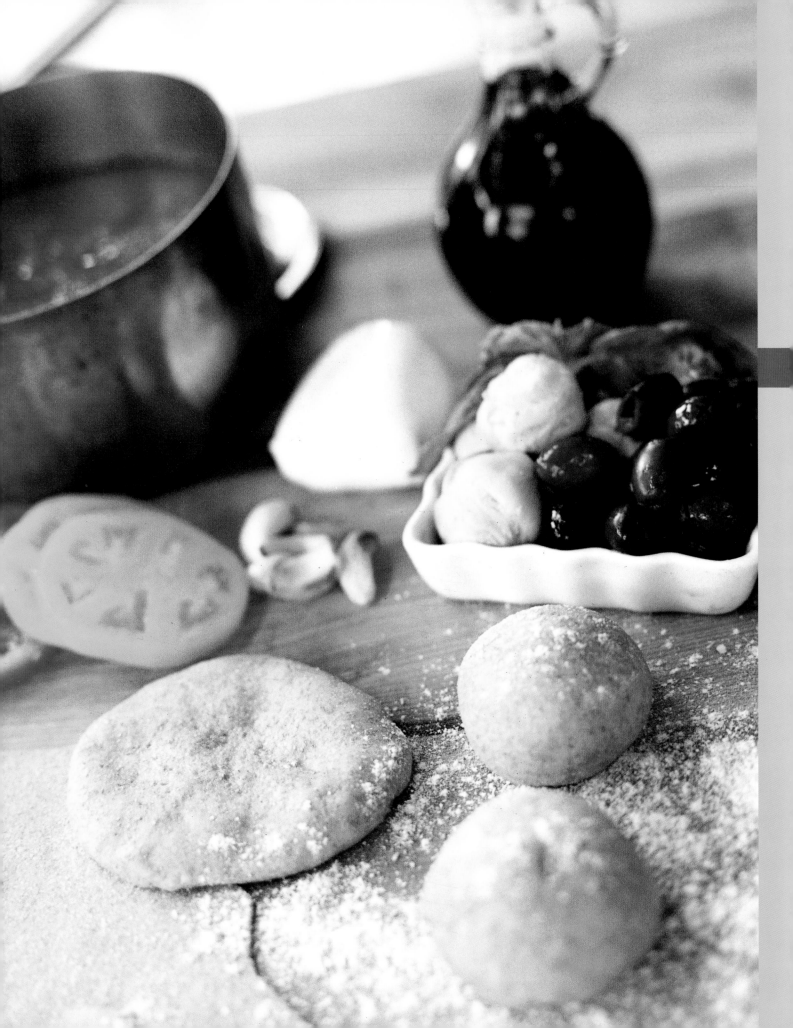

Miraval Favorites

Pictured at left: Flatbreads with Assorted Toppings

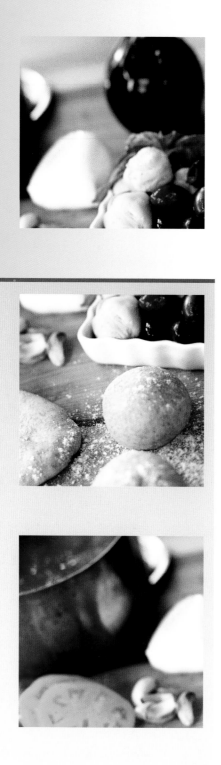

I had the good fortune to work at Miraval Life in Balance Resort and Spa for eight years. There I learned the underlying theme of mindfulness and the daily challenge of creating an oasis of well-being. It took me some time to understand and to fully embrace the idea of living in the moment. The premise of living in the moment grows on you, and you never want to let it go.

As a chef, I had trained my body and mind to work constantly, often never stopping to look at or appreciate what I had achieved. Twelve- to fourteen-hour days, six days a week, were common. Squeezing in moments with my family and friends whenever possible was the best that I could do, leaving very little time for myself. This was the lifestyle of my mentors, and I convinced myself that this was the only acceptable lifestyle for a master chef. Then my father passed away and so did my best friend, Bob Allen. What I saw and appreciated about both men was their earnest work efforts and dedication to their families.

Fortunately for me when I was grieving, I had a place to go within the grounds of Miraval—a most peaceful and spiritual place called the labyrinth. The labyrinth is a rock formation of concentric circles designed by the Tohono O'odham tribe located near the burial grounds of the Hohokam Indians and nestled on a picturesque peak of the Santa Catalina Mountains. A walk through the labyrinth is meditative and calming. There I found an overwhelming sense of thankfulness for the undeniable natural beauty around me and for the Creator of this beauty. This is where I found meaning in the life and death of my father and good friend. The labyrinth at Miraval is also where I found a renewed direction and purpose in my life. I'm no longer a slave to my career, but I'm experiencing greater joy in my efforts with continued success. I'm now more deliberate in my time spent with family, friends, and myself. In short, the ancient labyrinth helped me find myself.

Miraval's goal is to create an environment where guests can not only experience this oasis of well-being, but also take it home with them. The hope is that their visit to Miraval will be for them the beginning of a new, conscious way of life.

For this reason, unlike other spas, food is available at Miraval throughout the day and most of the night. The thought is to help teach guests how to make responsible and conscious choices when it comes to food, rather than build a false sense of reality where there are no tempting goodies. This chapter includes some of guests' favorite recipes that I created for Miraval. One of the most popular items by far the cookies served in the Palm Court Juice Bar, an example of nutritious foods that can be eaten on the run for those who insist that they are too busy to eat.

This chapter also includes recipes for vegetable spreads for bread that are ideal alternatives to butter or olive oil and have a multitude of other uses such as vegetable dips, flatbread toppings, and vegetarian fillings. There are about twenty different vegetable spreads to enhance the dining experience at Miraval, and guests love them. In addition, here are a few of Miraval's guests' favorite fruit preserves, compotes, and conserves.

Whole-Wheat Honey Flat Bread or Pizza Crusts

Flatbreads are extremely thin leavened or unleavened breads. I created this recipe for the wood-burning hearth oven at Miraval. Pizzas are typically a good source of nutrition because, between the toppings and the crust, each of the four food groups is represented. What can make pizza less good for you is over-indulgence in America's slice of Italy. At Miraval, we roll 2 ounces of this flavorful dough into an ultra-thin, 9-inch individual serving. We consciously choose less-processed grains to increase the dough's nutritional value. Photo on page 306.

Ingredients

Makes 12 servings.

1 cup warm water
1 tablespoon active, dry yeast
1/4 cup honey
2 tablespoons extra-virgin olive oil
2 cups whole-wheat flour
1 1/2 cups semolina flour
1 teaspoon sea salt
Suggested toppings: Marinara Sauce (see page 33), reduced-fat cream cheese, Basil Pesto (see page 37), vegetable spreads (pages 310–311), cheese, cooked vegetables, seafood, poultry, or baked tofu

Preparation

Use an electric mixer with a dough hook to mix the dough. Stir together the warm water, yeast, honey, and olive oil. Let the mixture stand until frothy, about 10 minutes. In another bowl, combine the flours and salt. With the mixer on low, slowly add the flours to the yeast mixture. Increase the speed to medium-high and mix until the dough is smooth and elastic, about 2 minutes.

Lightly oil a medium bowl. Add the dough and turn to coat lightly with oil. Cover the bowl with plastic wrap and allow to rise at warm room temperature (about 75°F, 25°C) until doubled, about 1 hour.

Preheat the oven to 400°F (205°C).

Punch down the dough and divide into 12 equal-size balls. Dust a cutting board with flour and roll out each ball to 1/4-inch thickness.

Add the topping of your choice. Bake for 5 to 7 minutes or until the pizzas are lightly browned, the cheese has melted, and the dough is crispy.

Artichoke Spread

Per 2 tablespoons:
Calories 20; Protein 1g; Total Fat 0g; Saturated Fat 0g; Carbohydrates 4g; Dietary Fiber 1g; Cholesterol 0mg; Sodium 220mg

To make this spread even better, season with truffle oil instead of the olive oil, and add a little chopped truffle. Truffle oil is available in most specialty food stores.

Ingredients
Makes 3 cups.

2 14-ounce jars water-packed artichoke
 hearts
1 1/2 teaspoons minced Roasted Garlic
 (see page 38)
1 teaspoon minced fresh garlic
1 tablespoon chopped fresh parsley
1 teaspoon chopped fresh oregano
1 teaspoon extra-virgin olive oil
1/4 teaspoon sea salt
1/8 teaspoon freshly ground black pepper

Preparation
Place all the ingredients into a food processor and process until smooth. The spread will keep for up to 1 week in an airtight container in the refrigerator.

Roasted Eggplant Spread

Per 2 tablespoons:
Calories 20; Protein 1g; Total Fat 0g; Saturated Fat 0g; Carbohydrates 4g; Dietary Fiber 1g; Cholesterol 0mg; Sodium 120mg

Filled with sunny Mediterranean flavors, this is awesome on crackers or as a topping for flatbreads or pizza. Photo on page 311.

Ingredients
Makes 2 1/2 cups.

2 large eggplants, peeled and chopped
 into 1-inch cubes
1 teaspoon sea salt
1/2 teaspoon freshly ground black pepper
1 teaspoon minced garlic
2 tablespoon fresh lemon juice
1 teaspoon extra-virgin olive oil
1/2 teaspoon cumin
1/2 teaspoon chopped fresh cilantro
2 tablespoons chopped green onions
1 cup Vegetable Stock (see page 152)

Preparation
Preheat the oven to 400°F (205°C). Place the eggplant on a baking sheet and spray with cooking spray. Sprinkle with 1/2 teaspoon of the salt. Bake for 20 to 25 minutes or until the eggplants are lightly browned and softened.

Combine the eggplant with the remaining ingredients in a food processor and process until smooth. The spread will keep for up to 1 week in an airtight container in the refrigerator.

Spinach, White Bean, and Tofu Spread

Per 2 tablespoons:
Calories 25; Protein 2g; Total Fat 0g; Saturated Fat 0g; Carbohydrates 4g; Dietary Fiber 1g; Cholesterol 0mg; Sodium 65mg

This spread serves as a wonderful dip for vegetable crudités, as well as a flavorful filling in the baked Vegetable Casserole (see page 264). You can substitute red beans or kidney beans for the white beans.

Ingredients
Makes 3 cups.

1 3/4 cups canned or cooked white beans (14-ounce can), drained

12.3-ounce package Mori-Nu extra-firm silken tofu

1/2 teaspoon minced garlic

1 cup packed fresh spinach

2 tablespoons seasoned rice wine vinegar

1/4 teaspoon sea salt

1/8 teaspoon freshly ground black pepper

Preparation

Combine all the ingredients in a food processor and process until smooth. The spread will keep for up to 1 week in an airtight container in the refrigerator.

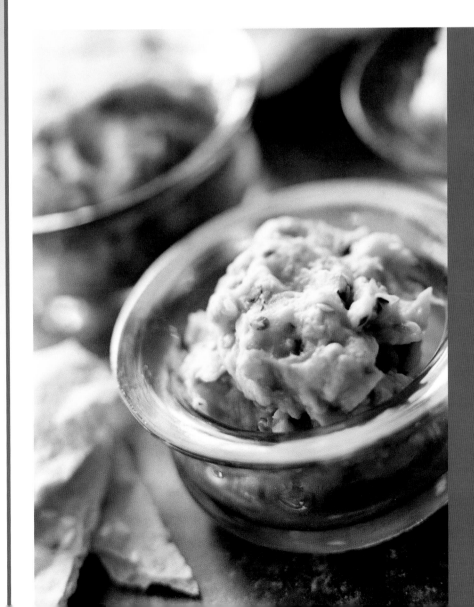

Pictured at right: (left to right) Spinach, White Bean, and Tofu Spread and Roasted Eggplant Spread

Hummus

Per 2 tablespoons:
Calories 50; Protein 2g; Total Fat 1.5g;
Saturated Fat 0g; Carbohydrates 7g; Dietary
Fiber 2g; Cholesterol 0mg; Sodium 60mg

This chickpea and sesame dip is a staple in Middle Eastern cuisine. It makes a great high-protein snack served with whole-grain crackers.

Ingredients
Makes 2 1/2 cups.

3 cups canned or cooked chickpeas
    (2 15-ounce cans), drained, liquid
    reserved
4 small garlic cloves, peeled
1/4 cup fresh lemon juice
2 teaspoons tahini (sesame seed paste)
1 teaspoon cumin
1/2 teaspoon sea salt
1/2 cup water or the reserved liquid from
    the chickpeas
2 1/2 teaspoons extra-virgin olive oil

Garnish
Paprika

Preparation
Place the chickpeas, garlic, lemon juice, tahini, cumin, and salt in the bowl of a food processor. Process until the beans start to break up, about 1 minute. Add the water and olive oil. Process until smooth and creamy, scraping down the sides to ensure that all the beans are pureed.

Transfer to a bowl, cover, and chill for 30 minutes before serving. The spread will keep for up to 1 week in an airtight container in the refrigerator.

Garnish with a sprinkle of paprika for extra flavor and color.

Variation
For a richer flavor and aroma, toast some whole cumin seeds in a dry sauté pan until browned and fragrant, about 1 minute. Cool and grind in a spice grinder. Use to season the hummus instead of preground cumin.

Fig-Apricot Conserve

Per 2 tablespoons:
Calories 50; Protein 1g; Total Fat 0g; Saturated Fat 0g; Carbohydrates 13g; Dietary Fiber 2g; Cholesterol 0mg; Sodium 0mg

Fresh figs are a real treat, but when they are not in season, I use dried figs. This recipe, created to accompany breakfast breads, is also wonderful with desserts or aged cheeses.

Ingredients
Makes 4 cups.

2 cups dried figs, cut in half
1 cup dried apricots, cut into quarters
1/2 teaspoon cinnamon
1/8 teaspoon nutmeg
1/4 teaspoon cardamom
2 1/2 cups unsweetened orange juice

Preparation

Combine all the ingredients in a small saucepan and bring to a boil over medium-high heat. Reduce heat to low and simmer, stirring occasionally, until the fruit has become soft and the mixture is thick and homogenous, about 20 minutes.

Pour into sterilized jars and seal. The conserve will keep for up to 2 weeks in the refrigerator. If you wish to keep it longer, be sure to follow standard canning instructions to prevent the growth of bacteria.

Peach Butter

If you are fortunate enough to enjoy fresh, ripe, organic peaches during the summer, I'm sure you will agree that it's hard to describe the outrageously sweet and juicy taste of the summer's best. This is a way to enjoy the pleasure of summer a little bit longer.

Ingredients
Makes 1 1/2 cups.

1/2 vanilla bean, split in half lengthwise
4 cups (20 ounces) fresh or frozen, sliced, peeled peaches
2 cinnamon sticks
1 tablespoon honey
1/4 cup unsweetened orange juice

Preparation

Scrape the seeds from the vanilla bean pod. In a medium saucepan, combine the vanilla bean pod and seeds with the remaining ingredients. Bring to a boil over medium-high heat. Reduce the heat and simmer, stirring occasionally, until the fruit has become very soft and the mixture is thick and homogenous, about 40 minutes. (It should be the consistency of apple butter.) Discard the cinnamon sticks and vanilla bean.

Pour into sterilized jars and seal. The peach butter will keep for up to 2 weeks in the refrigerator. If you wish to keep it longer, be sure to follow standard canning instructions to prevent the growth of bacteria.

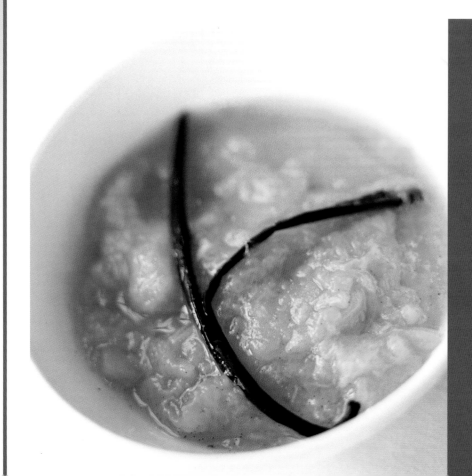

Apple-Cranberry Compote

Per 2 tablespoons:
Calories 25; Protein 0g; Total Fat 0g; Saturated
Fat 0g; Carbohydrates 7g; Dietary Fiber 0g;
Cholesterol 0mg; Sodium 0mg

The combination of tart Granny Smith apples and sweet dried cranberries forms a successful marriage of flavors and colors. This compote makes a fragrant and delicious treat served on waffles or pancakes.

Ingredients
Makes 9 cups.

1/2 cup honey
1 tablespoon minced fresh ginger
3 pounds chopped, peeled Granny Smith
    apples (about 12)
3 cups unsweetened apple juice or apple
    cider
2 tablespoons grated orange zest
1 cup fresh orange juice
1 teaspoon grated lime zest
1 teaspoon fresh lime juice
1 cup dried cranberries
1/2 teaspoon allspice
2 cinnamon sticks

Preparation

In a noncorrosive or stainless steel saucepan, simmer the honey and ginger together for 2 or 3 minutes. Add the apples and stir to coat with the honey mixture. Add the remaining ingredients and bring to a boil. Reduce the heat and simmer uncovered until the mixture is thick, with most of its liquid reduced down to a syrup, about 45 minutes. Stir occasionally to prevent scorching.

Cool, and discard the cinnamon sticks. The compote will keep for up to 1 week in an airtight container in the refrigerator.

Citrus Prunes

Per 2 tablespoons:
Calories 35; Protein 0g; Total Fat 0g; Saturated
Fat 0g; Carbohydrates 9g; Dietary Fiber 1g;
Cholesterol 0mg; Sodium 0mg

After years of being called "prunes," these dried fruits are now "dried plums" in an image remake. This recipe has been a favorite since the first day I served it.

Ingredients
Makes 3 cups.

1/2 vanilla bean, split in half lengthwise
30-ounce can (3 cups) pitted prunes in
    liquid
1 tablespoon grated orange zest
1 cup unsweetened orange juice
2 cinnamon sticks
1/4 teaspoon grated fresh ginger

Preparation

Scrape the seeds from the vanilla bean pod. In a medium saucepan, combine the seeds with the remaining ingredients. (The remaining pod can be put to another use such as flavoring vanilla sugar, see page xix.) Bring to a boil over medium-high heat. Reduce the heat and simmer, stirring occasionally, until the fruit has become soft and the mixture has thickened. Serve warm or chilled.

The prunes will keep for up to 1 week in an airtight container in the refrigerator.

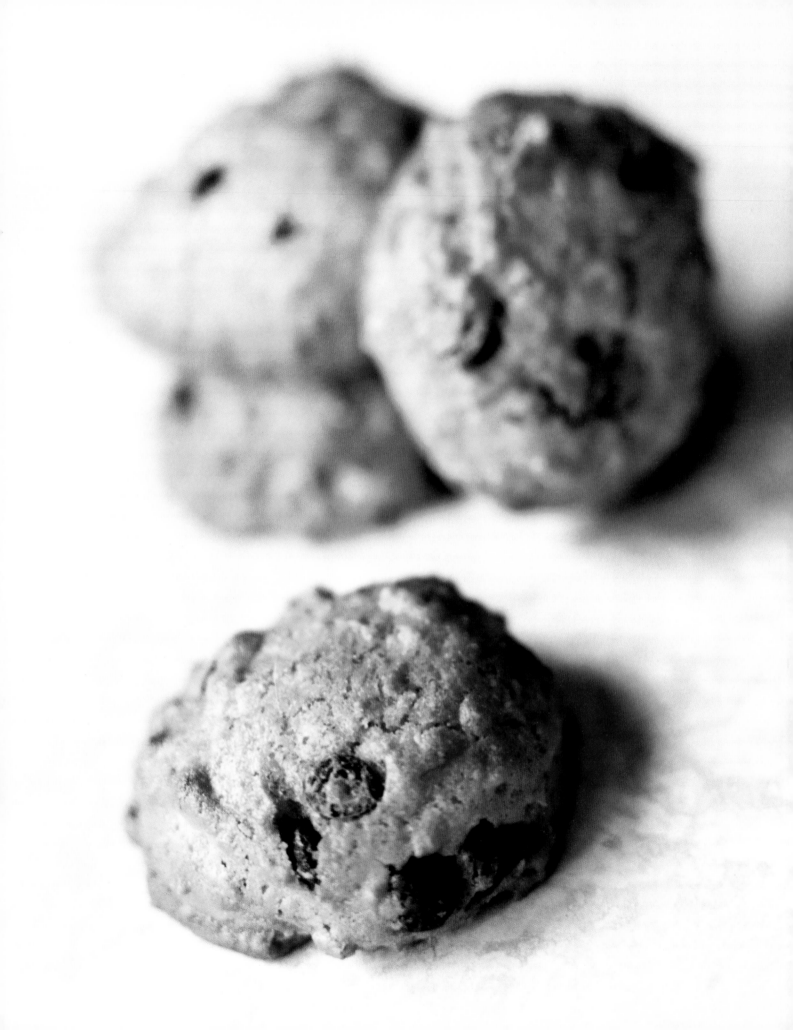

Banana-Chocolate Chip Cookies

When your bananas begin to darken, do not discard them—peel them, seal them in a plastic bag, and freeze them. The riper or darker a banana gets, the sweeter it becomes. The use of very ripe bananas in this recipe helps reduce the amount of sugar needed, and provides extra body that reduces the amount of butter or oil that's normally needed. Chocolate chips and bananas make a wonderful flavor combination that's good any time of the day.

Ingredients

Makes 8 dozen.

1/2 cup butter, softened
1/2 cup prune puree
   or unsweetened applesauce
1 cup raw cane sugar (Turbinado)
3 ripe medium bananas, mashed
2 large eggs
1 teaspoon pure vanilla extract
2 1/2 cups unbleached all-purpose flour
1 1/2 teaspoons baking soda
2 cups quick-cooking oats
1 cup semisweet chocolate chips

Preparation

Preheat the oven to 350°F (175°C). Coat 2 baking sheets with cooking spray and set aside.

In a mixing bowl, combine the butter and prune puree and beat with an electric mixer until creamy. Add the sugar, bananas, eggs, and vanilla. Beat until smooth. Gradually add the flour and baking soda. Stir in the oats and chocolate chips until incorporated.

Drop the dough by teaspoons onto the prepared baking sheets. Bake for 7 to 10 minutes or until golden brown. Transfer to a wire rack to cool.

Ginger Spice Cookies

These flavorful little gems have been a staple at Miraval since its first week of operation. The recipe has evolved to include less-processed flour and sugar. The wonderful flavor has remained the same.

Ingredients
Makes 65 cookies.

3/4 cup butter, softened
1/2 cups prune puree or unsweetened applesauce
1/2 cup pumpkin puree
1 cup molasses
1/4 cup egg whites (about 4 large egg whites)
1 1/2 cups unbleached all-purpose flour
1 cup whole-wheat pastry flour
1 teaspoon baking soda
1 1/4 teaspoon ginger
1 teaspoon cinnamon
1/2 teaspoon cloves
1/2 teaspoon nutmeg

Preparation
Preheat the oven to 350°F (175°C). Coat 2 baking sheets with cooking spray and set aside.

In a mixing bowl, beat the butter with an electric mixer until soft and creamy. Add the prune and pumpkin purees and mix well. Add the molasses and egg whites and beat until creamy.

In a separate mixing bowl, combine the flours, baking soda, ginger, cinnamon, cloves, and nutmeg. Stir the dry ingredients into the wet mixture until well combined.

Drop the dough by heaping teaspoons onto the prepared baking sheets. Bake for 12 to 15 minutes or until lightly browned. Transfer to a wire rack to cool.

Lemon-Raspberry Cookies

I'm the original cookie monster—a good cookie has always been my favorite choice for snack food. This is my favorite. The subtle flavors of lemon, raspberry, and, of course, white chocolate, make this cookie sensational.

Ingredients

Makes 5 dozen cookies.

3/4 cup butter, softened
1 cup raw cane sugar (Turbinado)
1 large egg
3 large egg whites
1/4 cup fresh lemon juice
1 teaspoon grated lemon zest
3 1/2 cups unbleached all-purpose flour
2 1/2 teaspoons baking soda
1/3 cup white chocolate chips
1/2 cup fresh raspberries

Preparation

Preheat the oven to 350°F (175°C). Coat 2 baking sheets with cooking spray and set aside.

In a mixing bowl, beat the butter and sugar with an electric mixer until creamy. Add the egg and egg whites and beat to incorporate. Mix in the lemon juice and zest.

In a separate mixing bowl, combine the flour and baking soda. Mix the dry ingredients into the butter mixture. Stir in the white chocolate chips and gently fold in the raspberries. Do not overmix or the raspberries will break up into small pieces.

Drop the dough by heaping teaspoons onto the prepared baking sheets. Bake for 7 to 10 minutes, or until lightly brown. Transfer to a wire rack to cool.

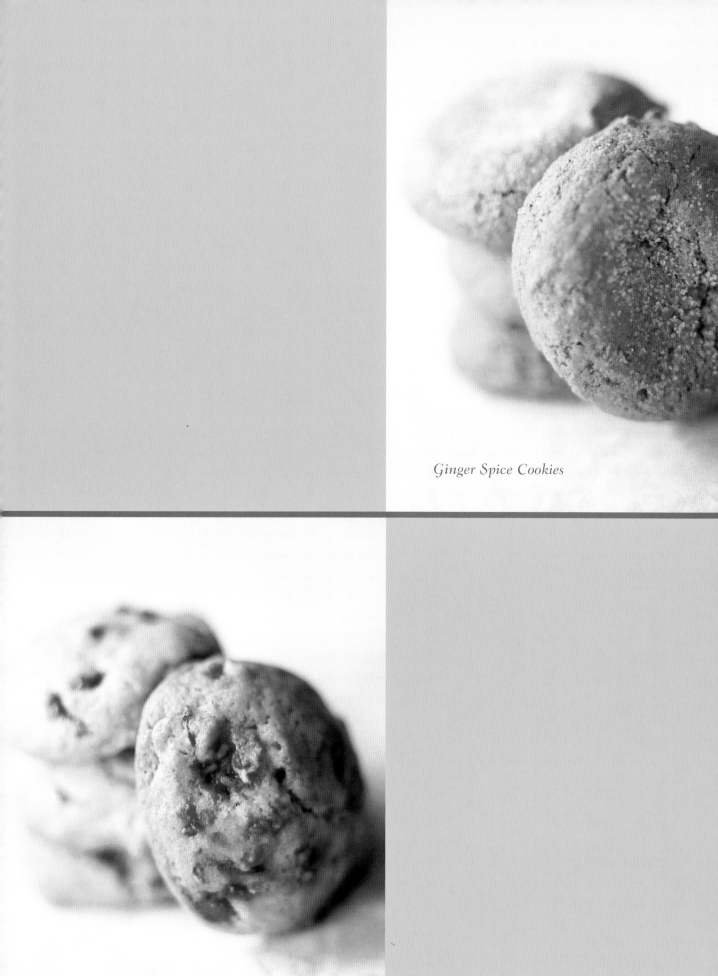

Ginger Spice Cookies

Lemon-Raspberry Cookies

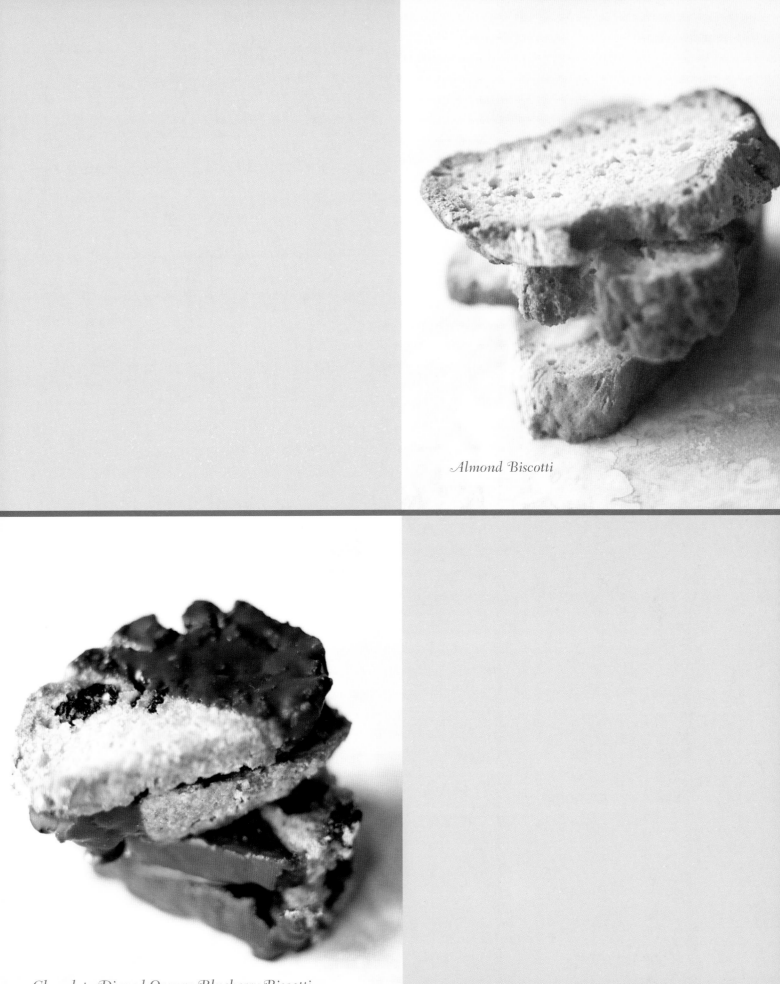

Almond Biscotti

Chocolate-Dipped Orange-Blueberry Biscotti

Almond Biscotti

Per 1 biscotti:
Calories 45; Protein 2g; Total Fat 1g; Saturated Fat 0g; Carbohydrates 7g; Dietary Fiber 0g; Cholesterol 0mg; Sodium 35mg

New to the basket of goodies offered at Miraval are these crisp biscotti, just begging to be dunked.

Ingredients

Makes 2 dozen biscotti.

1 cup unbleached all-purpose flour
1 teaspoon baking powder
1/3 cup raw cane sugar (Turbinado)
1/2 cup plain, dry bread crumbs
1/3 cup whole almonds, with skins
1/2 teaspoon pure vanilla extract
1/2 teaspoon pure almond extract
1 tablespoon unsweetened apple juice
2 large egg whites
1 large egg white, lightly beaten, for topping
1 teaspoon raw cane sugar (Turbinado), for topping

Preparation

Preheat the oven to 350°F (175°C). Coat a baking sheet with cooking spray and set aside.

In a mixing bowl, sift the flour with the baking powder. Add the sugar and bread crumbs and mix well. Stir in the nuts.

In a separate mixing bowl, whisk together the extracts, apple juice, and egg whites. Add the juice mixture to the dry ingredients and mix until combined, about 1 minute.

On a lightly floured board, shape the dough into a long, flat loaf about 2 inches wide and 12 inches long. Place the loaf on the prepared baking sheet. Brush the top with the beaten egg white and sprinkle with sugar. Bake for 20 to 25 minutes or until the top is browned. Cool the biscotti at room temperature for 1 hour.

Preheat the oven to 350°F (175°C). Diagonally cut the baked loaf into 24 slices. Arrange the slices in a single layer on the baking sheet. Bake for 10 to 12 minutes or until golden brown. Cool the cookies on a wire rack.

Chocolate-Dipped Orange-Blueberry Biscotti

Per 1 biscotti:
Calories 70; Protein 2g; Total Fat 1g; Saturated Fat 0.5g; Carbohydrates 14g; Dietary Fiber 0g; Cholesterol 0mg; Sodium 35mg

Chocolate, orange, and blueberries, oh my! Bake these for morning, afternoon, or evening snacks. They also make a terrific addition to gift baskets.

Ingredients
Makes 2 dozen biscotti.

1 cup unbleached all-purpose flour
1 teaspoon baking powder
1/3 cup raw cane sugar (Turbinado)
1/2 cup plain, dry bread crumbs
1 cup dried blueberries
1/2 teaspoon pure vanilla extract
1/2 teaspoon pure lemon extract
2 teaspoons grated orange zest
1 tablespoon unsweetened orange juice
2 large egg whites
1 large egg white, lightly beaten, for topping
1 teaspoon raw cane sugar (Turbinado), for topping
4 ounces dark chocolate, chopped and melted, for dipping

Preparation
Preheat the oven to 350°F (175°C). Coat a baking sheet with cooking spray and set aside.

In a mixing bowl, sift the flour with the baking powder. Add the sugar and bread crumbs and mix well. Gently stir in the blueberries.

In a separate mixing bowl, combine the extracts, zest, juice, and egg whites. Add the juice mixture to the dry ingredients and mix until combined, about 1 minute.

On a lightly floured board, shape the dough into a long, flat loaf about 2 inches wide and 12 inches long. Place the loaf on the prepared baking sheet. Brush the top with the beaten egg white and sprinkle with sugar. Bake for 20 to 25 minutes or until the top is browned. Cool the biscotti at room temperature for 1 hour.

Preheat the oven to 350°F (175°C). Diagonally cut the baked loaf into 24 slices. Arrange the slices in a single layer on the baking sheet. Bake for 10 to 12 minutes or until golden brown. Cool the cookies on a wire rack.

Dip half of each cookie into the melted chocolate. Place cookies on a wire rack until the chocolate is set.

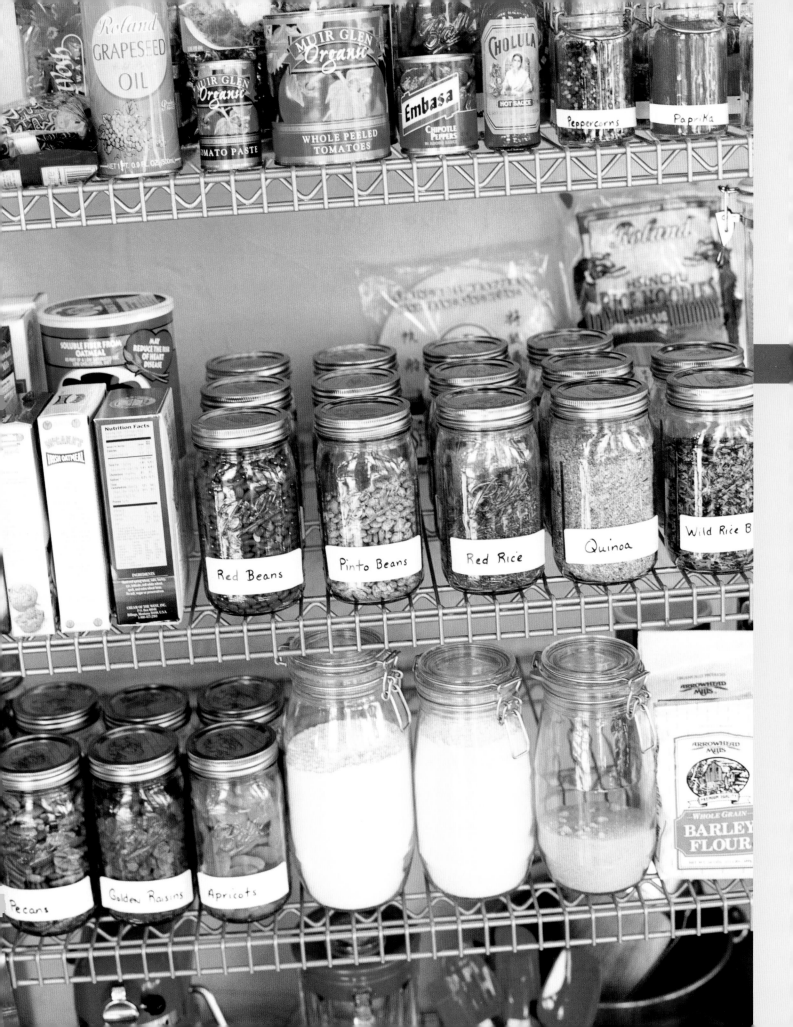

Pantry Resources

chapter 13

The chapter Kitchen Wisdom offers suggestions about stocking your pantry with good, wholesome foods: whole grains, flavorful oils and vinegars, least-processed sugars, whole spices, and dried fruits. Good food requires good ingredients.

Depending on the region, city, or state in which you live, you might find it quite easy or extremely difficult to find some of these nutritious and delicious ingredients. This convenient list of food manufacturers is compiled to assist you in your search for some of the best foods available for your health and wellness. By contacting these fine companies, you will have access to ingredients you may need when preparing some of the recipes. Remember, each ingredient was selected for its wholesomeness and its intense flavor properties. Be sure to ask the purveyor where you may find their products in stores near you. This will introduce you to new stores in your area offering other great finds.

Asian Specialty Products

Menlo Food Corporation
650-328-1107
Menlo wrappers, lumpia wrappers, and mu-shu pork wrappers.
Available in Asian markets.

Huy Fong Foods Inc.
5001 Earle Avenue
Rosemead, CA 91770
626-286-8328
www.huyfong.com
Asian hot sauces and Sriracha hot sauce.
Available in Asian markets, some natural food stores, grocery stores, and by mail order.

Culinary Instruction and Kitchen Equipment

Inspired Chef
800-528-1030
www.inspiredchef.com
A division of Kitchen Aid and Whirlpool Corporation specializing in premiere cooking equipment and tools and in-home, professional cooking classes. Products include Kitchen Aid mixers, blenders, food processors, Emile Henry, and Le Creuset.

Exotic Tea/Organic Coffee

Arbuckle Coffee Roasters
3498 South Dodge Blvd.
Tucson, AZ 85713
800-533-8278
www.arbucklecoffee.com
Exotic teas and organic coffee.
Available by phone, online, and in the Arizona store.

Fat Replacers

Sunsweet Growers Inc.
800-447-5218
www.sunsweet.com
Lighter bake, fat replacer made from prunes.
Available in select grocery stores and by mail order.

Gourmet Sauces and Stocks

More Than Gourmet
929 Home Avenue
Akron, OH 44310
800-860-9385
www.morethangourmet.com
Classically prepared reduced stocks.
Available online and by mail order.

Grains, Flours, and Pastas

Arrowhead Flours Inc.
Box 2059
Hereford, TX 79045
806-364-0730
Organic grains, flours, beans, and nut butters.
Available in most natural food stores, some grocery stores, by mail order, and online.

Bob's Red Mill Natural Foods Inc.
Milwaukie, Oregon 97222
800-349-2173
www.bobsredmill.com
Extensive selection of organic and natural grains, flours, cereals, and whole-grain foods.
Available in most natural food stores, some grocery stores, by mail order, and online.

Cream of the West Inc.
P.O. Box 80946
Billings, MT 59108
800-477-2383
Seven-grain cereal, roasted wheat cereal, ranch oats, and quick oats.
Available by mail order.

Lotus Foods
El Cerrito, CA
510-525-3137
www.lotusfoods.com
Assorted rice and rice flours, Bhutanese red rice.
Available in most natural food stores, some grocery stores, and online.

Lundberg Family Farms
5370 Church Street
Richvale, CA 95974-0369
530-882-4551
www.lundberg.com
Assorted varieties of organic brown and white rices and rice blends.
Available in most natural food stores, some grocery stores, and online.

Odlum Group Ltd.
www.mccanns.ie
McCanns steel-cut oats and Irish oatmeal.
Available in most natural food stores and some grocery stores.

Quinoa Corporation
P.O. Box 279
Gardena, CA 90248
310-217-8125
www.quinoa.net
Quinoa products, pasta, and flours.
Available in most natural food stores and online.

Lavender

Purple Haze Lavender
180 Bell Bottom Road
Sequim, WA 98382
888-852-6560
www.purplehazelavender.com
Organic lavender, herbes de Provence, lavender recipes, and other products.
Available online or by mail order.

Natural Sweeteners

Wax Orchards
22744 Wax Orchards Road
Vashon Island, WA 98070
800-634-6132
www.waxorchards.com
Fruit Sweet Syrup, fudge toppings, condiments, and fruit sweetened preserves.
Available in most natural food stores, by mail order, and online.

Wholesome Sweeteners
8016 Highway 90A
Sugarland, TX 77487
www.wholesomesweeteners.com
Organic sugar (evaporated cane juice).
Available in most natural food stores,
some grocery stores, and by mail order.

Nut Butters

Kettle Foods USA
503-364-0399
www.kettlefoods.com
Nut butters, potato chips, and tortilla
chips.
Available in most natural food stores,
some grocery stores, and online.

Organic Meat and Vegetable Products

Gold Label Meat
Danny and Lauri Martin
15401 South Empire Road
Benson, AZ 85602
520-586-7567
All natural, USDA-inspected beef.
Available by phone and mail order.

Niman Ranch
510-436-2320
www.nimanranch.com
Naturally raised beef, pork, and lamb.
Available online and in some natural
food stores.

Petaluma Poultry
707-763-1904
www.petalumapoultry.com
Certified organic chicken.
Available at most natural food stores and
specialty grocery stores.

VB Farms
P.O. Box 2581
Watsonville, CA 95077
www.sunshineorganic.com
831-728-9218
Organic strawberries, vegetables, jam,
and gift packs.
Available online.

Diamond Organics
P.O. Box 2159
Freedom, CA 95019
www.diamondorganics.com
888-674-2642
Organic vegetables.
Available online and by mail order.

Earthbound Farm
1721 San Juan Highway
San Juan Bautista, CA 95045
888-EAT-ORGANIC
www.ebfarm.com
Organic salads, fruits, and vegetables.
Available at natural food stores and
major grocery stores.

Specialty Pantry Items

ChefShop.com
877-337-2491
Specialty pantry items, organic, and
imported cocoa powders.
Available online.

Soy Products, Assorted Organic Products, and Rice Milk

Eden Foods
888-424-3336
www.edenfoods.com
Organic beans, soymilks, chips, crackers,
oils, vinegars, pastas, sweeteners, tomatoes, and sauerkraut.
Available in most natural food stores
and some grocery stores. Store locator
online.

White Wave Inc.
1990 North 57th Court
Boulder, CO 80301
www.silkissoy.com
Silk soymilk, Silk soy milk cream, Silk
cultured soy (yogurt), tofu, baked tofu,
tempeh, and seitan.
Available in most natural food stores
and some grocery stores.

Lightlife Foods
800-769-3279
www.lightlife.com
Soy products including smoky tempeh
strips.
Available in most natural food stores.

Mori-Nu
Morinaga Nutritional Foods Inc.
2050 West 190th Street #110
Torrance, CA 90504
800-NOW-TOFU
www.morinu.com
Nine varieties of silken tofu.
Available in most natural food stores,
grocery stores, and online.

Vitasoy USA Inc.
888-VITASOY
www.vitasoy-usa.com
Soy products, soymilk, tofu, veggie salad
dressing, and soy mayonnaise.
Available in most natural food stores
and some grocery stores.

Imagine Food Incorporated
1245 San Carlos Avenue
San Carlos, CA 94070
650-595-6300
www.imaginefoods.com
Rice Dream, Soy Dream, organic broths,
and soups.
Available in most natural food stores,
some grocery stores, and online.

Index

About the Author

Star Chef Cary Neff has established Conscious Cuisine as one of the nation's leading spa cuisines. In 2002, a *Condé Nast* reader's poll voted Conscious Cuisine the No. 1 spa diet/cuisine.

Trained in classic French kitchens, Chef Neff is a master at creating intense and vivid flavors, exploring gutsy Thai, Mediterranean, and southwestern cuisine. Throughout his career, he has earned national accolades for Arizona multimillion-dollar establishments, such as the Scottsdale Princess Resort, the Citadel, the historic Wrigley Mansion Club, the Wigwam Resort, and Miraval Life in Balance Resort and Spa. His cuisine has been featured in many major magazines, including *Bon Appetit*, *Gourmet*, *Food and Wine*, *New York Times Magazine*, and *Metropolitan Home*.

Cary Neff grew up on the south side of Chicago and discovered the joys of cooking in a high school home-economics class. He graduated from the prestigious Washburne Trade School in Chicago, Illinois, and began his culinary career in some of the city's most respected dining establishments, including the Ritz Carlton, Four Seasons, and Park Hyatt Hotels.

Chef Neff is an active member of the International Association of Culinary Professionals, Chef's Collaborative, and the American Culinary Federation's Apprentice Program.